DATE DUE

DEMCO, INC. 38-2931

AIDS &
ETHICS

AIDS & ETHICS

FREDERIC G. REAMER

EDITOR

COLUMBIA UNIVERSITY PRESS • NEW YORK

Columbia University Press
New York · Oxford

Copyright © 1991 Columbia University Press
All rights reserved

Library of Congress Cataloging-in-Publication Data
AIDS and ethics / Frederic G. Reamer, editor.
    p.   cm.
  Includes bibliographical references and index.
  ISBN 0-231-07358-5
  1. AIDS (Disease)—Moral and ethical aspects.   2. AID (Disease)—
Social aspects.   I. Reamer, Frederic G.
RA644.A25A34454   1991
362.1′969792—dc20   91-21477
                                                                CIP

∞

Casebound editions of Columbia University Press books are Smyth-sewn
and printed on permanent and durable acid-free paper.

Printed in the United States of America

c 10 9 8 7 6 5 4 3 2 1

For Deborah and Emma

▪ Contents

▪ Preface

ACQUIRED IMMUNE DEFICIENCY SYNDROME (hereafter AIDS) has given new meaning to the term *crisis*. The numbers alone are staggering, each new set of infection and mortality data often being outdated by the time they are printed.

But the AIDS crisis is exacting more than a death toll. It is also imposing disturbingly novel and provocative ethical questions. Under what circumstances is mandatory screening for this infectious disease warranted? What access should AIDS patients have to nonapproved therapies? Should pregnant AIDS patients be permitted to participate in randomized clinical trials? Should insurance companies be required to insure individuals who are seropositive? What are the limits of AIDS patients' right to confidentiality? Do physicians and other health care professionals have an obligation to treat AIDS patients?

By now, as we bring to a close the first decade of the disease's history, we have a good grasp of the most troubling and troublesome ethical questions. With respect to some, consensus on the answers is beginning to emerge. Few, for example, now argue for widespread or universal mandatory testing. It is also now widely believed that contact tracing should preserve, as much as possible, AIDS patients' privacy.

But with a number of other questions broached in these pages, the only thing clear is that the answers are murky. Do parents of a human immunodeficiency virus (HIV)-infected child have a duty to disclose this fact to parents of the child's playmates? Does a physician have an obligation to warn the spouse of an infected patient who wants this fact kept secret? Should rigorous methodological features that govern AIDS research be relaxed to enhance patients' access to nonapproved drugs?

AIDS and Ethics includes a series of original, seminal essays offering a systematic overview of these and other questions from the perspectives of scholars and practitioners trained in strikingly diverse disciplines and professions. Among the fields represented by the authors are law, medicine, philosophy, political science, religious studies, and social work.

In the first chapter, I explore the broad ethical implications of the AIDS crisis and speculate about the relevance of ethical inquiry, language, and concepts. In the end I conclude that, despite its well-known limitations, applied ethics has much to offer those of us who are troubled by and concerned about the normative dimensions of the disease and society's response to it. I also argue that professionals in the field must look beyond abstract and applied ethical theory and widen their lens to examine their personal moral commitment to work with the AIDS population.

The next several chapters explore the ethical features of a broad range of key policy debates related to AIDS. Ronald Bayer provides a valuable analysis of the shifting tension that has emerged between public health and civil liberties advocates. Bayer traces the evolution of this relationship, beginning with the emergence of AIDS in the early 1980s and continuing along its subsequent course. His insightful assessment offers a sobering look at the historical and political factors that influence the unstable balance between public health safeguards and civil liberties protections.

James Childress focuses specifically on the collection of debates concerning mandatory screening and testing of various populations. Following his presentation of a conceptual template for examining these issues, Childress considers and critiques, in turn, arguments that have been advanced concerning testing and screening of hospital patients, marriage license applicants, pregnant women, newborns, individuals in the state's custody, and international travelers.

Childress' analysis is followed by Carol Levine's comprehensive review of issues related to human subjects research. After her brief review of prevailing ethical standards in research, Levine identifies dilemmas posed by the AIDS crisis, focusing especially on the ethical dimensions of research design, access to nonapproved therapies, the duties of subjects and physicians involved in clinical trials, eligibility for participation in clinical research, and vaccine-related research. As Levine concludes, some of these issues have been largely resolved (such as the need for strict confidentiality safeguards) while others continue to be the subject of intense debate (such as the participation of pregnant women in clinical research on new drugs).

The AIDS crisis has also stimulated considerable debate about health insurance — in particular, emerging insurance industry underwriting practices. Gerald Oppenheimer and Robert Padgug offer a forceful argument that insurers' efforts to limit coverage of HIV-infected individuals and persons with AIDS constitutes a crisis of community. Following their historical review of insurers' shift from an inclusionary "community rating" approach to an exclusionary "experience rating" approach, Oppenheimer and Padgug lobby aggressively for universal and uniform health care coverage. For them, the distressing alternative to universal health care is a fragmented, unfair, and inefficient approach to health insurance that, in the final analysis, will not provide adequate protection to AIDS patients and those at risk for the disease.

One of the most enduring debates concerning AIDS pertains to the use of coercion to contain transmission of the disease. In recent years we have seen a variety of calls for the use of quarantine, isolation, mandatory notification of partners, and other social control measures in an effort to prevent the spread of AIDS. In her chapter on AIDS education, Nora Kizer Bell challenges claims that punitive and coercive measures are the most appropriate public response to the crisis. For Bell, rudimentary principles of democracy call for assertive and frank forms of education designed to prevent the spread of AIDS. Although AIDS may tempt us toward a variety of strict social control tactics, Bell argues that our democratic roots should lead us instead toward voluntary efforts to change attitudes and behavior among those with AIDS or at risk for the disease.

Much of the recent controversy concerning AIDS has focused on the adequacy of public funds dedicated to research, prevention, and treatment. For many, funding has been intolerably inadequate and research progress has been painfully slow. This frustration — along with concern about emerging public policy — has led to diverse forms of militancy and civil disobedience directed at public officials, researchers, religious leaders, and pharmaceutical companies. Courtney Campbell takes a hard, critical look at AIDS activism and assesses the moral warrant claimed by AIDS activists. Campbell explores the extent to which AIDS activists have met the burden of persuasion and the moral criteria that inhere in the tradition of civil disobedience.

Using different conceptual lenses, Robert Levine and Abigail Zuger then discuss vexing questions concerning health care professionals' duty to treat AIDS patients. From a phenomenological framework, Levine dismantles the physician-patient relationship into its component parts and speculates about why physicians ask the question "Do I have a duty to treat AIDS patients?" Levine's task is not to answer the question itself but rather to explain why physicians are moved to ask the question in the first place. Levine begins with the first "moment" of encounter between physician and patient and sheds light on the dynamics of the evolving relationship that account for this now-common query.

The answer to the question about the health care professional's duty to treat is left to Abigail Zuger. Following her brief historical insight into the behavior of physicians during a variety of plagues and epidemics, Zuger examines the ethical norms that have emerged within the medical profession and among individual health care practitioners. She concludes her discussion with a number of thought-provoking observations about health care professionals' moral duty to treat and what patients have the right to expect of them.

There is no question that issues of intimacy are prominent in any discussion of AIDS. Personal details abound concerning sexual activity, drug use, and test results. Not surprisingly, there is considerable controversy pertaining to privacy of information and limitations imposed on it. Ferdinand Schoeman offers us a systematic review of a broad range of privacy issues that have emerged within the AIDS context. Schoeman reviews the nature of privacy norms in general and discusses the various privacy issues that need to be addressed concerning AIDS. For Schoeman the most compelling questions pertain to therapists' obligations to disclose confidential information to protect third parties who may be at risk because of the behavior of an HIV-infected patient or client, the responsibility of an HIV-infected individual to warn others of his or her potential to transmit the disease, the right of health insurers to private information about applicants, and the responsibility of the state to trace sexual contacts of HIV-infected individuals.

It is difficult to examine this diverse collection of ethical issues without bumping into a variety of compelling legal conundra. By now there is a myriad of statutes and legal precedents on issues such as mandatory testing, privacy, employment and school-based discrimination, protection of third parties, the duty to treat, the use of quarantine, and civil liability. Donald Hermann reviews the range of legal issues and developments triggered by the AIDS crisis and alerts readers to fundamental tensions between protection of individual interests and the public's health. His discussion provides a useful perspective on the legal dimensions of the most prominent debates about AIDS and ethics.

This project could not have been completed without the able assistance of a number of colleagues. As is their custom, my editors at Columbia University Press, Ann Miller and Louise Waller, provided consistently constructive suggestions and encouragement. Louise deserves special credit for having the imagination that led to this project in the first place and for helping me map the book's content. I was especially impressed by her genuine commitment to the substantive issues addressed here. I also want to thank the Rhode Island College Council and Faculty Research Committee for their support.

It is hard to know how to express my appreciation to the authors themselves. These are among the brightest, most dedicated, and talented scholars with whom I have had the privilege to work. Their unique ability to mesh intellectual rigor with compelling prose — under an unusually tight deadline — impressed me continually. They were remarkably tolerant of my editorial suggestions and requests for yet another draft. I am confident that these authors' insights will provide an important lodestar (and lightning rod, perhaps) to those who care deeply about the AIDS crisis.

This has been a difficult project to complete. It has been simultaneously exciting to forge new intellectual paths that are so important and depressing to face the unrelentingly morbid facts produced by AIDS. No other research has forced me to examine, in so intense a fashion, my own ethical beliefs. The nature of this subject is such that one must confront his or her most basic values and biases. I have learned a great deal in the process.

In this regard, I offer my most heartfelt thanks to my wife, Deborah, and daughter, Emma, who help me to understand what the term *virtue* means.

Frederic G. Reamer

▪ Contributors

RONALD BAYER is associate professor in the School of Public Health, Columbia University. He received his Ph.D. from the University of Chicago. Currently Bayer is a member of the Committee to Monitor the Social Impact of AIDS, National Research Council, and consultant to the World Health Organization, Global Programme on AIDS. Formerly he was associate for policy studies at The Hastings Center. Bayer is the author of *Private Acts, Social Consequences: AIDS and the Politics of Public Health* (Free Press, 1989) and *Homosexuality and American Psychiatry: The Politics of Diagnosis* (Basic Books, 1981), editor of *The Health and Safety of Workers: The Politics of Professional Responsibility* (Oxford University Press, 1988), and coeditor of *In Search of Equity: Health Needs and the Health Care System* (Plenum Press, 1983).

NORA KIZER BELL is professor of philosophy at the University of South Carolina (Columbia), where she is Chair of the Department of Philosophy. She received her Ph.D. from the University of North Carolina. Bell serves as a medical ethicist at the University of South Carolina School of Medicine, adjunct associate professor at the University of South Carolina School of Public Health, adjunct associate professor at the University of South Carolina School of Medicine (Department of Family and Preventive Medicine), and was an Exxon Fellow in Ethics and Medicine at the Baylor College of Medicine. She is the editor of *Who Decides? Conflicts of Rights in Health Care* (Humana Press, 1982) and is the author of a number of journal articles on medical ethics.

COURTNEY S. CAMPBELL is assistant professor in the Department of Religious Studies, Oregon State University. He received his Ph.D.

from the University of Virginia. Formerly he was the editor of the *Hastings Center Report* and associate for religious studies, The Hastings Center. Campbell is the author or coauthor of a number of publications on health care ethics, including "The Moral Meaning of Religion for Bioethics," *Boletin de la OPS;* "At the Edges of Life," *This People;* "Plague, Piety, and Policy," *Second Opinion;* "Ethics, Technology, and Resource Allocation in Health Care," *Michigan Hospitals;* "Patients Who Refuse Treatment in Medical Offices," *Archives of Internal Medicine;* and "AZT: The Ethical Debate," *BioLaw.*

JAMES F. CHILDRESS is the Edwin B. Kyle Professor of Religious Studies and professor of medical education at the University of Virginia, where he is also chairman of the Department of Religious Studies and principal of the Monroe Hill Residential College. He received his Ph.D. from Yale University. Childress is a fellow of the American Academy of Arts and Sciences and of The Hastings Center. He is the author of numerous articles and several books on biomedical ethics, including *Principles of Biomedical Ethics* (with Tom L. Beauchamp, 3d ed., Oxford University Press, 1989); *Priorities in Biomedical Ethics* (The Westminster Press, 1981); and *Who Should Decide?* (Oxford University Press, 1982).

DONALD H. J. HERMANN is professor of law and professor of philosophy as well as director of the Health Law Institute at DePaul University College of Law. He received his J.D. from Columbia University and his Ph.D. in philosophy from Northwestern University. Hermann is editor of the *Journal of Health and Hospital Law* and a fellow of the American Academy of Hospital Attorneys. He is coauthor of *Legal Aspects of AIDS* (Callaghan and Co., 1990) and *AIDS Law in a Nutshell* (West, Publishing Co., 1990) and coeditor of *AIDS: Cases and Materials* (John Marshall Publishing Co., 1989). He is also the author of "Torts: Private Lawsuits About AIDS," in *AIDS and the Law.*

CAROL LEVINE is executive director, Citizens Commission on AIDS. She completed her graduate education in public law and government at Columbia University. Formerly Levine was editor of *The Hastings Center Report* and associate for publications, The Hastings Center. She currently serves as managing editor of *IRB: A Review of Human Subjects Research,* and is a member of the Scientific Committee, American Foundation for AIDS Research. Levine is editor of *Taking Sides: Clashing Views on Controversial Bioethical Issues* (3d ed., Dushkin Publishing Group, 1989) and *Cases in Bioethics from the Hastings Center Report* (2d. ed., St. Martin's Press, 1989) and the author or coauthor of numerous articles on the AIDS crisis, including

"Has AIDS Changed the Ethics of Human Subjects Research?" *Law, Medicine, & Health Care;* "The Ethics of Screening for Early Intervention in HIV Disease," *American Journal of Public Health;* and "HIV Antibody Screening: An Ethical Framework for Evaluating Proposed Programs," *Journal of the American Medical Association.*

ROBERT J. LEVINE is professor of medicine and lecturer in pharmacology at Yale University School of Medicine. He received his M.D. from George Washington University School of Medicine. He is a fellow of The Hastings Center and of the American College of Physicians, a member of the American Society for Clinical Investigation, and president of the American Society of Law and Medicine. Levine, former editor of *Clinical Research,* is editor of *IRB: A Review of Human Subjects Research.* He is the author of numerous publications, including *Ethics and Regulation of Clinical Research* (2d ed., Urban and Schwarzenberg, 1986). Levine teaches medical ethics at Yale University.

GERALD M. OPPENHEIMER is associate professor in the Department of Health and Nutrition Sciences, Brooklyn College, City University of New York. He received his Ph.D. from the University of Chicago. Oppenheimer has authored or coauthored a number of publications on AIDS, including "AIDS and Health Insurance: Social and Ethical Issues," *AIDS and Public Policy Journal;* "AIDS: The Risk to Insurers, The Threat to Equity," *Hastings Center Report;* "AIDS in the Workplace," *Business and Health;* "Causes, Cases, and Cohorts: The Role of Epidemiology in the Historical Construction of AIDS, 1980–1989," in *AIDS: Contemporary History;* and "AIDS in the Workplace: The Ethical Ramifications," in *AIDS: Ethics and Public Policy.*

ROBERT A. PADGUG is director of health policy, Empire Blue Cross and Blue Shield. He received his Ph.D. from Harvard and formerly served on the faculty of Rutgers University. Padgug is the coeditor of *Passion and Power: Sexuality in History* (Temple University Press, 1989) and is the author or coauthor of numerous journal articles on AIDS, including "AIDS, Private Health Insurance, and the Crisis of Community," *Notre Dame Journal of Law, Ethics, and Public Policy;* "More Than the Story of a Virus: Gay History, Gay Communities, and AIDS," *Radical America;* "AIDS and Health Insurance: Social and Ethical Issues," *AIDS and Public Policy Journal;* and "AIDS: The Risk to Insurance, the Threat to Equity," *Hastings Center Report.*

FREDERIC G. REAMER is professor in the School of Social Work, Rhode Island College. He received his Ph.D. from the University of Chicago. Reamer is the author of *Ethical Dilemmas in Social Service* xviiiCONTRIBUTORS

(2d. ed., Columbia University Press, 1990) and coauthor of *The Teaching of Social Work Ethics* (The Hastings Center, 1982). He is also the author of numerous other publications on professional ethics, including "AIDS, Social Work, and the 'Duty to Protect,' " *Social Work;* "Toward Ethical Practice: The Relevance of Ethical Theory," *Social Thought;* "Social Work: Calling or Career?" *Hastings Center Report;* "The Emergence of Bioethics in Social Work," *Health and Social Work;* "Value and Ethics," *Encyclopedia of Social Work;* and "The Concept of Paternalism in Social Work," *Social Service Review.* Reamer is editor-in-chief of the *Journal of Social Work Education.*

FERDINAND SCHOEMAN is professor of philosophy at the University of South Carolina (Columbia). He received his Ph.D. from Brandeis University. Schoeman is the editor of *Philosophical Dimensions of Privacy: An Anthology* (Cambridge University Press, 1984) and *Responsibility, Character, and the Emotions: New Essays in Moral Psychology* (Cambridge University Press, 1987). Schoeman is the author of a number of additional publications on the subject of privacy, including "Privacy," *Encyclopedia of Ethics;* "Adolescent Confidentiality and Family Privacy," *John Marshall Law Review;* "Privacy: Philosophical Dimensions," *American Philosophical Quarterly;* and "Privacy and Criminal Justice Policies," *Criminal Justice Ethics.*

ABIGAIL ZUGER is assistant professor of medicine at Albert Einstein College of Medicine. She is also attending physician in the AIDS Center and director of the Infectious Diseases Clinic at Montefiore Medical Center. Zuger received her M.D. from Case Western Reserve University. She was also a fellow in the Center for Clinical Medical Ethics at the University of Chicago Medical Center. Zuger's most recent publications include "Physicians, AIDS, and Occupational Risk: Historic Traditions and Ethical Obligations," *Journal of the American Medical Association;* "AIDS on the Wards: A Residency in Medical Ethics," *Hastings Center Report;* and "Heterosexual Transmission of Human Immunodeficiency Syndrome," *AIDS Update.*

La vertu refuse la facilité pour compagne . . .
elle demande un chemin âpre et épineux.

Virtue shuns ease as a companion. . . . It demands
a rough and thorny path.

— Michel de Montaigne

AIDS &
ETHICS

1. AIDS: The Relevance of Ethics

FREDERIC G. REAMER

AT A RECENT conference I sat on a panel of professionals who are knowledgeable about AIDS. This interdisciplinary panel was convened to consider a variety of ethical issues related to the disease. During the discussion this group was presented with a series of case scenarios that raise complex ethical issues related to the AIDS pandemic. Among them was a case involving a young man with AIDS who refused to inform his girlfriend (his regular sexual partner) about his AIDS status. This fellow was unwilling to disclose details about his illness because he feared unpleasant recriminations and humiliation. He also feared that his partner would leave him at a time when he needed her support.

The panel was asked to consider whether the patient's physician should disclose confidential information to ensure that the patient's girlfriend learns of his AIDS diagnosis so that she can protect herself. We were to assume that every effort already had been made to get the patient to share this information on his own.

This case scenario, which is now distressingly familiar to those involved in the AIDS crisis, is characteristic of a wide variety of ethical choices practitioners are facing. It contains a classic clash of duties and rights, in this instance among the patient's ordinary right to privacy and confidentiality, his obligation toward his girlfriend, and the girlfriend's right to protection from harm. We can add into the mix the corollary tension between the physician's duty to respect confidentiality and her duty to protect third parties.

The panel's discussion of this troubling case had several striking features. First, it was clear that ethical norms related to AIDS are shifting, sometimes rapidly. Most of the panelists acknowledged that *at some point* the physician may be obligated to disclose confidential information to protect the patient's girlfriend. Even as recently as three years ago, I think such a diverse group of experts would not have reached this conclusion. While we disagreed some about where the line should be drawn and what steps should be taken before disclosure, most of the panelists agreed that, in principle, professionals may have an obligation to breach confidentiality. Our discussion provided a compelling example of how ethical bearings can float over time, moved in part by rapid changes in the public's understanding of the magnitude of a problem, its etiology, associated risks, and the effectiveness of available responses.

This case also captures what makes so many of the ethical issues related to AIDS so difficult. It contains what ethicists have dubbed *hard choices*, choices among rights and duties that clash.

As this book makes clear, the AIDS crisis is producing a staggering number of hard choices. To what extent should the rights of others prevail over the privacy rights of AIDS patients? Do the benefits of mandatory screening of newborns justify the intrusiveness that such procedures entail? Should the rights of persons with AIDS to use nonapproved drugs take precedence over the need to conduct carefully controlled clinical trials? Is it always unethical for health care professionals to refuse to treat persons with AIDS? Can militant activities, such as violent protest, be justified if they lead to meaningful change in funding for AIDS prevention, treatment, and research? Should employers and insurance companies be prohibited from screening for AIDS under any circumstances?

What was also striking about the panel's discussion was the influence of the various lenses through which we viewed the case. It became clear that our arguments and conclusions were shaped in part by the nature of our respective professional training; the language and conceptual frameworks we use to understand, interpret, and explain the worlds in which we work; our current affiliations; our political leanings; and our personal values (whatever we take this vague phrase to mean). A congresswoman on the panel clearly was alert to the political ramifications of her opinions, given the large numbers of gay constituents in her California district. The positions of an AIDS activist on the panel and a senior Blue Cross/Blue Shield official reflected their contrasting loyalty to their respective organizations and divergent missions. The views of the panel's two ethicists were grounded in their deep-seated beliefs about fundamental rights and duties.

As the group's discussion proceeded, however, it became clear that all of us were aware of the ethical dimensions of the debate. Some of us used more technical jargon than others, but we were all speaking the language of ethics. We talked of rights, duties, and obligations, and we speculated about justice, fairness, and equity. Although we stayed away from formal philosophical apparatus, all of us were drawn to basic ethical constructs.

This was not a surprising outcome. After all, it is difficult to discuss AIDS-related issues without venturing quickly into issues of right and wrong, and duty and obligation. Matters of life and death have an easy way of riveting one's attention to such rudimentary concepts.

The Nature of Ethical Discourse

As with most crises, the professions' response to AIDS is developing in stages. We have begun to grasp the enormity of the problem and now have a more mature understanding of constructive prevention strategies than we did in the early 1980s, when the disease was first identified. We also have a realistic understanding of the likelihood that researchers will imminently develop effective treatments.

More recently we have generated a rather comprehensive roster of the critical ethical choices that face us. We understand the need to examine complex issues related to privacy, mandatory screening, civil liberties, health care financing, research on human subjects, AIDS activism, treatment, and the obligations of professionals. We are just beginning, however, to formulate sophisticated analyses of the ethical features of these issues, much less clear answers to the questions they pose.

Those of us who study, talk about, and write about ethics seem to be assuming that the discipline's concepts and methods can be applied fruitfully to the AIDS crisis. After all, for centuries ethicists have been exploring the moral dimensions of a wide range of contemporary problems, ranging from abortion to suicide. Should not we be able to load another problem onto the line? Does not the AIDS crisis merely present us with a variation on the theme established by controversies surrounding issues such as fetal tissue research, frozen embryos, artificial organs, organ transplantation, and euthanasia? Or is there something special about AIDS, such that the familiar ethics template we have been using needs to be refashioned?

Relatively few of us question the general value of ethical analysis, although there certainly is a handful of detractors. (For an overview of critical commentary, see Macklin (1988).) Since Socrates, at least, we have recognized the importance of moral inquiry, of a systematic examination of the moral features of life. Hence, our shelves are filled with the statements of major and minor philosophers on subjects such as justice, equality, and fairness.

Most recently, as philosophers have moved away from a preoccupation with metaethics—the study of the meaning of ethical terms and the abstract analysis of moral concepts—the field has, to a great extent, shifted its attention toward the application of ethics to contemporary problems (Rachels 1980). The burgeoning interest in applied ethics has occurred for several reasons. Well-publicized scandals in government and the private sector have done much to fuel interest in applied ethics. Technological advances in a number of fields, particularly health care, have also brought with them a host of complex ethical puzzles and have forced us to acknowledge the limits of science. In addition, the turbulence of the 1960s introduced millions to the concept of rights as they pertain to the mentally ill, criminals, consumers, welfare recipients, and the public at large. All of this, combined with the maturation of the professions themselves, has led to the emergence of applied ethics as a discrete specialty (Reamer and Abramson 1982).

Can ethics help us with the problems posed by the AIDS crisis? I think so, although we must be realistic about our claims.

Let us take as an example the case with which we started. Here we have a physician who is caring for an AIDS patient who has refused to disclose his status to his girlfriend. The physician is caught on the horns of a dilemma. If she respects the patient's traditional right to privacy, she would fail to take steps that might protect the life of a third party, the girlfriend. Yet, if she takes steps to protect this third party, she may violate the sacred trust that ordinarily characterizes the physician-patient relationship.

So what does ethics have to say about all of this? For one thing, ethics can help us identify the critical questions. In this instance, there are several questions that pertain to the central ethical concepts of rights and duties: (1) Do persons with AIDS possess certain basic rights, and is confidentiality one of them? (2) Do persons with AIDS have certain basic obligations, and is protection of third parties one of them? (3) Do physicians have certain basic obligations, and is respecting patient confidentiality one of them? (4) Is protecting third parties another one of these obligations? If we believe, as most people seem to, that persons with AIDS ordinarily have a right to confidentiality *and* have an obligation to protect third parties, and that physicians also have an obligation to respect confidentiality *and* to protect third parties, we are led inevitably to a new question: (5) When various rights and duties conflict, how are we to reconcile them?

The Use of Ethical Theory

The form of these questions is a familiar one. Ethicists can offer a wide range of frameworks for addressing them, particularly with respect to the problem of conflicting rights and duties. The classic utilitarian position, the most common form of consequentialism, is that the physician ought to choose the course of action that produces the greatest good. There are several ways, however, for a utilitarian to "calculate" all of this. An *act* utilitarian would be interested primarily in the consequences of the physician's decision in this particular case. Hence, the physician ought to weigh the risks and benefits associated with respecting her patient's confidentiality versus breaching confidentiality to protect the girlfriend. Factors such as the value of privacy, the physician's reputation, the patient's right to self-determination, the girlfriend's assumption of risk, and the value of her life ought to be entered into the equation. Putting aside the age-old problem of quantification once the list of factors has been identified (which is not so easy to do, in fact), the task here is to carry out a calculus that enables one to determine the tradeoffs and net result of the physician's options.

A *rule* utilitarian, on the other hand, would be less interested in the consequences of the physician's decision in this one case. Rather, he or she would want to speculate about the long-range consequences of the physician's decision. For example, a rule utilitarian might want to know the likelihood that this one breach of confidentiality would lead to a more general practice of breaches that, ultimately, would seriously threaten the sanctity of the physician-patient relationship and diminish the public's trust in physicians. Thus, it is not hard to imagine that an act and rule utilitarian might disagree. An act utilitarian might conclude that confidentiality must be breached in this case to protect the patient's girlfriend, while a rule utilitarian might argue that this would be shortsighted. The act utilitarian might want to avoid naive "rule worship" (Smart 1971:199) while the rule utilitarian might claim that the long-range damage that would result from a confidentiality breach (e.g., possibly discouraging persons with AIDS from seeking medical attention) would outweigh the more immediate threat to the patient's girlfriend.

One can imagine how the act and rule utilitarian perspectives might pertain as well to other AIDS-related issues. Consider, for example, the debate about whether physicians have a right to refuse to treat AIDS patients (Zuger and Miles 1987). An act utilitarian might argue that the greatest good would result by allowing an individual physician who is keenly uncomfortable treating persons with AIDS to refuse to treat, based on a belief that the costs associated with the physician's discomfort and the risk to patients who might be served by a reluctant practitioner outweigh the benefit of whatever coercion might be involved in the physician's treatment of AIDS patients. A rule utilitarian might argue, however, that this one precedent might result in large numbers of physicians refusing to treat AIDS patients, with the eventual consequences that AIDS patients would be without adequate numbers of caretakers and that the risk to practitioners would be concentrated unfairly among physicians willing to treat persons with AIDS.

Similarly, one can imagine how an act utilitarian might argue that the greatest good would result by allowing an individual AIDS patient to have access to a nonapproved drug; considering the seriousness of the patient's illness, such a course of action would at least provide a slim measure of hope in the face of an otherwise bleak prognosis. A rule utilitarian would likely argue, however, that widespread access to nonapproved drugs would undermine researchers' ability to recruit patients for clinical trials and, ultimately, would limit the effectiveness of research designed to provide the greatest benefit to the greatest number (Rothman 1987; Freedman et al. 1989).

This general utilitarian framework contrasts with the conventional deontological perspective, which rejects the claim that the rightness of an action is determined by the goodness of its consequences. For a deontologist, one ought to engage in certain actions because it is right to do so as a matter of principle. Thus, a deontologist might not be interested in the practical consequences of a confidentiality breach. Instead, he or she might be concerned about the inherent importance of keeping a promise concerning confidentiality or about the inherent value of a life.

The problem with deontology is, of course, that it too is capable of producing conflicting claims about what one ought to do. It is not hard to imagine one deontologist who dwells on the value of privacy or promise-keeping while a second emphasizes the duty to protect life. In the end, despite our use of these theoretical perspectives, we may still be faced with clashing conclusions.

Applying Ethics to AIDS

The tension between utilitarian and deontological perspectives—ethical theory's principal schools of thought—is already emerging in organized discourse about AIDS. Consider, for instance, debate about the morality of civil disobedience and militancy. Are forms of protest engaged in by AIDS activists—including sabotage of pharmaceutical research, disruption of scientific meetings, occupying corporate offices, or demonstrating during a Catholic Mass—defensible on moral grounds? A traditional deontological position opposes illegal disobedience because it challenges the sanctity of the law (Bedau 1969; Wasserstrom 1975). The utilitarian position, in contrast, typically holds that disobedience—in the form of property destruction, say—is justifiable because of the long-term benefits that result when such pressure leads to constructive changes in public policy, funding, research priorities, and so on. As Carl Cohen notes in his essay on AIDS activism, "the justification of indirect symbolic disobedience is generally utilitarian in form. Agitation, it is thought, will bring public education and eventual legislative reform" (1989:24).

The tension between deontological and utilitarian perspectives is a familiar one in public health. Although the terminology may be absent, scores of public health policies and related court decisions are products of efforts to balance these two points of view. For example, the Constitution provides states with the power to take necessary action to promote public health and welfare, yet the exercise of this power is subject to constitutional protection of individual rights (Merritt 1986; Brandt 1987:40–41; Gostin 1987:48–49; Bayer 1989). Through the Bill of Rights, the Constitution established basic (read *deontological*) rights that cannot be infringed upon by the federal government, e.g., freedom of speech and religion, freedom from unreasonable searches and seizures, and the insistence that life, liberty, and property cannot be abridged without due process of law.

Not surprisingly, however, these basic individual rights sometimes come into conflict with the rights of the majority, as when an individual with a communicable disease is isolated against his or her will. In these cases courts essentially balance deontological against utilitarian concerns, that is, individuals' basic constitutional rights against the consequences for the general public. As Lawrence Gostin observes:

> Whenever individuals (or classes of persons) assert in litigation that their rights have been abridged by the act of a local, state, or federal government, they are implicitly asking the court to undo the will of the majority as expressed through the executive or the legislature. Given this reality, it is not surprising that rights are rarely regarded as absolute. . . . No matter how reluctant a judge is to get involved in deciding whether a challenged health measure is a good idea, if the measure tends to abridge constitutionally protected rights, he or she must inevitably evaluate the measure's propriety, its *utility,* and its necessity (1987:49; emphasis added).

This line of reasoning was prevalent in landmark judicial decisions around the turn of the century—in response to epidemics of venereal disease, scarlet fever, cholera, tuberculosis, smallpox, leprosy, and bubonic plague—and it is prevalent in today's AIDS cases (Fox 1988).

Returning to our opening vignette, for example, we find that courts and ethicists face very much the same challenge and that neither has a corner on easy solutions. Although their methods of analysis and conceptual foundations differ, each has a deep-seated tradition of attempts to reconcile conflicting obligations. For instance, over the years a number of courts have sought to develop guidelines to balance individuals' right to privacy in a therapeutic context with protection of third parties threatened by these clients or patients. The best known precedent is *Tarasoff v. Regents of the University of California* (1976). In *Tarasoff,* Prosenjit Poddar, a graduate student at the University of California at Berkeley, sought counseling at the student health clinic. During a session with his therapist, Poddar indicated that he was having thoughts about killing a woman who did not return his affections, Tatiana Tarasoff. The therapist notified campus security who, after interviewing Poddar and obtaining his promise to stay away from Tarasoff, released Poddar. The police concluded that Poddar did not pose an imminent threat. Following Poddar's release, the director of the health clinic asked the police to return all correspondence related to the case, in order to preserve Poddar's right to confidentiality. Approximately two months later, Poddar murdered Tarasoff.

Tarasoff's parents sued the counselor and other state officials for their failure to detain Poddar and their failure to warn their daughter of Poddar's threat. The case was initially dismissed in the original court, was appealed, and was heard again by the California Supreme Court. The appeals court ruled that professionals do have a duty to protect a potential victim or others likely to have contact with the victim when the professional determines, or should determine, that such action is necessary to protect third parties. Specifically, the court concluded that:

> We recognize the public interest in supporting effective treatment of mental illness and in protecting the rights of patients to privacy and the consequent public importance of safeguarding the confidential character of psychotherapeutic communication. Against this interest, however, we must weigh the public interest in safety from violent assault. ... We conclude that the public policy favoring protection of the confidential character of patient-psychotherapist communications must yield to the extent to which disclosure is essential to avert danger to others.

now we know that she was essentially mistaken. While some analysts have strayed too far in the direction of intellectual gymnastics that have little bearing on modern-day problems, there is no question that to date the net result of applied ethics—despite its limitations—has been significant. Although ethicists have not produced definitive guidelines to resolve enduring issues related to every complex dilemma, and should not be expected to, there can be no doubt that their assessments have done much to illuminate critical issues and to suggest practical options and alternatives. One needs only to look at the emerging literature on issues such as organ allocation, fetal research, psychosurgery, drug screening, frozen embryos, and termination of life support. Our thinking about these phenomena is becoming increasingly mature and insightful, and this is partly due to the work of ethicists (certainly others, such as theologians and policy analysts, have contributed much as well). Our efforts to shed light on important ethical issues related to AIDS are also productive.

Noble *was* right to suggest, however, that ethics has been oversold somewhat. In a sense, we have shot ourselves in the foot whenever we have suggested to impressionable audiences that ethicists are capable of producing all-purpose or one-stop theories that can resolve complicated, seemingly intractable problems. We have invited disappointment by heightening expectations for the arrival of a messianic ethical theory.

Fortunately, most of us are past that sort of hubris, and our goals are more modest. As Ruth Macklin has concluded, "Rarely does bioethics offer 'one right answer' to a moral dilemma. Seldom can a philosopher arrive on the scene and make unequivocal pronouncements about the right thing to do. Yet, despite the fact that it has no magic wand, bioethics is still useful and can go a long way toward 'resolving the issues,' once that phrase is properly interpreted" (1988:52).

In this respect, attempts to produce grand ethical theory have had the unfortunate consequence of producing moral skeptics and relativists. Too many have been sold a bill of goods about the clarity and efficacy of ethical theory. As Annette Baier astutely observes:

> The obvious trouble with our contemporary attempts to use moral theory to guide action is the lack of agreement on which theory we are to apply. The standard undergraduate course in, say, medical ethics, or business ethics, acquaints the student with a variety of theories, and shows the difference in the guidance they give. We, in effect, give courses in comparative ethical theory, and like courses in comparative religion, their usual effect in the student is loss of faith in *any* of the alternatives presented. We produce relativists and moral skeptics, per-

sons who have been convinced by our teaching that whatever they do
in some difficult situation, some moral theory will condone it, another
will condemn it. The usual, and the sensible, reaction to this confrontation with a variety of conflicting theories, all apparently having some
plausibility and respectable credentials, is to turn to a guide that speaks
more univocally, to turn from morality to self-interest, or mere convenience (1988:26).

What, then, can we expect ethics to offer with respect to the AIDS
crisis? Several things. First, ethical inquiry can greatly enhance our
understanding of the moral issues pertaining to AIDS. Policies related
to phenomena such as mandatory screening of hospital patients, prostitutes, international travelers, newborns, prisoners, and pregnant
women, for example, require more than consideration of relevant clinical dimensions. Although it is essential to take into account available
technical knowledge concerning the epidemiology and transmission of
disease, we must also examine mandatory screening proposals from
the point of view of relevant moral concepts, such as *rights* (of those
who would be subjected to screening and contact tracing and of those
who may be at risk of future infection), *duties* (of government officials
who are charged with protecting and enhancing public health), *justice*
(for all parties involved), and so on. In order to grapple adequately with
such hard choices, it is helpful to enumerate the various moral duties
and rights involved in such policy formulation and the ways in which
they compete with each other (Childress 1987). It is also helpful to ask
what constitutes a duty and a right in the first place, and these are
traditional questions of ethics.

The same holds true for debate about AIDS activism. It is helpful
to consider the arguments of AIDS activists and their critics in light of
age-old commentary on the ethics of civil disobedience and militancy.
These arguments have been worked out in great depth, and there is
no sense reinventing the wheel. As Peter Singer argues, it is important
to have "some understanding of the nature of ethics and the meaning
of moral concepts. Those who do not understand the terms they are
using are more likely to create confusion than to dispel it, and it is only
too easy to become confused about the concepts used in ethics"
(1988:153).

In addition, ethical inquiry can acquaint practitioners with the ethical traditions of their respective professions and of their implications
for the AIDS crisis. Take, for instance, the controversy concerning, and
obligation of physicians to treat, AIDS patients. The bioethics literature
is replete with discussions of physicians' duty to treat during public
health crises and epidemics throughout history (Cipolla 1977; Loewy

1986; Zuger and Miles 1987; Arras 1988; Emanuel 1988; Fox 1988; Friedlander 1990; Jonsen 1990). It is important for practitioners to know what ethical norms have evolved during the profession's history, the nature of debate about these norms, and their possible relevance to the AIDS crisis.

It is particularly useful for practitioners to have at least a rudimentary grasp of ethical theories, speculation about their validity and value, and possible connections to AIDS-related policy. It is true, for example, that deontological and utilitarian theories come up short when it comes to providing clear guidance in controversy concerning the limits of confidentiality in AIDS cases. Careful consideration of these two classic perspectives—along with others that focus on rights, duties, and virtue—can produce a series of conflicting conclusions. What, one might reasonably ask, is the point? The point is that these theoretical schools of thought contain elements that many people find compelling or intuitively appealing, and it is important to consider their implications and their merits and demerits. The final outcome may be that reasonable people will disagree, but the process of debate and scrutiny of these perspectives is likely to produce the kind of thoughtful judgment that is always more valuable than simplistic conclusions reached without the benefit of careful, sustained reflection and discourse. Moreover, such thorough analysis very often leads to appropriate and principled shifts in opinion. As Ruth Macklin claims:

> As long as the debate between Kantians and utilitarians continues to rage and as long as the Western political and philosophical tradition continues to embrace both the respect-for-persons principle and the principle of beneficence, there can be no possible resolution of dilemmas traceable to those competing theoretical approaches. But the inability to make a final determination of which theoretical approach is ultimately "right" does not rule out the prospect for making sound moral judgments in practical contexts, based on one or the other theoretical perspective.
>
> The choice between utilitarian ethics and a deontological moral system rooted in rights and duties is not a choice between one moral and one immoral alternative. Rather, it rests on a commitment to one moral viewpoint instead of another, where both are capable of providing good reasons for acting. Both perspectives stand in opposition to egoistic or selfish approaches, or to a philosophy whose precepts are grounded in privileges of power, wealth, or the authority of technical experts (1988:66–67).

It is helpful to remember that in the final analysis the Darwinistic forces of the intellectual marketplace will determine which theoretical perspectives are most helpful and persuasive. Pushing competing points of view to their respective limits, in dialectical fashion, helps to reveal the strengths and weaknesses of a position, and eventually helps the fittest arguments survive. Jan Narveson makes the point nicely:

> [I]f some ethical theory would prove to be genuinely indeterminate at some point where determination is needed, then there is nothing to say except that it is a fatal objection to that theory as it stands. It would have to be supplemented, patched up, or discarded. If, for example, it could be established that the whole idea of cardinal utility is in principle incoherent, then that is a blow from which utilitarianism, as usually understood, could not recover. The point here is that we must not identify the whole enterprise of moral philosophy with any particular theory within it. But why should there not be progress? Old theories will fall into disuse or simply die from fatal conceptual diseases; new theories will replace them. So it goes. None of this has any tendency to establish that the enterprise is unfounded or that we can never expect any definite results (1988:104).

James Nickel offers a particularly useful framework for assessing the value of ethics (1988:139–148). According to the "strong" version of applied ethics, some particular ethical theory is considered to be true, well founded, or authoritative, and it is possible in principle to settle policy issues by deriving a prescription from that theory. Thus, someone who accepts Rawls' theory of justice would use it to determine appropriate levels of funding for AIDS prevention, research, and treatment. One would draw on Rawls' concepts related to the *veil of ignorance, original position, difference principle,* and *the least advantaged* to determine the most just allocation of scarce health care resources.

As I noted earlier, however, few embrace the "strong" version of applied ethics. As A. J. Ayer observed several decades ago, "It is silly, as well as presumptuous, for any one type of philosopher to pose as the champion of virtue. And it is also one reason why many people find moral philosophy an unsatisfactory subject" (in Singer 1988:149).

Instead, most contemporary ethicists prefer what Nickel calls the "weak" version of applied ethics, where ethical concepts and theory are used mainly to illuminate policy issues and their moral features. According to the weak version, it is helpful to survey available concepts and theories (and to formulate new ones) to try to shed light on compelling issues and to consider them from various, and often competing, perspectives. Thus, it is useful to examine civil liberties issues related to the mandatory segregation of persons with AIDS from various versions of deontological theories, utilitarian theories, and other theories that do not fall neatly into these two categories. Weak applied ethics does not assume that any one theory is completely adequate. As Nickel concludes,

> I am open-minded about the future prospects of moral theorizing, but I doubt that we have much moral theory in hand that can be offered with confidence as a guide to policy in hard cases. As guides to policy, I am much more comfortable with middle-level moral principles that are widely accepted than with grand principles such as the principle of utility or Rawls's difference principle (1988:148).

Moral Worth and Responsibility

Thus far I have commented on the need for professionals concerned about AIDS to draw on relevant ethical concepts and theory. Unfortunately, the implication here may be that mastery of ethical concepts and theory will suffice. However, all of this inappropriately ignores another essential element: the personal moral frameworks or values of the professionals involved with AIDS cases, particularly the influence of professionals' beliefs about the morality and culpability of persons with AIDS.

Throughout history, professionals have had to make decisions about their duty to treat during an epidemic. Historical accounts suggest that during most epidemics most physicians have treated most of the patients who sought their help. Apparently this was the case during a wide range of epidemics, including the Black Death that began in Italy in the fourteenth century, the outbreak of yellow fever in various U.S. locations in the eighteenth and nineteenth centuries, and cholera epidemics in New York City in the nineteenth century (Fox 1988).

It is tempting to believe, as some have argued (Fox 1988:9), that AIDS does not pose a new challenge in this respect. It may be that most health care professionals will commit themselves to treating persons with AIDS, at some risk to themselves, just as they have fulfilled their duties during past public health crises. I fear, however, that the AIDS crisis adds a novel variable to the equation, one that may substantially affect the willingness of practitioners to treat.

Historically, health care professionals have generally viewed victims of epidemics as just that: *victims*. With few exceptions, victims of infectious diseases have been regarded as innocent, vulnerable people who have had the misfortune to contract a dreaded illness. Generally speaking, they have not been viewed as morally suspect or as individuals who were culpable for their susceptibility to illness.

In contrast, persons with AIDS are often viewed as morally defective and blameworthy. Unlike most other epidemic victims, persons at high risk for AIDS are often viewed as marginal members of society. It is well known among health care professionals that the majority of persons with AIDS are gay or bisexual men, or intravenous (IV) drug users, individuals whose life-styles placed them at higher risk for contracting AIDS. My conversations with health care professionals suggest that there is a disturbing tendency for some of them to view persons with AIDS as individuals who chose, by virtue of their own free will, to engage in a variety of high-risk activities, and that this has some bearing on (1) their rights, e.g., to privacy, health care and social service resources, jobs, housing, and (2) professionals' duty, e.g., to treat persons with AIDS, respect their confidentiality.[1] Moreover, the fact that the poor and minorities of color are overrepresented among persons with AIDS may also influence professionals' willingness to treat. Discriminatory attitudes related to race, ethnicity, and poverty may exacerbate judgmental attitudes toward gay and bisexual men and toward IV drug users.

Debate about the extent to which persons with AIDS are morally responsible for their status certainly has precedents. Treatment of populations such as criminals, the poor, mentally ill, abused, and alcoholic has also been, to a great extent, a function of professionals' perceptions of their clients' culpability for their problems. With these populations too, professionals' judgments about the morality of their clients tend to get entangled with their beliefs about their duty to aid.

In philosophical terms, debate among professionals about the relevance of client culpability has focused on the concepts of free will and determinism (Frankfurt 1973; Reamer 1983). Professionals repeatedly make assumptions about the determinants of people's problems and shape interventions and treatment plans accordingly. For instance, some forms of mental retardation, we may conclude, are a result of certain chromosomal abnormalities and thus are amenable to only a limited range of treatments. Some might argue that poverty stems from structural problems in our economy that need to be addressed (e.g., high unemployment or unfair tax structures) while others believe that poverty must be attacked by discouraging sloth. And with respect to AIDS we find equally diverse opinion. In the minds of some, AIDS can be prevented primarily by discouraging immoral activities engaged in by people who are without rectitude. For others, the disease will not be prevented until we acknowledge that persons with AIDS are victims of a variety of structural defects in the culture related to inadequate education, oppression, and discrimination. How we respond to these problems—whether we focus our attention on environmental determinants or individual character—frequently depends on assumptions we make about the extent to which people's problems are the result of factors over which they have control.

Further, the conclusions professionals reach about the causes of people's problems frequently lead to assumptions about the extent to which they *deserve* assistance. If we conclude that a person is chronically depressed because of a series of unforeseen, tragic events in her life, we may be more inclined to offer solace and support than we would be if we decide that her depression is a calculated, willful, protracted, and self-serving attempt to gain sympathy and attention. If we conclude that an individual has difficulty sustaining employment because of a congenital learning disability that he has tried persistently to overcome, we may be more willing to invest our professional time and energy than we would with an individual who is fired from jobs repeatedly because he resents having to arrive for work at 8:30 A.M. every day. A dentist who contracts AIDS as a result of a needle stick may elicit more sympathetic, humane, and comprehensive care than an AIDS patient who was infected by a prostitute.

An alternative to extreme views of either free will or determinism, but which contains elements of both schools of thought, has become known in philosophical circles as the "mixed view" or "soft determinism." This view seems most prevalent with respect to persons with AIDS. According to this mixed view, although people's problems are sometimes caused by antecedent circumstances over which they have little or no control, voluntary behavior is nonetheless possible and, in the absence of coercion, is brought about by the individual's own decisions, choices, and preferences (Taylor 1963:43–44). From this perspective, AIDS is viewed as the consequence of both (1) deterministic antecedents (e.g., the consequence of inadequate education provided to low-income and oppressed groups, homophobia and discrimination against gay and bisexual men, rampant IV drug use that is the by-product of a capitalistic nation that has a vested interest in sustaining an underclass) *and* (2) voluntary choice (e.g., individuals *choose* to engage in unprotected sexual activity, individuals *choose* to share needles). The exception would be, of course, the individual who is perceived as a "pure" victim of the AIDS disease, e.g., the surgical patient who is transfused with contaminated blood, the wife of a prostitute-visiting husband, the newborn whose mother is infected, the physician who contracts AIDS as a result of a needle stick or blood splash.

The mixed view of the free will-determinism debate is based on what philosophers refer to as the compatibility argument, according to which these two concepts are not, contrary to first impressions, necessarily mutually exclusive. Rather they are complementary. This is a view that has been espoused by such diverse luminaries as Thomas Hobbes, David Hume, and John Stuart Mill (Ginet 1962:49–55). It is also a view that reflects the enduring tension between professionals' desire to understand and respond to human tragedy by uncovering complex causal connections and their wish to see people as autonomous individuals who are not subject entirely to intrapsychic, biological, and environmental forces that lie beyond their control. As Tolstoy said,

> The problem lies in the fact that if we regard man as a subject for observation from whatever point of view—theological, historical, ethical, or philosophic—we find the universal law of necessity to which he (like everything else that exists) is subject. But looking upon man from within ourselves—man as the object of our own inner consciousness of self—we feel ourselves to be free (in Kenny 1973:89).

The kind of assistance that health care professionals choose to offer persons with AIDS is significantly influenced by the degree to which they hold infected persons responsible for contracting the disease. In this respect, there is a close relationship between the concepts of moral responsibility and moral desert. That is, the extent to which professionals assist or shun persons with AIDS is likely to be a function of beliefs about the degree to which infected persons are morally responsible for contracting the disease.

We must be particularly concerned about the tendency among professionals to understand intellectually the causes of AIDS and still regard persons with AIDS as blameworthy (just as professionals sometimes understand the causes of poverty, alcoholism, and crime and yet still blame the poor, alcoholic, and criminal for their difficulties). Ultimately, it is this sort of bias that may impede efforts to provide humane care to persons with AIDS. Harry Frankfurt noted this general tendency in his important essay on the relationship between coercion and moral responsibility:

> We do on some occasions find it appropriate to make an adverse judgment concerning a person's submission to a threat, even though we

recognise that he has genuinely been coerced and that he is therefore not properly to be held morally responsible for his submission. This is because we think that the person, although he was in fact quite unable to control a desire, ought to have been able to control it (1973:79).

The Place for Ethics

Clearly, our analysis and understanding of ethical concepts can contribute in a large way to the formulation of a moral response to the AIDS crisis. We face critical questions concerning conflicts of professional duty and the delivery of services to persons with AIDS. Ultimately, our answers to these questions should rest on conclusions we reach about such central ethical concepts as justice, fairness, respect, equity, rights, and duties.

The AIDS crisis poses a very special challenge for applied ethics. The life-and-death stakes are high, and this, of course, adds a sense of urgency. But the *ethical* stakes are high too, in that the AIDS crisis is testing the moral mettle of professionals in a way perhaps that no prior public health crisis has. In the final analysis, the answers we provide to the ethical questions that face us will say a great deal about what we mean when we use the term *professional*.

How shall we go about the task of applying ethics to AIDS? For one thing, we must quicken our efforts to acquaint health care professionals with the relevant ethical issues. This can be done through a variety of existing mechanisms, including instruction in graduate and professional training programs, and through in-service training in health care settings. Bioethics is an increasingly secure fixture in contemporary health care settings, and ethical issues related to AIDS can be added to the impressive list of topics that are covered currently in bioethics education.

The growing number of institutional ethics committees (IECs) can also be used to help focus professionals' attention on the ethical dimensions of the AIDS crisis. The concept of IECs emerged most prominently in 1976, when the New Jersey Supreme Court ruled that Karen Anne Quinlan's family and physicians should consult an ethics committee in deciding whether to remove her from life-support systems (although a number of hospitals have had something resembling ethics committees since at least the 1920s). The court based its ruling in part on a seminal article that appeared in the *Baylor Law Review* in 1975, in which a pediatrician advocated the use of ethics committees in cases when health care professionals face difficult ethical choices (Teel 1975).

Ethics committees typically perform several functions that can be focused on AIDS-related issues. Among the most important functions is that of educating staff about ethical issues. Thus, in health care settings, training sessions might be devoted to the topics of confidentiality and privacy, the professional's right to refuse to treat, screening of pregnant women and newborns, participation in research projects, access to nonapproved treatments, the use of isolation, and the relevance of ethical theory and concepts.

A related function concerns the review and formulation of agency policies and guidelines for use by staff members who encounter ethical dilemmas (Cranford and Doudera 1984; Cohen 1988). Thus, an ethics committee might develop detailed guidelines concerning the release of information to outside parties, obtaining informed consent, health care coverage, or mandatory testing.

Finally, in some instances staff members may wish to call on an ethics committee for advice and consultation regarding a specific case. A large percentage of existing ethics committees provides nonbinding ethics consultation from an interdisciplinary group that typically includes some combination of physicians, nurses, clergy, social service professionals, ethicists, administrators, and attorneys. An ethics committee can offer an opportunity for staff members to think through case-specific issues with colleagues who have knowledge of ethical issues as a result of their experiences, familiarity with relevant concepts and literature, and specialized training. Although IECs are not always able to provide definitive, consensus-based opinions about the complex issues that are frequently brought to their attention (nor should they be expected to), they can provide a valuable forum for thorough and critical analyses of troublesome dilemmas.

Note, however, that while cognitively oriented training in and discussion of ethics can be enormously helpful, no amount of it can substitute for an innate sensitivity to matters of justice, right and wrong, and duty and obligation. At some point we are dealing with the moral fiber of professionals themselves, not just with their intellectual grasp of an intriguing collection of ethical theories and concepts. As Albert Jonsen astutely argues, ethics guidelines "are not the modern substitute for the Decalogue. They are, rather, shorthand moral education. They set out the concise definitions and the relevant distinctions that prepare the already well-disposed person to make the shrewd judgment that this or that instance is a typical case of this or that sort, and, then, decide how to act" (1984:4).

We are, after all, seeking a certain form of virtue here, one that is informed by reason. Virtue can certainly be taught but probably not so well in university classrooms, hospital conference rooms, insurance company board rooms, or in legislative subcommittee meetings. Most of us got whatever virtue we now possess long before we walked into those rooms, and it is this deep-seated virtue that is essential if we are to respond ethically to the AIDS crisis. As C. S. Lewis observed some years ago:

> It still remains true that no justification of virtue will enable a man to be virtuous. Without the aid of trained emotions the intellect is powerless against the animal organism. I had sooner play cards against a man who was quite skeptical about ethics, but bred to believe that "a gentleman does not cheat," than against an irreproachable moral philosopher who had been brought up among sharpers (1947:3–4).

The AIDS crisis and the field of applied ethics are burgeoning together. There is probably more than coincidence at work here, but that is the subject of a different essay. What is important to note for our purposes is that one of humankind's greatest public health challenges—accompanied by all of its troubling moral dimensions—has emerged at a time when professionals' ability to identify and grapple with complex ethical issues is maturing in an unprecedented way.

But we should not take too much comfort in this. At best, the field of applied ethics is moving from childhood to adolescence, and we all know what adolescence entails. It is characterized by turmoil, identity issues, and a search for bearings. And this is about where we are with applied ethics. To be sure, during the first two decades of the field's life, we have seen tremendous growth. Professionals are now much more aware of the ethical elements of their work, they are much better able to reason about moral matters, and all sorts of policies and guidelines have been produced to help professionals navigate. We are more self-conscious about ethics, and that is good.

But how well equipped are we to face the sort of intimidating ethical challenges posed by AIDS? Certainly we have available all manner of moral concepts and principles to help us take positions on issues of mandatory screening, AIDS education, research design, allocation of limited resources, AIDS activism, and confidentiality. Certainly we have the tools to engage in protracted rational discourse about the merits of competing arguments on the ethics of this or that policy.

What seems to be missing, however, is sustained discourse about professionals' *commitment* to do the right thing once a decision has been reached about the right thing to do. It is not surprising that MacIntyre (1981:179–181) describes courage as one of life's principal virtues. It is one thing to engage in a depersonalized, stripped-down, yet intellectually sophisticated discussion of complex moral matters related to AIDS without displaying one's own personal beliefs, anxieties, and biases. It is quite another to take seriously the question, Why be moral in the first place?

To answer this question satisfactorily, we must deal with people who are genuinely concerned about persons with AIDS, those who minister to them, and members of the broader commonweal. We cannot afford to regard AIDS as just another intellectual puzzle that mainly provides intriguing grist for the heuristic mill or opportunity for one's own career advancement. Rather, we are talking about fundamental questions of right and wrong and of duty and obligation that strike at the core of what we mean by ethics. Motive is relevant. We must move beyond the sterile analysis of theory and concept (while continuing to incorporate both) to focus on why people do or do not care about doing what is right with respect to AIDS. For this to happen, we need to broaden our lens to include issues of commitment and caring to complement our concern with grand ethical guidelines and principles, and to include what Leon Kass has described as the " 'small morals' that are the bedrock of ordinary experience and the matrix of all interpersonal relations" (1990:8). With customary insight, Kass goes on to conclude that: "Perhaps in ethics, the true route begins with practice, with deeds and doers, and moves only secondarily to reflection on practice. Indeed, even the propensity to *care* about moral matters requires a certain *moral disposition,* acquired in practice, before the age of reflection arrives. As Aristotle points out, he who has 'the that' can easily get 'the why.' "

The AIDS crisis is important in and of itself because of the nature of this public health pandemic. However, if ethical thinking is to make a meaningful difference in the AIDS crisis—and in any comparable crisis—it must help us balance our concern about abstract reasons for right action with a concern about what moves people to care about right action. But AIDS also provides a severe test of our commitment to the most basic of human values. How we respond to this crisis will teach us a great deal about our virtue and the relevance of ethics.

NOTE

1. Recently I had a conversation with a prominent oral surgeon in which we discussed the risks to dentists who treat AIDS patients. Without hesitation and with considerable conviction, this practitioner argued that *gay* dentists should assume the primary responsibility for treatment of persons with AIDS, since "they are all

members of the same high-risk community." This dentist's comments demonstrate the depth of the challenge involved in educating professionals about the AIDS crisis and confronting their homophobic and other discriminatory beliefs. For discussion of health care professionals' attitudes and biases toward AIDS patients, see Ghitelman 1987; Searle 1987; Imperato et al. 1988; Link et al. 1988; Arnow et al. 1989).

REFERENCES

Arnow, Paul M., Lawrence A. Pottenger, Carol B. Stocking, Mark Siegler, and Henry W. DeLeeuw. 1989. Orthopedic Surgeons' Attitudes and Practices Concerning Treatment of Patients with HIV Infection. *Public Health Reports* 104(2):121–129.

Arras, John D. 1988. The Fragile Web of Responsibility: AIDS and the Duty to Treat. *Hastings Center Report* (April/May), Special Suppl. 18(2):10–20.

Baier, Annette. 1988. Theory and Reflective Practices. In David M. Rosenthal and Fadlou Shehadi, eds., *Applied Ethics and Ethical Theory*, pp. 25–49. Salt Lake City: University of Utah Press.

Bayer, Ronald. 1989. *Private Acts, Social Consequences: AIDS and the Politics of Public Health*. New York: Free Press.

Bedau, Hugo Adam, ed. 1969. *Civil Disobedience: Theory and Practice*. Indianapolis: Bobbs-Merrill.

Brandt, Allan M. 1987. A Historical Perspective. In Harlon L. Dalton, Scott Burris, and the Yale AIDS Law Project, eds., *AIDS and the Law*, pp. 37–43. New Haven: Yale University Press.

Childress, James F. 1987. An Ethical Framework for Assessing Policies to Screen for Antibodies to HIV. *AIDS and Public Policy Journal* (Winter), 2:28–31.

Cipolla, Carlo M. 1977. A Plague Doctor. In Harry A. Miskimin, D. Herlihy, A. L. Udovitch, eds., *The Medieval City*. New Haven: Yale University Press.

Cohen, Carl. 1989. Militant Morality: Civil Disobedience and Bioethics. *Hastings Center Report* 19(6):23–25.

Cohen, Cynthia B. 1988. Ethics Committees. *Hastings Center Report* 18:11.

Cranford, Ronald E. and Edward Doudera, eds. 1984. *Institutional Ethics Committees and Health Care Decision Making*. Ann Arbor, Mich.: Health Administration Press.

Emanuel, Ezekiel J. 1988. Do Physicians Have an Obligation to Treat Patients with AIDS? *New England Journal of Medicine* 318(25):1686–1690.

Fox, Daniel M. 1988. The Politics of Physicians' Responsibility in Epidemics: A Note on History. *Hastings Center Report* (April/May), Special Suppl., 18(2): 5–10.

Francis, Donald D. and James Chin. 1987. The Prevention of Acquired Immunodeficiency Syndrome in the United States. *JAMA* 257:1357–1366.

Frankfurt, Harry G. 1973. Coercion and Moral Responsibility. In Ted Honderich, ed., *Essays on Freedom of Action*, p. 79. London: Routledge and Kegan Paul.

Freedman, Benjamin and the McGill/Boston Research Group. 1989. Nonvalidated Therapies and HIV Disease. *Hastings Center Report* (May/June), 19(3):14–20.

Friedlander, Walter J. 1990. On the Obligation of Physicians to Treat AIDS: Is There a Historical Basis? *Reviews of Infectious Diseases* 12(2):191–203.

Gewirth, Alan. 1978. *Reason and Morality*. Chicago: University of Chicago Press.

Ghitelman, David. 1987. AIDS. *MD* (January), 91–100.

Ginet, Carl. 1962. Can the Will Be Caused? *Philosophical Review* 71:49–55.

Gostin, Larry. 1987. Traditional Public Health Strategies. In Harlon L. Dalton, Scott Burris, and the Yale AIDS Law Project, eds., *AIDS and the Law*, pp. 47–65. New Haven: Yale University Press.

Gray, Lizbeth A. and Anna K. Harding. 1988. Confidentiality Limits with Clients Who Have the AIDS Virus. *Journal of Counseling and Development* (January), 66(5):219–223.

Hare, R. M. 1986. Why Do Applied Ethics? In Joseph de Marco and Richard M. Fox, eds., *New Directions in Ethics*, pp. 225–237. London: Routledge and Kegan Paul.

Imperato, Pascal James, Joseph G. Feldman, Kamran Nayeri, and Jack A. DeHovitz. 1988. Medical Students' Attitudes Towards Caring for Patients with AIDS in a High Incidence Area. *New York State Journal of Medicine* 88(5):223–228.

Jonsen, Albert R. 1984. A Guide to Guidelines. *American Society of Law and Medicine: Ethics Committee Newsletter* 2:4.

Jonsen, Albert R. 1990. The Duty to Treat Patients with AIDS and HIV Infection. In Lawrence O. Gostin, ed., *AIDS and the Health Care System*, pp. 155–168. New Haven: Yale University Press.

Kain, Craig D. 1988. To Breach or Not to Breach: Is that the Question? *Journal of Counseling and Development* 66(5):224–225.

Kass, Leon R. 1990. Practicing Ethics: Where's the Action? *Hastings Center Report* (January/February), 20(1):5–12.

Kenny, Anthony. 1973. Freedom, Spontaneity, and Indifference. In Ted Honderich, ed., *Essays on Freedom of Action*, p. 89. London: Routledge and Kegan Paul.

Lamb, Douglas H., Claudia Clark, Philip Drumheller, Kathleen Frizzell, and Lynn Surrey. 1989. Applying *Tarasoff* to AIDS-Related Psychotherapy Issues. *Professional Psychology: Research and Practice* 20(1):37–43.

Lewis, C. S. 1947. *The Abolition of Man*. New York: Macmillan.

Lewis, Marjorie B. 1986. Duty to Warn Versus Duty to Maintain Confidentiality: Conflicting Demands on Mental Health Professionals. *Suffolk Law Review* 20(3):579–615.

Link, R. Nathan, Anat R. Feingold, Mitchell H. Charap, Katherine Freeman, and Steven P. Shelov. 1988. Concerns of Medical and Pediatric Officers About Acquiring AIDS from Their Patients. *American Journal of Public Health* 78(4):455–459.

Loewy, Erich H. 1986. Duties, Fears, and Physicians. *Social Science and Medicine* 12:1363–1366.

Macklin, Ruth. 1988. Theoretical and Applied Ethics: A Reply to the Skeptics. In David M. Rosenthal and Fadlou Shehadi, eds., *Applied Ethics and Ethical Theory*, pp. 50–70. Salt Lake City: University of Utah Press.

MacIntyre, Alasdair. 1981. *After Virtue*. South Bend, Ind.: University of Notre Dame Press.

Merritt, Deborah Jones. 1986. The Constitutional Balance Between Health and Liberty. *Hastings Center Report* (December), Special Suppl. 16(6):2–10.

Narveson, Jan. 1988. Is There a Problem About "Applied" Ethics? In David M. Rosenthal and Fadlou Shehadi, eds., *Applied Ethics and Ethical Theory*, pp. 100–115. Salt Lake City: University of Utah Press.

Nickel, James W. 1988. Philosophy and Policy. In David M. Rosenthal and Fadlou Shehadi, eds., *Applied Ethics and Ethical Theory*, pp. 139–148. Salt Lake City: University of Utah Press.

Noble, Cheryl N. 1982. Ethics and Experts. *Hastings Center Report* (June), 12(3):5–9.

Rachels, James. 1980. Can Ethics Provide Answers? *Hastings Center Report* (June), 10:32–40.

Rawls, John. 1971. *A Theory of Justice*. Cambridge, Mass.: Harvard University Press.

Reamer, Frederic G. 1983. The Free Will-Determinism Debate and Social Work. *Social Service Review* 57(4):626–644.

Reamer, Frederic G. 1990. *Ethical Dilemmas in Social Service*. 2d ed. New York: Columbia University Press.

Reamer, Frederic G. and Marcia Abramson. 1982. *The Teaching of Social Work Ethics*. Hastings-on-Hudson, N.Y.: The Hastings Center.

Ross, W. D. 1930. *The Right and the Good*. Oxford: Clarendon Press.

Rothman, David J. 1987. Ethical and Social Issues in the Development of New Drugs and Vaccines. *Bulletin of the New York Academy of Medicine* 63(6):557–568.

Searle, E. Stephen. 1987. Knowledge, Attitudes, and Behaviour of Health Professionals in Relation to AIDS. *Lancet* 1:26–28.

Singer, Peter. 1988. Ethical Experts in a Democracy. In David M. Rosenthal and Fadlou Shehadi, eds., *Applied Ethics and Ethical Theory*, pp. 149–161. Salt Lake City: University of Utah Press.

Smart, J. J. C. 1971. Extreme and Restricted Utilitarianism. In Samuel Gorovitz, ed., *Mill: Utilitarianism*, p. 199. Indianapolis: Bobbs-Merrill.

Tarasoff v. Board of Regents of the University of California. 1976. 17 Cal. 3d 425, 551 P.2d 334, 131 *California Reporter* 14.

Taylor, Richard. 1963. *Metaphysics*. Englewood Cliffs, N.J.: Prentice-Hall.

Teel, Karen. 1975. The Physician's Dilemma: A Doctor's View: What the Law Should Be. *Baylor Law Review* 27(6):9.

Wasserstrom, Richard. 1975. The Obligation to Obey the Law. In Richard Wasserstrom, ed., *Today's Moral Problems*. New York: Macmillan.

Zuger, Abigail and Steven H. Miles. 1987. Physicians, AIDS, and Occupational Risk: Historic Traditions and Ethical Obligations. *JAMA* (October 9), 258(14):1924–1928.

2. AIDS, Public Health, and Civil Liberties: Consensus and Conflict in Policy

RONALD BAYER

WHEN AIDS FIRST made its appearance in the early 1980s, thereby shattering the illusion that advanced industrial societies had placed behind them the threat of infectious disease, it became necessary once again for the United States to consider the role of public health as a defense against the threat of epidemic disease. Among the profoundly important questions posed by AIDS was whether a liberal society with a hard-won commitment to privacy could effectively confront an epidemic spread in the context of intimate relationships. That was a question that would compel a consideration of the tension between the protection of the public health and communal welfare on the one hand and of civil liberties on the other (Bayer 1989).

The ethos of public health and that of civil liberties are radically distinct. At the most fundamental level, the ethos of public health takes the well-being of the community as its highest good and would, in the face of uncertainty—especially where the risks are high—and to the extent deemed necessary, limit freedom or place restrictions on the realm of privacy in order to prevent morbidity from taking its toll. The burden of proof against proceeding from this perspective rests upon those who assert that the harms to liberty would, from a social point of view, outweigh the health benefits to be obtained from a proposed course of action.

From the point of view of civil liberties, the situation is quite the reverse. No civil libertarian denies the importance of protecting others from injury. The "harm principle" enunciated by John Stuart Mill is, in fact, the universally acknowledged limiting standard circumscribing individual freedom. For twentieth-century liberals and civil libertarians that principle has typically accorded considerable latitude to measures taken in the name of public health—indeed more so than some contemporary civil libertarians find comfortable. But since from a libertarian point of view the freedom of the individual is the highest good of a liberal society, measures designed to restrict personal freedom must be justified by a strong showing that no other path exists to protect the public health. When there are doubts, a heavy burden of proof must be borne by those who would act to impose restrictions.

These two abstractions, liberty and communal welfare, are always in a state of tension in the realm of public health policy. How the balance between the two is struck in a particular historical moment is a function of the relationship among political forces, the dominance of ideological commitments, and the contour of the threat—both social and biological—posed by a particular epidemic.

If AIDS had struck at a different moment in American political history, the balances struck, indeed the very questions asked, would have been far different from those that emerged in the first years of the epidemic. AIDS posed its challenge to the polity at a unique juncture. For almost twenty years the courts had been deepening and extending the scope of the constitutionally protected realm of privacy (Karst 1980). Paralleling these developments, and drawing upon the same reformist spirit, the courts had redefined the standards of due process against which all measures that could limit fundamental rights would be judged. And although there were only limited indications of how those changes would affect the tradition of deference to the decisions made by officials acting to protect the public health, it was almost certain that their exercise of authority would not remain unchallenged (Merritt 1986).

AIDS, a lethal disease transmitted in the most private settings, would test the vitality of the jurisprudence of privacy, the durability of commitment to due process, and the capacity of those responsible for the defense of the public health to adjust their professional traditions —the authoritarian measures that defined the historical repertoire of responses to epidemic threats—of public health to a social milieu far different from those that gave rise to and endowed them with legitimacy. How would the linkage of intimacy and lethality serve to inform debates about the protected realm of privacy? Would coercion be used to identify those who were infected with human immunodeficiency virus (HIV)? How would the claim of confidentiality be balanced against those of the public health that might require disclosure? Would the power to quarantine ever be used to restrict individuals whose behaviors posed a threat of HIV transmission?

The answers given to each of these questions would inevitably be affected by the unique social character of the American AIDS epidemic. Primarily a disease of the socially marginal—gay men, intravenous (IV) drug users and their sexual partners—one in which poor blacks and Hispanics were overrepresented, AIDS might well have provoked a response within which privacy rights would have been subordinated. That was not the case in great measure because of the extraordinary skill and energy of organizations representing white middle-class gay men who fiercely defended the rights of privacy in the face of AIDS. In doing so they fundamentally shaped the course of public debate and practice in the epidemic's first years.

As public health officials, gay activists, and civil liberties advocates faced the questions posed by AIDS, there emerged a broad consensus on how AIDS was to be confronted. The very privacy of the acts linked to HIV transmission imposed practical limitations on what could be done. The importance of eliciting the cooperation of those most at risk for infection imposed political limitations on what should be done. The centrality of civil liberties to American political culture imposed ideological limitations on what ought to be done. Pragmatic and philosophical considerations thus dictated the adoption of a course within which the defense of the public health and respect for privacy were joined.

Supported by the nation's leading public health officials, including the Surgeon General, associations of health care professionals, liberal political figures, representatives of the gay community, and proponents of civil liberties, a consensus emerged that was voluntarist at its core, that rejected recourse to coercion in favor of strategies designed to motivate mass behavioral change. This remarkable consensus, achieved at a moment of national anxiety, when the prospects for therapeutic intervention with those with HIV disease were very poor, suggested to some that the historic tension between advocates of civil liberties and public health had been dissolved. Many who had been fearful of how AIDS could provide the context for the imposition of a harsh regimen in the name of communal protection claimed that at least in context of AIDS the defense of the public health and that of civil liberties were not only compatible but interdependent. But by the end of the epidemic's first decade the alliances that had forged the voluntarist consensus and that had seemed so secure had begun to unravel. A changing epidemiological picture, rapid advances in the clinical management of HIV-related diseases, and, beginning in 1989, the promise of early therapeutic intervention to slow the progression of disease in those who were asymptomatic set the stage for the reemergence of public health traditionalism. What had appeared to be a new ethos of public health was revealed to be the achievement of a particular historical moment, a political solution reflecting a unique confluence of forces.

The inherent tension between public health and civil liberties had thus reemerged and with it inevitable public controversies necessitating new political solutions.

In this essay, the rise and decline of the unusual alliance between proponents of civil liberties and public health is traced through a schematic discussion of several key moments in the evolution of AIDS policy in the United States. In each case the interplay of gay activists, civil liberties organizations, public health professionals, and the broader political system will demonstrate that the making of public health policy entails far more than the application of scientific knowledge to the resolution of epidemiological threats.

The Rise of the Voluntarist Consensus: 1983–1989

Even before the discovery of HIV, public health officials had been compelled to recognize that the struggle against AIDS would require the adoption of a strategy designed to reassure those most at risk about the benign intentions of state agencies that had been perceived as antagonistic. For gay men who suffered the legacy of official repression and social exclusion, such efforts would necessitate a willingness to negotiate differences rather than impose solutions. For intravenous drug users, policies of AIDS control would have to be radically distinct from repressive drug control programs. For Haitians, who in the early days of the epidemic were perceived as being at increased risk, it was necessary to create reassurances that the strategy of public health would be untainted by efforts of the immigration authorities to locate undocumented aliens. In all, the emerging campaign against AIDS would have to display a respect for confidentiality and privacy (Bayer, Levine, and Murray 1984). Yet even in the epidemic's first phase, tensions emerged between public health officials, gay activists, and civil liberties organizations. Nowhere was this more obvious than in the bitter debates over whether to close or regulate quasi-public commercial establishments where gay and bisexual men engaged in sexual activity linked to the spread of AIDS.

The Bathhouse Debates

On October 9, 1984, Mervyn Silverman, director of public health in San Francisco, issued the following announcement:

> The [gay bathhouses] that I have ordered closed today have continued in the face of this epidemic to provide an environment that encourages

and facilitates multiple unsafe sexual contacts, which are an important contributory factor in the spread of this deadly disease. When activities are proven to be dangerous to the public and continue to take place in commercial settings, the Health Department has the duty to intercede and halt the operation of such establishments (Silverman 1984 press statement).

Thus did San Francisco's liberal chief health official reject the claims of those who sought to protect the gay bathhouse by the invocation of the principles governing the state's relationship to private sexual behavior between consenting adults. The very commercial nature of the establishments involved removed, for him, the protective mantle and provided the warrant for intervention. Responding to those who he knew would charge that his actions represented a profound assault on the interests of gay men and a reversal of the social and legal advances attained by San Francisco's homosexual community, Silverman ended his statement by declaring, "Make no mistake about it. These fourteen establishments are not fostering gay liberation. They are fostering disease and death." In so moving, Silverman, who had gained the support of some gay leaders, brought to an end almost a year of heated political debate over the course he should follow in facing the persistence of behavior linked to the spread of AIDS in public settings. The debate posed in stark form the clash between the values of privacy and public health.

Very early in the epidemic, the limitation of the perspective focusing solely on the decisions about sexual conduct made by gay men as private individuals became apparent. This was the context in which the question of the bathhouses, those bold expressions of an unfettered gay sexuality, had become the subject of an acrimonious controversy that divided the gay community and forced a confrontation over privacy, sexual behavior, and limits of state intervention in the name of public health. "Could [it] be," wrote the publisher of the *Advocate*, a West Coast gay newspaper, "that the sex palaces which encourage orgies and lack adequate showers are public health hazards? . . . I shudder at the political implications of this notion" (*Advocate*, March 18, 1982, p. 6).

Despite occasional suggestions that the gay community might have to collaborate with public health officials to regulate the bathhouses or to limit the activity permitted to occur within them, the dominant ideological voice projected by the gay press was antistatist. It was hostile to the claims that the defense of public health by government officials might rightfully entail restrictions on commercial establishments serving the sexual desires of their gay clientele, hostile to the suggestion that the gay community act to force changes in the institutions providing the setting for anonymous sexual encounters that could lead to the spread of AIDS.

Having so recently emerged from long, bitter struggles against statutory prohibitions on homosexuality and the socially sanctioned pattern of discrimination that made privacy so central to the struggle for survival, it is not surprising that gay political thought was so libertarian in its orientation. Indeed, despite the language of community that filled the columns of the gay press, a radical individualism inspired much of the early rhetoric about the bathhouses.

One of the most forceful and principled defenses of the importance of shielding the right of adults to conduct their sexual lives free of state interference, even in the face of decisions that could lead to illness and death, came from Neil Schram, president of the American Association of Physicians for Human Rights, a gay-health professional organization (Schram letter to Silverman, April 2, 1984). Drawing on the antistatist and individualistic themes of gay political thought and the ever-present concern that sodomy laws might be reenacted, Schram linked the debate over the bathhouses to those that had raged over other behaviorally related diseases—those caused by smoking, alcohol consumption, and overeating, and to the risks associated with motorcycle riding without helmets.

Since personal freedom was at stake, only a posture of laissez-faire was tolerable, Schram said. Physicians had an obligation to educate and warn about high-risk behavior, but it was not for the medical community or the state in its public health role to enforce behavioral norms. "The closing of the businesses to protect people from themselves cannot be accepted. . . . Ultimately each individual is responsible for himself," stated Schram. To permit the closure of the bathhouses would be to permit an assault on an institution "where it is safe to meet other gay people without fear of arrest and harassment" and would represent the "beginning of the end." An ineluctable course led from the public bathhouse to the private bedroom. The memories of oppression were all too fresh. Repeating the leitmotiv of virtually every pronouncement in the organized gay medical community, Schram concluded that though he and his association sought to discourage sexual behavior that might increase the risk of AIDS, "we cannot and will not support any effort to enforce that viewpoint."

These views were echoed by Thomas Stoddard, then serving as the legislative director of the New York Civil Liberties Union (letter, April 10, 1984). For him any effort to regulate conduct in the bathhouse had to be viewed as antithetical to the principles of civil liberties. "There

are two principles at stake here: the right of sexual privacy and the
right of gay people to the equal protection of the laws." Acknowledging
that the bathhouse might indeed promote conduct implicated in the
spread of AIDS, he nevertheless underscored his opposition to state
interference. "To admit that we confront a problem of grave significance, disease related sexual conduct at public bathhouses is not the
same issue as whether government should be the means by which we
solve the problem. That is, it seems to me, a fundamental precept of
civil liberties. . . . Civil libertarians are naturally distrustful of government. . . . Therefore, they turn to the state only when there is no real
alternative." Action on the part of the gay community, picket lines
outside the bathhouses, would be an acceptable method of pressing
the bathhouses to change. For Stoddard, as for Schram, the specter of
sodomy statutes was ever present. "With the history [of sodomy laws]
and with consensual sodomy still a crime in nearly half the states, it
hardly seems appropriate to invite the state to regulate private sexual
conduct when now it does not."

Some gay medical professionals, however, viewed the baths as threats
to the health of gay men and supported severe restrictions, even closure of such establishments. Haunted by visions of their dying patients
and by the toll AIDS was taking, these professionals saw the bathhouse
as a unique environment in which the disease could spread. Some
were moved by the knowledge that their own patients, acting as agents
of further infection, continued to attend the baths. Hopes that the
threat of transmitting a lethal disease would result in a radical modification of behavior had for some at that moment met with bitter disappointment. There was no alternative; the claims of privacy and civil
liberties had to be subordinated to the demands of the public's health.

Ultimately public health officials in a number of cities, including
New York (Stoddard, letter, April 10, 1984), moved to close or severely
regulate the bathhouses, the way having been led by San Francisco.
That they, as well as others, had not moved more forcefully in the first
years of the AIDS epidemic was in part a consequence of the political
constraints imposed by having to chart a course compatible with a
policy of cooperation with gay men, who viewed all agencies of the
state with profound suspicion. Public health officials were also re-
strained by the impact of liberal political values since the centers of the
AIDS epidemic were cosmopolitan cities with political cultures of relative tolerance in which sexual privacy was a preeminent concern.
Finally, officials recognized that bathhouse behavior was but a very
small part of the vaster problem of a pattern of sexual behavior that
occurred in settings beyond the reach of the state.

Viewed from the perspective of the history of public health measures designed to control the spread of infectious diseases, the decision to close the baths was not remarkable. Had not periodic raids closed houses of prostitution during panics about venereal disease (Brandt 1985)? What was remarkable was the prudence and restraint that characterized such moves. The closing of the baths could thus be seen as at once reflecting the traditional orientation of public health and the new sensitivity to matters of civil liberties, reflecting the impact not only of the jurisprudence of privacy but also of the recognition that the practice of public health necessitated political compromises.

Thunder on the Right and the Consolidation of the Voluntarist Consensus

Despite the bitter aftermath of the bathhouse wars the political processes of conflict, negotiation, and compromise in the epidemic's first phase produced a rather uniform series of understandings and agreements on how best to limit the spread of HIV infection. By 1986 the essential elements of the voluntarist consensus on how to meet the challenge of AIDS were in place. With its stress on education (Institute of Medicine and National Academy of Sciences 1986), voluntary HIV testing (ASTHO 1985), confidentiality (CDC, December 6, 1985:721–726, 731–732), protection against discrimination (*Surgeon General's Report* 1986), and a rejection of coercive or intrusive public health measures (USPHS, July–August 1986, pp 341–348), the program had broad support, which was all the more significant since social anxiety and the failure of firm national leadership permitted a pattern of egregious practices to emerge. To those who viewed this consensus as too soft, as lacking an aggressive commitment to the control of the epidemic, the voluntarist consensus represented a capitulation to those who placed the claims of privacy, civil liberties, and gay rights above the common good. The most striking challenge to the consensus was to come from the extremist political front aligned with Lyndon LaRouche. What made it so significant was the reaction it provoked. In that response the strength and depth of the opposition to repressive public health measures was revealed.

In October 1985 the National Democratic Policy Committee—the political arm of Lyndon LaRouche's extreme movement—began a campaign to place an initiative before the voters of California that would have rejected the essential elements of the voluntarist consensus. To protect the people of California from what the legislature had already declared a "serious and life-threatening" challenge to "men and women from all segments of society," the initiative would have required that AIDS be defined as an "infectious, contagious and communicable disease" and that the condition of being a carrier of the HIV virus be defined as an infectious, contagious, and communicable condition. Both were to be listed by the Department of Health Services among the reportable diseases and conditions covered by existing relevant state statutes. To preclude any recapitulation of what was portrayed as the failure of state officials to protect residents of California from AIDS, the proposition mandated the enforcement of all relevant public health statutes and administrative provisions (California, State of n.d. mimeo).

Late in 1985, the Civil Liberties Union of Southern California undertook its first analysis of what might follow from the application to AIDS of extant statutes and regulations concerning communicable disease (ACLU, Southern California Branch, April 10, 1986 mimeo). Seropositive schoolchildren would be barred from school, together with all others who had communicable diseases. Antibody-positive individuals "could be" excluded from jobs that entailed food handling. Public funerals for those with AIDS or infected with HIV "might be" prohibited. Those who tested positive for antibodies to the AIDS virus not only would be reported to state health officials but also would be subject to "discretionary quarantine by local health authorities."

Such a reading of Proposition 64 presupposed that public health officials would apply the relevant statutes and regulations governing communicable diseases in general in an inflexible way, with little tailoring to what was known about the transmission of HIV. But given the risk that such an interpretation might be put forth by some local health officials, "it appears that all the more Draconian general provisions . . . might be applied to all [HIV] positive individuals." For the Civil Liberties Union there was no question but that the "ultimate intent of the initiative appears to be to subject [HIV] carriers to serious deprivations of civil liberties."

Opposition to the referendum came from the entire medical establishment, including the California Medical Association, the California Nurses' Association, and the California Hospital Association. In a statement to the voters, the three associations stressed the irrationality of a proposal that assumed the existence of casual transmission of HIV in the schools, the workplace, or restaurants. Only those who were expert in the scientific and clinical dimensions of AIDS were qualified to fashion public health policy, not those driven by politically motivated "partial truths and falsehoods" (CMA, CNA, and CHA n.d. mimeo).

The deans of the four schools of public health in the state—the University of California at Berkeley and Los Angeles, San Diego State, and Loma Linda University—signed a joint statement declaring, "Proposition 64 would foster the inaccurate belief that AIDS is a highly contagious disease, easily spread through food or by coughing, sneezing, touching or other types of casual contact" (*New Scientist,* September 25, 1986, p. 30). The actions that would follow from the initiative were "scientifically unwarranted [and] would do nothing to curtail the spread of AIDS." James Chin, chief of infectious disease of the state's Department of Health Services, characterized the initiative as "absurd," "stupid," and "disastrous" (California AIDS Task Force 1986 minutes). Finally, the state's AIDS Task Force found the proposition both dangerous and "utterly without merit as a public health measure" (California AIDS Task Force 1986 minutes).

Joining the state's medical establishment in opposition to what was officially called Proposition 64 was a broad spectrum of social organizations, the state's political elite, as well as its major newspapers (*Los Angeles Times,* August 14, 1986, part 5, p. 4; *San Francisco Chronicle,* June 27, 1986, p. 76; *San Francisco Examiner,* June 29, 1986, p. A12).

While opponents of Proposition 64 characterized the political consequences of its passage in dire terms, its proponents sought to argue that its passage would merely require public health officials to treat AIDS like any other major public health threat. "What we are doing in the process of this initiative is forcing the state to take those proven standard public health measures which are already law, in fact, in this state, in every other state, and in fact are generally the law in every advanced country around the world and now implement those public health laws with respect to AIDS" (*Los Angeles Times,* August 24, 1986, p. 30). In short, the supporters of the proposition sought to portray themselves as defending the tradition of public health intervention against the restraint and passivity of those who had failed to safeguard the people of California.

So ambiguous was Proposition 64 that the state's legislative analyst could not determine with any degree of certainty the ultimate fiscal impact if the initiative were to be approved by the voters (California Legislative Analyst, July 21, 1986, mimeo). Everything would depend "on what actions are taken by health officers and the courts to implement the measure." If existing laws and regulations governing the control of communicable diseases were applied and health officials continued to exercise professional discretion in determining the appropriate forms of intervention, "few, if any, AIDS patients, [or] carriers of the AIDS virus would be placed in isolation or under quarantine.

Similarly, few, if any, persons would be excluded from school or food-handling jobs." If, however, Proposition 64 were interpreted so as to place new requirements on health officers, the results would be far different, involving a massive expansion of testing, the exclusion of infected individuals from schools and food-handling positions, and the imposition of isolation.

With so ill defined a situation before the voters, with the proposition's opponents suggesting that dire and Draconian measures would follow from voter approval, and with the proposition's proponents insisting that the implications of approval would be limited and appropriate, what could the November referendum signify? At a minimum, given the political alliance that had materialized in opposition to Proposition 64, a "yes" vote could be read only as a rejection of the claims of the medical and public health establishments that they were, in fact, doing everything within reason to limit the spread of AIDS and that voluntarist strategy that respected civil liberties was compatible with the protection of the public health. Further, a "yes" vote would be an expression of distrust and profound frustration. A "no" vote would have much broader implications. It would represent not only an expression of confidence in the state's health leadership and its policies but also a rejection of the Draconian alternative—mandatory testing, the reporting by name of those who were infected to public health registries, workplace and school exclusions, and reliance on threats of isolation and quarantine.

On election day close to seven million voters cast ballots on Proposition 64. Seventy-one percent opposed it; 29 percent favored it (No on 64, November 30, 1986, mimeo). A stunning defeat, it was nevertheless a hard-won victory. Two and a quarter million dollars had been spent. The organization of the cultural, social, medical, and political elites in opposition to the proposition had required an enormous expenditure of energy. And so, despite the success, there was a darker side to this story. The referendum had revealed how popular discontent might be exploited in the years ahead as the absolute numbers of AIDS cases mounted. It had also demonstrated the existence of a popular base that could be mobilized for a repressive turn in public policy. Nevertheless, the California referendum revealed the existence of a firm alliance between public health officials and proponents of civil liberties in the face of authoritarian challenges to the voluntarist consensus.

Screening for HIV Infection

The strength of that alliance was both tested and affirmed in the debates that began in mid-1985 when the capacity to screen for the presence of the etiological agent responsible for AIDS became technologically possible. Despite profound disagreements about the role that antibody testing could play in the overall strategy of mass behavioral change, and the question of whether those who were tested had a right to remain ignorant of their test results, there was widescale agreement that compulsory programs to identify the presence of HIV infection were, in general, unacceptable (Bayer, Levine, and Wolf 1986:1768–1774). The scope of that agreement was revealed in 1987 at a meeting called by the Centers for Disease Control (CDC).

In early February 1987 the CDC announced that it would host a conference of public health officials and those concerned about civil liberties to discuss the future role of HIV-antibody testing in the overall strategy to control AIDS. A furor was touched off because two among the many proposals to be considered would entail mass mandatory screening: the testing of all applicants for marriage licenses (though not the prohibition of marriage by those found seropositive) and of all hospital admissions. Proposals for premarital testing were not new. But no one had ever before proposed the testing of all hospital admissions, regardless of age or diagnosis. In a front page *New York Times* story, Lawrence Altman, the medical correspondent, predicted that the ensuing discussion and the CDC meeting "would bring clashes over attempts to protect civil liberties as opposed to protecting public health" (Altman 1987:1). In fact, the debate over the next month would reveal that both public health officials and the defenders of civil liberties found little to recommend in the proposals for mandatory screening.

Despite the presence at the conference of public health officials with very different perspectives on such matters as the importance of reporting positive antibody test results to health departments and voluntary contact tracing, a remarkable consensus emerged against the mandatory testing of those considered the primary targets of such proposals—patients attending drug abuse programs and clinics for sexually transmitted diseases, persons seeking family planning services, and pregnant women (Conference on the Role of AIDS Virus Antibody Testing 1987 mimeo). The two proposals—mandatory premarital testing and universal hospital admission screening—received virtually no support. For those whose primary concern was the protection of privacy and civil liberties, such screening was unwarranted,

given the obvious costs and the very remote prospect that either mandatory program would make a contribution to the protection of the
public health. For those whose analysis was based on the importance
of the efficient exercise of public health power, neither proposal, if
adopted, would have resulted in a rational expenditure of resources,
given the very low rates of infection among those who would be tested.

Despite the opposition to mandatory testing, there was—especially
among public health officials at the conference—a perceptible shift
toward the aggressive promotion of voluntary testing among high-risk
groups, when appropriate pretest and posttest counseling could ensure
the assimilation of the significance of serological findings and provide
the necessary psychological support to those found to be positive. For
those concerned about how rapidly expanded testing could, perhaps
inadvertently, provide the basis for discrimination and social isolation,
the critical question remained as it had been since mid-1985, when
testing first became available, whether an aggressive program of voluntary testing was compatible with the protection of civil liberties and
the social interests of the infected.

One issue did not emerge as a matter of debate, even of discussion:
the use of blinded or anonymous screening for epidemiological purposes. From mid-1985 the CDC had begun to encourage the testing of
blood samples drawn for purposes other than HIV screening as a way
of tracking the prevalence and incidence of infection in the United
States. Because such samples were stripped of any personal identifiers,
a broad consensus existed that consent was not required for such
testing. Because of the importance of the data to be generated by such
studies, there was widespread accord about the acceptability of a procedure that, by definition, precluded the possibility of notifying individuals about their serostatus. Just how remarkable this consensus was
would be revealed only when efforts to launch similar studies in the
United Kingdom and the Netherlands provoked fierce opposition from
those committed to the protection of the rights of privacy and of the
principle of informed consent.

What did draw the attention of those brought together by the CDC
was the centrality of the protection of confidentiality and the importance of protections against discrimination. Both followed naturally
from the rejection of mandatory testing and from the appreciation of
the role of voluntary testing in the modification of sexual practices and
drug-using behavior linked to the transmission of HIV infection. Only
if the threats to privacy and the hazard of discrimination were forcefully addressed would it be possible to induce large numbers to be
tested. It was on this common ground that the defenders of public

health, civil liberties, and the rights of those most at risk for AIDS could find themselves in agreement. The imprint of the meeting's broad consensus was to be found in the follow-up recommendations issued by the CDC (April 30, 1987 mimeo).

Despite the fact that the federal government had initiated a program of mandatory testing in the military, the Job Corps, and the Foreign Service, and despite the exclusionary policies that were linked to such screening, the CDC acknowledged the importance, from the perspective of public health, of protecting the confidentiality of HIV-antibody test results and the social and economic interests of those found to be infected. Not only were exclusionary policies directed at the infected unnecessary for the protection of the public health; they would subvert the efforts of public health officials to win the confidence of those at risk.

> The ability of health departments, hospitals, and other health care providers to assure confidentiality of patient information and the public's confidence in that ability are crucial to efforts to increase the number of persons requesting or willing to undergo counseling and testing for HIV antibody. But of equal or even greater importance is the public perception that persons found to be positive will not experience unfair treatment as a result of being tested (CDC, April 30, 1987 mimeo).

The care with which the issues of confidentiality and discrimination were addressed is striking. State governments were called upon to review current procedures for the protection of medical records and to determine their adequacy. The Public Health Service was urged to "seek national AIDS confidentiality legislation and/or to work with its state and local health constituencies to develop model confidentiality legislation appropriate to the AIDS situation." Similarly, states were called upon to enforce relevant antidiscrimination statutes—generally those applying to the handicapped. The Public Health Service was asked to emphasize the absence of any justification for routine or mandatory screening as a condition of employment or admission to school, housing, or other public accommodations. Finally, the Department of Health and Human Services was urged to review the adequacy of antidiscrimination protections under federal law and to propose additional protections if necessary. In these recommendations the most nearly fully developed expression of a public health strategy that was compatible with a respect for the privacy and civil liberties of those infected with HIV could be found.

Reflecting the impact of such concerns, states have moved to extend protections against discrimination to individuals with AIDS and HIV infection. All fifty states have laws that protect individuals with handicaps against unjustified discrimination. More than half have extended the scope of such statutes to include those with HIV infection. In addition, the attorney generals of many states, as well as state human rights commissioners, have declared HIV-related discrimination to be a violation of the law. On a federal level, the most significant action occurred in 1990 as the Congress enacted the Americans with Disabilities Act, which extends civil rights protections to handicapped individuals who face discrimination in both the public and private sectors. Individuals with HIV infection are explicitly included.

Despite such enactments, discrimination has remained a critical issue. A survey undertaken by the American Civil Liberties Union found more than 13,000 complaints of HIV-related discrimination from 1983–1988 (ACLU 1990). In 1988 the ACLU found that the number of such reports increased by 50 percent following an increase of 87 percent in 1987. More sanguine in its conclusion was a study undertaken by the AIDS Litigation Project under the direction of Larry Gostin (1990), a strong proponent of efforts to protect those with HIV infection. Gostin found a shifting pattern of discrimination reflecting the effectiveness of efforts to combat crude exclusions. The early cases often involved discriminatory practices by employers based on prejudice or fears of transmission in the workforce. Employers now appear much less likely to exclude employees from ordinary workplaces. The significance of such discrimination may only increase as greater numbers of individuals with HIV infection seek care because of the promise of early therapeutic intervention.

The Resurgence of Public Health Traditionalism — 1989

In mid-1989, clinical trials revealed the efficacy of early therapeutic intervention in slowing the course of illness in asymptomatic but infected persons and in preventing the occurrence of *Pneumocystis carinii* pneumonia (PHS, June 15, 1989).

With the promise of early therapeutic intervention came the unraveling of the alliances that had been forged in the first phase of the epidemic. On issue after issue, divisions began to surface on matters of public health policy. Those whose primary commitment was to civil liberties increasingly found themselves at odds with public health officials. In the debates over policy and practice with regard to HIV testing, the resurgence of traditional public health values was dramatic.

norms, the realization that some patients could pose a grave threat to unsuspecting partners, and the increasing importance of early therapeutic intervention have led to modifications of early confidentiality restrictions. Although often opposed on principled grounds by those who believed that physician-patient communications should never be violated and by those who argued that such breaches of confidentiality would have the counterproductive consequence of reducing patient candor, thus limiting the capacity of clinicians to effectively counsel and persuade individuals who might harm their partners, such modifications in the standard of strict confidentiality have been given strong support in a number of state legislatures and by the American Medical Association (AMA 1989) and the Association of State and Territorial Health Officials (ASTHO 1988).

As of 1990, no state had imposed upon physicians a duty to warn unsuspecting partners. But about a dozen had adopted legislation granting physicians a "privilege to warn or inform," thus freeing physicians from liability for either warning or not warning those at risk (Intergovernmental Health Policy Project 1990:3).

The question of how to respond to individuals whose behavior represented a threat to unknowing partners inevitably provoked continued discussion of the public health tradition of imposing restrictions on liberty in the name of communal welfare. The specter of quarantine has haunted all such discussions, not because there was any serious consideration in the United States of the Cuban approach to AIDS (Bayer and Healton 1989:1022–1024)—which mandates the isolation of all persons infected with HIV regardless of their behaviors—but because of fears that even a more limited recognition of the authority to quarantine individuals whose behavior posed a risk of HIV transmission would lead to egregious intrusions upon privacy and invidiously imposed deprivations of freedom (Gostin 1989:1041). How would evidence about threatening behavior be gathered? How would such cases be adjudicated? How would predictions of future dangerousness be arrived at? For how long and under what conditions would those adjudged a danger to the public health be subjected to control? It was such concerns, as well as principled opposition to the intrusion of the state into matters of sexuality, that had led the American Civil Liberties Union to oppose all coercive personal control measures in the context of AIDS.

Soon after he resigned as commissioner of health in New York City at the end of 1989, Stephen Joseph bluntly made the case for the careful exercise of the power of quarantine (*New York Times*, February 10, 1990, p. 25). He did so on the occasion of the continuing uproar

As pressure to identify those with HIV infection mounted, efforts to loosen the requirements for specific consent to testing intensified. Nowhere was this clearer than in the emergence of a powerful movement supported by obstetricians and pediatricians for the routine screening of pregnant women who could transmit HIV to their offspring and the mandatory screening of infants at high risk for infection. In the case of the former, the public health practice of testing for syphilis and hepatitis B served as a model. In the latter instance, it was the widescale and broadly accepted tradition of screening for congenital conditions such as phenylketonuria (PKU) that served as the standard. The promise—with little evidentiary base—that early intervention might protect the fetus or at least enhance the life prospects of babies at risk for HIV infection had begun to override concerns about the coercive identification of infected women, most of whom were black or Hispanic, as well as about the potential burdens of exclusion from housing, social services, and health care itself that might be imposed on those so identified.

The erosion of the alliance that had resisted the application of traditional public health practices could be seen also in the shifting trends on the issue of whether to report the names of those infected with HIV to confidential public health department registries. Such reporting requirements had been fiercely resisted by gay groups and civil liberties organizations because of concerns about privacy and confidentiality and opposed by public health officials in areas with large numbers of AIDS cases because of the potential impact on the willingness of individuals to seek voluntary HIV testing and counseling (Bayer 1989:116–123). As a consequence, they had become policy in only a handful of states, typically those with few cases. It was thus a great setback for those who opposed reporting that the Presidential Commission on the HIV Epidemic—appointed by President Reagan and skillfully chaired by Admiral James D. Watkins—urged in its mid-1988 final report that HIV infection be made a reportable condition (Presidential Commission, June 1988).

Ultimately more significant were the fissures that had begun to appear in the alliance opposing named reporting in those states where the prevalence of HIV infection was high and where gay communities were well organized. In New York, for example, four medical societies sought to compel the commissioner of health to declare AIDS a sexually transmitted disease so that HIV infection could be made a reportable condition (*New York State Society of Surgeons, New York State Society of Orthopedic Surgeons, New York State Society of Obstetricians and Gynecologists and the Medical Society of New York v. David*

Axelrod.) What made the suit so remarkable was the posture of the opposing sides. Historically, clinicians had resisted efforts by public health officials to require the reporting by name of individuals with infectious diseases, arguing that such policies represented an intrusion upon the doctor-patient relationship (Fox 1986:11–16). In this instance the representatives of clinical medicine were asserting that reporting was critical to the public health while the state's chief health official resisted such a perspective. That apparent paradox can be explained only by the unique political alliances that had been created early in the epidemic between gay organizations, civil liberties groups, and public health officials. But the impact of therapeutic advances was to expose such alliances to increasing stress.

In June 1989 in an address that was met with cries of protest, Stephen Joseph, commissioner of health in New York City, told the Fifth International Conference on AIDS that the prospect of early clinical intervention necessitated "a shift toward a disease control approach to HIV infection along the lines of classic tuberculosis practices" (Joseph 1989 mimeo). A central feature of such an approach would be the "reporting of seropositives" to ensure effective clinical follow-up and the initiation of "more aggressive contact tracing." Joseph's proposals opened a debate that was only temporarily settled by the defeat of New York's Mayor Edward Koch in his bid for reelection. When newly elected Mayor David Dinkins selected Woodrow Myers, formerly commissioner of health in Indiana, to replace Joseph, his appointment was almost aborted, in part because he had supported named reporting. The festering debate was ended only by a political decision on the part of the mayor, who had drawn heavily on support within the gay community, to stand by his appointment while promising that there would be no named reporting in New York.

In New Jersey, which shares with New York a relatively high level of HIV infection, the commissioner of health also supported named reporting, but in that case the politics that surrounded the issue were very different. There both houses of the state legislature endorsed, without dissent, a confidentiality statute that included named reporting of cases of HIV infection. New Jersey simply exemplified a national trend (*Newark Star Ledger,* January 5, 1990). For, although only nine states at the end of 1989 required named reporting without any provision for anonymity, states increasingly were adopting policies that required reporting in at least some circumstances (Intergovernmental Health Policy Project 1989). And always the arguments were the same. New therapeutic possibilities provided the warrant for reestablishing a standard of traditional public health practice.

The move toward reporting was linked only in part to the argum that state health departments needed the names of individuals to sure adequate clinical follow-up. As important was the assertion fr public health officials that effective contact tracing, now more criti than ever because of the need for early clinical intervention, could undertaken only if those with HIV infection but who were not diagnosed as having AIDS could be interviewed. Despite its cent and well-established role in venereal disease control, the notification the sexual and needle-sharing partners in the context of AIDS h been a source of ongoing conflict between gay groups and civil liberti organizations on the one hand and public health officials who ha proposed such a strategy in the early years of the epidemic on the othe (Bayer 1989). Always predicated on the willingness of those with sex ually transmitted diseases to provide public health workers with th names of their partners in exchange for a promise of anonymity, thi standard disease control measure had been viewed by AIDS activists civil liberties groups, and their political allies as a threat to confidential ity and as a potentially coercive intervention. Indeed, opponents of contact tracing typically denounced it as "mandatory."

With time and a better understanding of how contact tracing func- tioned in the context of sexually transmitted diseases, some of the most vocal opponents of tracing yielded their principled opposition, at least in private meetings and discussions, and instead centered their con- cerns on the cost of so labor-intensive an intervention (ASTHO 1988). Those who did not yield their opposition to tracing were increasingly isolated, for support for such efforts was ultimately to come from the Institute of Medicine and the National Academy of Sciences (Institute of Medicine 1988), the Presidential Commission on the HIV Epidemic of Medicine 1988), the Presidential Commission 1988:76), the American Bar Association (ABA (Presidential Commission 1988:76), the American Medical News 1988), and the American Medical Association (*American Medical News* 1988:4).

In part, both the early and the lingering resistance to partner notifi- cation can be explained by the conflation of the standard public health approach to sexually transmitted disease control with policies and prac- tices that are rooted in a very different tradition, entailing a "duty to warn" or protect those who might be threatened by individuals with communicable conditions.

The early and strict confidentiality rules surrounding HIV screening and medical records in states like New York and California all but precluded physicians from acting to warn the unsuspecting partners of those with HIV infection. The recognition that such limitations placed physicians in a position that sometimes violated professional ethical

surrounding the appointment of Woodrow Myers as his successor. Gay and civil liberties groups opposed Myers, in part, because he had supported quarantine legislation in Indiana and had reportedly exercised the authority then granted him under state law. They demanded that such policies never be pursued in New York. No such pledge could or should be made, stated Joseph in an editorial written for the *New York Times*. Among his last formal acts had been the signing of a detention order for a woman with infectious tuberculosis because of her repeated unwillingness to take the medication that would render her noninfectious. "It is virtually certain that at some point, a New York City Health Commissioner will be faced with an analogous situation concerning the transmission of the AIDS virus. When all lesser remedies have failed, can anyone doubt what would be the proper course of action for the Commissioner to take, faced with . . . an infected individual who knowingly and repeatedly sold his blood for transfusion?" When and if a treatment became available that would render HIV-infected persons less infectious, "would there not then be a clear obligation to take all reasonable measures to ensure that the infected take their medication, thus protecting others?"

Although fierce opposition has surfaced to all efforts to bring AIDS within the scope of state quarantine statutes, more than a dozen states had done so between 1987 and 1990 (based on a review of all AIDS-related legislation in the files of the Intergovernmental Health Policy Project, Washington, D.C.), typically using the occasion to modernize their disease control laws to reflect contemporary constitutional standards, which detail procedural guarantees, and to require that restrictions on freedom represent the "least restrictive alternative" available to achieve a "compelling state interest."

The enactment of statutes criminalizing the knowing transmission of HIV infection has paralleled the political receptivity to laws extending the authority of public health officials to control individuals whose behavior posed a risk of HIV transmission. On *theoretical* grounds such statutes have been viewed as less troubling than public health control measures by those concerned about civil liberties (Field and Sullivan 1987:46–60). Bounded by the procedural protections surrounding criminal prosecutions, by the requirement that the court determine whether the accused committed a clearly defined crime rather than make judgments about future dangerousness, and by the time-limited feature of criminal sentencing, such measures have been thought, in principle, to pose a relatively smaller risk to the right of the accused. Nevertheless, the specter of criminalizing sexual behavior has led most proponents of civil liberties to react with alarm to all such measures.

Recourse to the criminal law to punish the knowing transmission of
HIV, broadly endorsed by the Presidential Commission on the HIV
Epidemic (Presidential Commission 1988:76), called upon a tradition
of state enactments that made the knowing transmission of venereal
disease a crime. Though they were almost never enforced, the existence of these older laws served as a rationale for new legislative
initiatives. Between 1987 and 1989 (based on a review of all AIDS-
related legislation in the files of the Intergovernmental Health Policy
Project, Washington, D.C.), twenty states enacted such statutes, the
vast majority of which defined the proscribed acts as felonies despite
the fact that older statutes typically treated knowing transmission as a
misdemeanor. As important, aggressive prosecutors have relied on laws
defining assaultive behavior and attempted murder to bring indict-
ments even in the absence of AIDS-specific legislation. Individuals
have been charged for such offenses as biting, spitting, splattering/
donating blood, or having sexual intercourse.

In the epidemic's first years, when little could be done for those with
HIV infection, the central points of public policy debate centered on
questions of privacy, confidentiality, and the role of coercive state
interventions. Now that the prospects of therapeutic intervention have
improved, debate increasingly centers on the question of equity. How
will the United States choose to act in terms of ensuring access to life-
extending therapies? But the increasing importance of the political
conflict over justice and access to treatment has not eliminated the
earlier set of issues. Indeed, many of the controversies in the next
years may center on clashes over rights within the context of medicine.
Under what conditions should people be screened? Should physicians
be permitted to refuse to care for HIV-infected persons? Should infected physicians be permitted to engage in invasive procedures that
pose an extremely small, but nevertheless real, risk to patients? What
methods should be employed to protect uninfected psychiatric patients
from sexual encounters with infected patients during hospitalization?

That the emergence of public health traditionalism has resulted in
sharp debates over some elements of the strategy to combat AIDS
forged in the epidemic's first years only makes manifest what periods
of broad consensus tend to mask: that public health policy, like all
public policy, is essentially political, reflecting a balance of ethical,
social, and ideological forces, that socially critical health policy is never
simply the result of decisions made by public health professionals
drawing on their own traditions but is rather the result of the interplay

on much broader interests and institutions. Public strategies can, of course, be more or less irrational, more or less compatible with what science reveals about the world. But within the parameters established by the "facts" there must always remain a realm of uncertainty and of irreducible choice. Recourse to claims about "scientifically justified policy"—typical of all parties to disputes about public health policy—merely deflects attention from the inherent role of competing social values in the charting of appropriate strategies of social action.

Now that the "natural" alliance between proponents of civil liberties and the public health has been ruptured, it will be necessary to confront openly questions posed by Lawrence Tribe, the liberal theorist of jurisprudence, about policy in the face of epidemic challenges. "Who is being hurt? Who benefits? By what process is the rule imposed? For what reasons? With what likely effect on precedent" (Tribe 1978:891)? How these questions are answered and with what relative weight given to security and safety on the one hand and to privacy and autonomy on the other will determine the shape of AIDS policy and will have significant implications for the contours of the United States as a liberal society in the next years.

REFERENCES

Advocate, March 18, 1982, p. 6.
Altman, Lawrence. 1987. *New York Times*, February 4, p. 1.
ABA (American Bar Association) AIDS Coordinating Committee. Chicago: August 1988. ABA Policy on AIDS.
ACLU (American Civil Liberties Union). New York: 1990.
ACLU, Southern California Branch. 1986. LaRouche Initiative and Existing Laws. April 10. Mimeo.
AMA (American Medical Association). Board of Trustees. Chicago: December 1989.
American Medical News, July 8–15, 1988, p. 4.
ASTHO (Association of State and Territorial Health Officials). 1985. *ASTHO Guide to Public Health Practice: HTLV-III Antibody Testing and Community Approaches*. Washington, D.C.: Public Health Foundation.
ASTHO. National Association of County Health Officials, U.S. Conference of Local Health Officers. 1988. *Guide to Public Health Practice: HIV Partner Notification Strategies*. Washington, D.C.: Public Health Foundation.
Bayer, Ronald. 1989. *Private Acts, Social Consequences: AIDS and the Politics of Public Health*. New York: Free Press.
Bayer, Ronald and Cheryl Healton. 1989. Controlling AIDS in Cuba. *New England Journal of Medicine* (April), 321:1022–1024.
Bayer, Ronald, Carol Levine, and Thomas Murray. 1984. Guidelines for Confidentiality in AIDS Research. *IRB* (November–December), pp. 1–7.

48   **RONALD BAYER**

Bayer, Ronald, Carol Levine, and Susan Wolf. 1986, HIV Antibody Screening: An Ethical Framework. *JAMA* 258:1768–1774.
Brandt, Alan. 1985. *No Magic Bullet: A Social History of Venereal Diseases in the United States from 1880.* New York: Oxford University Press.
California, State of. n.d. Initiative Measure to Be Submitted Directly to Voters. Mimeo.
California AIDS Task Force Minutes. August 13, 1986.
California Legislative Analyst. Acquired Immune Deficiency Syndrome (AIDS) Institute. July 21, 1986. Mimeo.
CMA (California Medical Association), CNA (California Nurses' Association), and CHA (California Hospital Association). n.d. Rebuttal Argument Against Proposition 64. Mimeo.
CDC (Centers for Disease Control). 1985. Recommendations for Assisting in the Prevention of Perinatal Transmission of Human T-Lymphotropic Virus Type III/Lymphadenopathy-associated Virus and Acquired Immunodeficiency Syndrome. *MMWR,* December 6, pp. 721–26, 731–32.
CDC (Centers for Disease Control). 1987. Recommended Additional Guidelines for HIV Antibody Counseling and Testing in the Prevention of HIV Infection and AIDS. April 30. Mimeo.
Conference on the Role of AIDS Virus Antibody Testing in the Prevention and Control of AIDS. 1987. Reports from the Workshops, Transcript of the Proceedings. February 24–25. Mimeo.
Field, Martha A. and Kathleen M. Sullivan. 1987. AIDS and the Criminal Law. *Law, Medicine, and Health Care* (Summer), pp. 46–60.
Fox, Daniel. 1986. From TB to AIDS: Value Conflicts in Reporting Disease. *Hastings Center Report* (December), pp. 11–16.
Gostin, Larry. 1989. The Politics of AIDS: Compulsory State Powers, Public Health, Civil Liberties. *Ohio State Law Review* 49(4):1041.
Gostin, Larry. 1990. The AIDS Litigation Project: A National Review of Court and Human Rights Commission Decisions. Part II: Discrimination. *JAMA* 263:2086–2093.
Institute of Medicine and National Academy of Sciences. 1986. *Confronting AIDS.* Washington D.C.: National Academy Press.
Institute of Medicine and National Academy of Sciences. 1988. *Confronting AIDS: Update 1988.* Washington D.C.: National Academy Press.
Intergovernmental Health Policy Project. 1989. HIV Reporting in the States. *Intergovernmental AIDS Reports* (November–December).
Intergovernmental Health Policy Project. 1990. 1989 Legislative Overview. *Intergovernmental AIDS Reports* (January), p. 3.
Joseph, Stephen C. 1989. Remarks at the Fifth International Conference on AIDS. June 5. Mimeo.
Karst, Kenneth L. 1980. The Freedom of Intimate Association. *Yale Law Review* 89:624–692.
Los Angeles Times, August 14, 1986, part 5, p. 4.
Los Angeles Times, August 24, 1986, p. 30.
Merritt, Deborah Jones. 1986. Communicable Disease and Constitutional Law: Controlling AIDS. *New York University Law Review* 61:739–799.
New Scientist, September 25, 1986, p. 30.
New York State Society of Surgeons, New York State Society of Orthopedic Surgeons, New York State Society of Obstetricians and Gynecologists and the Medical Society of New York v. David Axelrod.
New York Times, February 10, 1990, p. 25.
Newark Star Ledger, January 5, 1990.

No on 64. 1986. Campaign Report. November 30. Mimeo.

Presidential Commission on the Human Immunodeficiency Virus Epidemic. 1988. Report (June), p. 76.

PHS (Public Health Service). U.S. Department of Health and Human Services. 1989. Guidelines for Prophylaxis Against *Pneumocystis Carinii* Pneumonia for Persons Infected with Human Immunodeficiency Virus. *MMWR* (June 15), Suppl. 5.

San Francisco Chronicle, June 27, 1986, p. 76.

San Francisco Examiner, June 29, 1986, p. A12.

Schram, Neil. 1984. Letter to Mervyn Silverman, April 2.

Silverman, Mervyn. 1984. Press Statement, October 9.

Stoddard, Thomas. 1984. Letter to Dorothy Ehrlich of the Northern California Civil Liberties Union, April 10.

Surgeon General's Report on Acquired Immune Deficiency Syndrome. 1986. Washington, D.C.: U.S. Government Printing Office.

Tribe, Lawrence. 1978. *American Constitutional Law.* Mineola, N.Y.: Foundation Press.

USPHS (United States Public Health Service). Department of Health and Human Services. 1986. Public Health Service Plan for the Prevention and Control of AIDS and the AIDS Virus. *Public Health Reports* (July–August), pp. 341–348.

3. Mandatory HIV Screening and Testing

JAMES F. CHILDRESS

FACED WITH EPIDEMICS, societies frequently curtail individual rights and liberties, often in ways later considered to be excessive and unnecessary. Even liberal societies have protected the public health by such measures as compulsory screening and testing, quarantine and isolation, and contact tracing. For a liberal society—that is, a society that recognizes and protects individual rights and liberties—the difficult question is, When does the public health justify overriding these rights and liberties? For several years—roughly from the late 1950s to the early 1980s—the United States considered itself largely immune to major public health crises; even though debates lingered about policies to control sexually transmitted diseases, these diseases were not viewed as major threats to individual or communal survival. During the same period, law, public policy, and social practice, including health care, provided additional protections for various individual rights and liberties. Then came AIDS with its threat to the public health, and, with the development in mid-1985 of tests for antibodies to the human immunodeficiency virus (HIV), calls to use these diagnostic tools to identify seropositive individuals through consensual and/or mandatory screening and testing (Osborn, 1987). Numerous bills were introduced in state legislatures to require testing in various contexts, such as applicants for marriage licenses, and the federal government instituted mandatory screening of immigrants, inmates in federal prisons, military personnel, etc.

Advocates of mandatory screening and testing, who often invoke the metaphor of war against AIDS, frequently leave unclear what actions would follow from the identification of HIV-antibody-positive individuals. Yet it is not possible to isolate mandatory (or even consensual) screening and testing from other possible interventions because, in contrast to vaccines, they have no impact on an epidemic. What is done with the information and with the people who test positive will determine the effect on the AIDS epidemic. Hence, a first question for all proposed HIV-antibody tests is, Why is the information wanted and what will be done with that information (as well as with the people who test positive)? There have been debates about whether sexual contacts should be traced, whether current sexual partners should be warned, whether certain employers should be notified, whether seropositive individuals should be quarantined, etc. Such questions provide the backdrop for much of the debate about mandatory screening and testing (Walters, 1988).

In this essay I assume the social ethics or political morality of a liberal society and then try to determine when such a society, under the threat to the public health from AIDS, may justifiably resort to mandatory screening and testing for HIV antibodies, thereby overriding some of its important principles and rules. After sketching the major presumptive or prima facie principles and rules that may constrain public health efforts in a liberal society, I identify some conditions that need to be met to justify infringing those principles and rules in the pursuit of public health. Then I develop a typology of screening/testing policies, and examine the issues raised by different policies. I stress throughout this discussion the central role of analogical reasoning, and I conclude with an analysis of the impact of the metaphor "war against AIDS" on our society's debates about mandatory screening and testing.

An Ethical Framework for Assessing Policies of Screening and Testing

It is not necessary to belabor why control of HIV infection and AIDS is a public health concern, rather than a private, individual matter. AIDS is an infectious disease; people may be infected and infectious for many years before they are aware of their condition; there is no known cure for AIDS, which has an extremely high death rate; the suffering of AIDS patients and others is tremendous; the cost for AIDS patients is very high; and so on. Protection of the public health, including health of individuals, is a legitimate moral concern—even a moral imperative—based on the fundamental moral principles affirmed by a liberal society, including beneficence, nonmaleficence, and justice, as well as respect for persons and their autonomy (Bayer, Levine, and Wolf 1986; Beauchamp and Childress 1989; Levine and Bayer 1989). "Public health is what we, as a society, do collectively to assure the conditions in which people can be healthy. This requires that continuing and emerging threats to the health of the public be successfully countered" (Committee 1986:1). AIDS is a paradigm instance of the public health threats that must be effectively countered.

If the goal of controlling AIDS is a strong moral imperative for the society, as well as for individuals, we still have to determine which measures may and should be adopted to achieve this goal. "The AIDS virus has no civil rights"—that rhetoric often suggests that the moral imperative to control AIDS cancels all other moral imperatives. Of course, few who use this rhetoric try to justify compulsory universal screening accompanied by mass quarantine or even mass slaughter. Even so, their position rarely takes seriously enough other significant moral principles and rules. I examine some of those principles and rules and sketch what they imply for public policies to control this infectious disease. This argument hinges on the best available medical information, including evidence that the spread of AIDS usually involves consensual, intimate contact, in the form of sexual activity or sharing intravenous (IV) drug needles and syringes, and that casual contact is not a mode of transmission. A different set of facts could justify different screening and testing policies.

The principle of respect for persons is a primary principle in the ethical framework of a liberal society (Childress 1982a,b, 1987, 1990). It implies that we should not treat people merely as means to ends. From this principle (and others) we can derive more specific rules that also direct and limit policies. Three such rules are especially important for this analysis: rules of liberty, including freedom of association; rules of privacy, including bodily integrity and decisional space; and rules of confidentiality. The principle of respect for persons and its derivative rules can be stated as individual rights or as societal obligations and duties—for example, the individual's right to privacy or the society's obligation not to violate an individual's privacy. Even if some of these rules are independent rather than derived, they are closely related to personal autonomy, for the individual can autonomously waive the rights expressed in the rules or, perhaps more accurately, can exercise those rights by yielding liberty or privacy or by granting access to previously confidential information. Furthermore, in a liberal society, overriding the principle or respect for autonomy and these rules can be justified more easily to protect others than to protect the agent himself or herself. Thus, there is a strong suspicion of paternalism, which infringes these principles and rules to protect the agent rather than others (Childress 1982a). (Of course, the goals of intervention are often mixed.) Rather than offer a theoretical foundation for the principle of respect for autonomy and the various derivative rules, I assume that they can be discerned in our constitution, laws, policies, and practices—in short, in the social ethics or political morality of a liberal society.

Conditions for Overriding Prima Facie Principles and Rules

My task is to try to determine which, if any, policies of mandatory screening and testing for HIV antibodies can be ethically justified in a liberal society in view of the moral imperative to control AIDS and these other moral principles and rules. We have to determine both what these principles and rules mean and how much weight they have relative to other principles and rules. (For brevity I sometimes use "principles" or "rules" to cover both principles and rules.) Some apparent violations of rules may not really be violations; upon closer inspection they may turn out to be consistent with the rules properly interpreted. And none of these rules is absolute; each one can be justifiably overridden in order to protect the public health under some conditions. However, in a liberal society these rules are more than mere maxims or rules of thumb, which yield to any and every utilitarian objection. If these rules are not absolute or mere maxims, is there an alternative conception of their weight or stringency? They may be construed as *prima facie* binding; that is, in and of themselves they have heavy moral weight or strong binding power. Because they are prima facie binding, it is necessary to justify any departures from them, and the process of justification involves meeting a heavy burden of proof (see Beauchamp and Childress 1989).

At least five conditions must be met to justify infringements of these rules (see Childress 1987, from which some of this discussion has been drawn). These conditions, which are called *justificatory conditions,* are effectiveness, proportionality, necessity, least infringement, and explanation and justification to the parties protected by the rules. These conditions express the logic of prima facie duties or rights, i.e., how principles and rules with such weight or stringency are to be approached, as well as the substance of the liberal principles and rules. A presupposition of these conditions is that the goal—both expressed and latent—is to protect public health, that is, the health of the community and the individuals within it, rather than to express moralistic judgments about individuals and their conduct or to exclude seropositive individuals from the community by subjecting them to discrimination or denying them access to needed services (Field 1990:54; see also Bayer, Levine, and Wolf 1986; Levine and Bayer 1989).

First, it is necessary to show that a policy infringing these rules will probably realize the goal of protecting public health. This first condition is one of effectiveness. A policy that infringes the moral rules but is ineffective simply has no justification; it is arbitrary and capricious. An ineffective policy to control HIV infection that infringes no moral rules may be wasteful, unwise, and even stupid, but if it infringes moral rules, there is a decisive moral argument against it.

Second, it is necessary to show that the probable benefits of a policy infringing rules outweigh both the moral rule(s) infringed and any negative consequences. This condition, which may be called proportionality, is complex, for it involves considering not only the weight of the infringed moral rule but also other harms, costs, and burdens that may flow from the infringement. For example, it is necessary to consider not only the weight of the rule of privacy but also other probably negative effects, such as discrimination, that may befall the one whose privacy is infringed. (As I argue later, to justify policies that *impose* community, it may also be essential to *express* community through protections against such negative consequences. Indeed, if community is expressed through such protections, imposition may be less necessary.)

Third, it is not sufficient to meet the first two conditions of effectiveness and proportionality and thus to show that infringement of these rules will produce better consequences for more people. As prima facie binding, these rules direct us to seek alternative ways to realize the end of public health, short of infringing the rules. For example, if it is possible to protect the public health without infringing liberty and privacy (and other moral rules), then the society should do so. This condition is one of necessity, last resort, or lack of a feasible alternative. Priority belongs to policies that do not infringe the rules of liberty, privacy, and confidentiality. For example, policies that seek to educate people about acting in certain ways have moral priority over policies that force people to act in certain ways. Under some circumstances, however, where coercive policies would be effective and proportionate, they can be justified if they are also necessary means to protect the public health. Many of the proposed policies of mandatory screening fail this third test.

Fourth, even when a liberal society is justified in infringing its moral rules to protect the public health, it is obligated to seek policies that least infringe its rules, for only the degree or extent of infringement that is necessary to realize the end that is sought can be justified. For example, when liberty is at stake, the society should seek the least restrictive alternative; when privacy is at stake, it should seek the least intrusive and invasive alternative; and when confidentiality is at stake, it should disclose only the amount and kind of information needed for effective action. This fourth condition may be called that of least infringement.

Finally, even when a public policy that infringes one or more moral rules satisfies all four prior conditions, the principle of respect for persons may generate additional requirements. This principle may require that the society inform those whose liberty, privacy, and confidential relations have been infringed. In many cases, such as coercive screening for HIV antibody, the infringements will be evident to the parties affected, but this may not be true in all cases, especially if secrecy or deception is involved. As Sisselal Bok (1978) notes, in some contexts, secret or deceptive actions may be more disrespectful and insulting to the parties affected than coercive actions. Hence, the society may have a duty to disclose, and even to justify, the actions to the person and even in some contexts to undertake compensatory measures. Even if it is essential to infringe a person's rights in order to protect the public health, that person should not be reduced to a mere means to the goal of public health. The crucial point can also be stated through an image drawn from Robert Nozick (1968): Overridden moral principles and rules leave "moral traces." They do not evaporate or simply disappear when they are overriden; they are outweighed, not canceled.

As is true of much moral, political, and legal reasoning, this process of reasoning about the justification of mandatory HIV-antibody tests is to a great extent analogical. The principle of universalizability or formal justice requires treating similar cases in a similar way. Hence it is necessary to consider the relevant similarities and differences among candidate targets for screening, not only for HIV antibodies but also for other conditions, such as genetic ones. Reasoning in a liberal society not only considers precedent cases—for example, the relevant similarities and differences between HIV-antibody screening and other mandatory screening policies that have been held to be justifiable—but also the precedents mandatory HIV-antibody screening would create. As Margaret Somerville (1989) argues, "HIV and AIDS must not be treated in isolation; comparison with analogous situations is mandatory."

Major Types of Screening/Testing Policies

In order to apply the principle of respect for personal autonomy and its derivative rules, all conceived as prima facie binding, along with the conditions for justifying their infringement, it is necessary to identify the range of proposed policies of mandatory screening and testing for HIV antibodies. The following chart indicates some of the most important options: policies of screening/testing may be consensual or compulsory and universal or selective.

Screening/Testing Policies

		Degree of Voluntariness	
		CONSENSUAL	COMPULSORY
	UNIVERSAL	1	2
Extent of Screening			
	SELECTIVE	3	4

The term "screening" usually refers to testing groups, while the term "testing" usually refers to testing individuals. However, even in mass screening, the individual is tested as part of the targeted group. Thus, I continue to use both terms as appropriate without drawing a sharp distinction between them. A more important distinction concerns the *scope* of the screening or testing: Is it universal or selective.

Universal Screening

There is simply no adequate justification for *universal screening*, whether voluntary or compulsory (numbers 1 and 2). Even serious proposals for widespread screening usually fall short of universal screening. For example, Rhame and Maki (1989: 1253) recommend "HIV testing vigorously to all U.S. adults under the age of sixty regardless of their reported risk history." Universal screening is not necessary to protect the public health; HIV infection is not widespread outside groups engaging in high-risk activities; screening in groups or areas with low seroprevalence produces a high rate of false positives; universal screening would be very costly and would not be cost effective—the funds could be spent more effectively on education; and its potential negative effects, including discrimination, would outweigh any potential benefits. It is not even justifiable to encourage everyone to be tested.

If universal consensual screening is not justifiable, there is, a fortiori, no justification for universal compulsory screening, which would also violate respect for autonomy and rules of liberty, privacy (and probably confidentiality), without compensating benefit. The main rationale for compulsory universal screening is that seropositive individuals can then reduce risks to others. There is evidence of some individual behavioral change following disclosure of seropositivity, especially with counseling (Cates and Handsfield 1988; McCusker et al. 1988), but there is no evidence that mandatory testing would produce the same level of voluntary changes in risk taking and risk imposition (Field 1990:58–59; Gostin 1987:9–10).

Identification of and disclosure to the individuals who are seropositive do not necessarily translate into benefits for others, apart from additional interventions. And appropriate education and counseling, apart from mandatory testing, could be effective ways to realize the same end, especially because universal precautions are recommended whether the individual is seropositive or seronegative (for a survey of published reports, see Becker and Joseph 1988). In view of the current scientific and medical evidence, compulsory universal screening fails to meet the five conditions identified earlier for justified breaches of the relevant moral principles and rules. Universal precautions, pursued through education, are morally preferable to mandatory universal screening, and the latter is not demonstrably more effective and would produce serious negative consequences.

Selective Screening

Consensual or voluntary selective screening may appear to pose no moral problems, but who should be encouraged to be tested, who should bear the costs, what sort of pretest and posttest counseling should be provided, and what conditions make the decision to have the test a rational one? Individuals making rational choices will consent to testing only when they perceive a favorable risk-benefit ratio. And "more than most medical tests, HIV screening has major benefits and harms that must be weighed" (Lo et al. 1989:730). In all risk-benefit analyses, including assessments of policies, the comparison is between the probability of a harm of some magnitude and the probability of a benefit of some magnitude (O'Brien 1989). Since "risk" is a probabilistic term, while "benefit" is not, the necessity of determining both probability and magnitude of both benefits and harms is sometimes neglected.

If we assume the accuracy of the test results, the possible *benefits* of testing to *seronegative* individuals include reassurance, the possibility of making future plans, and the motivation to make behavioral changes to prevent infection, while the possible *benefits* to *seropositive* individuals include closer medical follow-up, including prognoses of various stages, earlier use of azidothymidine (AZT) (and other treatments), prophylaxis or other care for associated diseases, protection of loved ones, and clearer plans for the future. There appears to be a very *low risk* of harm to *seronegative* individuals, even though there have been occasional reports of discrimination against individuals who have voluntarily taken the HIV-antibody test but with negative results. There are, however, *major risks* to *seropositive* individuals. (For these risks and possible benefits, see Lo et al. 1989). These risks may be identified as psychological and social (with considerable overlap and interaction). The psychological risks include anxiety and depression—followed by a higher rate of suicide than for the population at large (Marzuk et al. 1988)—while the social risks include stigma, discrimination, and breaches of confidentiality.

Clearly the society can have a major impact on the risk-benefit analyses of potential candidates for voluntary testing. On the one hand, the medical benefits are possible only if seropositive individuals can gain access to them. Hence, even on the benefit side, the problem is not merely medical because of the social problem of access to health care. On the other hand, the risks can be greatly reduced by societal decisions to allocate funds and to establish strong rules to protect individual rights and liberties. The society should provide resources for pretest and posttest counseling both to help the individual and also to reduce risks to others, and it should protect seropositive individuals from breaches of privacy and confidentiality and from discrimination in housing, employment, insurance, health and social services, etc. Without societal support and protection, the social risks may outweigh the benefits, including any medical benefits, of the test for rational individuals.

If voluntary or consensual testing of selected groups can be effective, in some contexts, then there is no justification for compulsory screening of those groups. The liberal justificatory framework imposes this necessary condition: moral principles and rules are not to be infringed if the same important ends—in this case, the public health—can be realized without their infringement. Furthermore, the society may even have to bear additional costs to protect its important principles and rules.

The requirement, expressed by the terms "mandatory" and "compulsory," may be imposed on the one to be tested or on the tester or on both. For example, in the context of screening donated blood for transfusions, the term "mandatory" refers in the first instance to the obligation imposed on the organizations collecting blood. And such "mandatory" screening may be imposed or permitted by the state. The one area of mandatory selective screening that is morally settled and uncontroversial is screening all donated (or sold) blood, organs, sperm, and ova, in part because recipients cannot take other measures to protect themselves. In this area universal precautions cannot work without screening and testing.

As is evident in programs of screening donated blood, many policies of screening are actually mixes of voluntary actions and compulsory actions. While individuals can choose to donate blood or not, their blood will be tested if they do donate. Another good example is the policy of screening recruits into the military (Bayer 1989:158–161). The U.S. armed forces consist of volunteers, who are tested for HIV antibodies upon entry (and then again at least once a year). It could be argued that volunteers for the armed forces consent to HIV testing, because they voluntarily enter an institution where screening is compulsory, and that the mandatory screening thus does not violate any of the volunteers' rights. This argument has merit, but it does not adequately address the question whether the society can justify its policy by the conditions identified earlier. The major express rationale is that each member of the armed forces is a potential donor of blood for transfusions on the battlefield; hence the rationale is comparable to the one that governs screening donated blood. Even if this rationale is solid, along with the rationale of protecting HIV-infected people from live virus vaccines used in the armed forces, there is also reason to suspect that the military's homophobia was a factor in the decision. Furthermore, there is concern about the precedent this mandatory screening creates, especially in the invocation of the cost of future health care (Bayer 1989:160).

Voluntariness may be compromised in various ways. We tend to think of coercion as the major compromise of voluntariness—for example, forcing someone to undergo a test for HIV antibody. However, conditional requirements—if you want X, then you have to do Y—may also be morally problematic. For example, requiring HIV antibody testing as a condition for obtaining some strongly desired benefit, such as a marriage license, may constitute an undue incentive, even if it is not, strictly speaking, coercive because the person can choose to decline the benefit (for an important discussion of coercion, see Wertheimer 1987). One important question then is whether it is fair to impose the condition, even if the person is free to take it or leave it. This question expresses the important general point that selection of targets for mandatory screening—or even for voluntary screening—is in part a matter of justice in the distribution of benefits and burdens (see Fletcher

1987) and that not all important moral issues are reducible to voluntary choices. The justificatory conditions identified earlier serve as important selection criteria.

Nevertheless, because of the centrality of the principle of respect for personal autonomy in a liberal framework, it is not surprising that consent plays such an important role in the analysis and assessment of screening policies. When an individual gives valid consent to testing, there is no violation of his or her personal autonomy and liberty of action. Nor does consensual testing violate the rule of privacy, for the individual voluntarily chooses to surrender some of his or her privacy. And, finally, if a person grants others access to information about his or her HIV-antibody status, the rule of confidentiality is not violated. In a liberal framework, valid consent creates rights that did not previously exist. I use the terms "voluntary" testing and "consensual" testing interchangeably to refer to testing with the individual's voluntary, informed consent. It is irrelevant whether he or she requested a test or only accepted a recommended test.

What counts as consent? This question becomes important because people have been held to consent in various ways, not simply by express oral or written statements. And some varieties of consent have been invoked to override a person's express wishes and choices. I discuss this topic in the context of selective screening of hospital patients for HIV antibodies. The question is whether the institutional rules of consent should be structured to authorize HIV antibody testing without express, specific consent.

Varieties of Consent in the Context of Screening Hospital Patients

The term "routine" often covers several types of screening and testing. However, this term is seriously misleading without further qualification, for its ethical significance is unclear until we can determine whether the screening will be done routinely, without notice or the possibility of refusal, or whether it will be offered routinely with the possibility of refusal (see Walters 1990).

When a hospital patient consents to HIV-antibody testing after being informed about the risks and benefits of the test—including whether the intended benefits are primarily for the patient or for the caregivers —there is no breach of moral principles. But are there forms of consent in addition to express and specific oral or written consent that can create rights on the part of hospitals to test patients?

First, *tacit consent,* a favorite tool of political theorists in the contract tradition, is expressed silently or passively by omissions or by failure to indicate or signify dissent (see Simmons 1976; for an analysis of varieties of consent in bioethics, see Childress 1982a). If a newly admitted hospital patient is silent when told that the HIV-antibody test will be performed, along with other tests, unless he objects, his silence may constitute valid (though tacit) consent, if there is understanding and voluntariness—the same conditions that are important for express oral or written consent. But if the question is not asked, the patient's failure to dissent from the test, without any notice or additional information, is *presumed* to be consent on the basis of a presumed general understanding of hospital testing policy. And its validity as consent is suspect, despite the patient's right to dissent or opt out.

Whereas tacit consent or presumed consent is expressed through failures to dissent, *implied* or implicit consent is, in part, inferred from actions. Consent to a specific action may be implied by general consent to professional authority or consent to a set of actions. Does a person's voluntary admission to the hospital imply consent to the HIV-antibody test without express consent? Again much will depend on the patient's understanding. However, rather than rely on general consent or consent to several tests, hospitals should be obligated to seek specific express consent for HIV-antibody tests because of the psychological and social risks of the tests and their results.

There are two major reasons for specific disclosure and explicit consent. On the one hand, the diagnostic or therapeutic procedure may be invasive—e.g., drawing blood. But if a patient has consented to blood drawing for various tests to determine his or her medical condition, there is no additional invasion of his or her body to test that blood for HIV antibodies. Then the second major reason for specific disclosure and consent enters—the risk to the patient. Even where the blood has already been drawn, the test has the psychological and social risks noted above, and explicit, specific consent should be sought (Swartz 1988). (This argument does not exclude the possibility and justifiability of unlinked testing of blood samples in the hospital in order to determine seroprevalence as part of epidemiological studies because of the absence of psychological and social risks.)

A recent Virginia law (Virginia Code 32.1–45.1) invokes "deemed consent" in permitting a health care provider to test a patient's blood, without specific consent, following the provider's exposure to the patient's body fluids under circumstances where HIV infection might be spread. In that case, "the patient whose body fluids were involved in the exposures shall be deemed to have consented to testing for infection with human immunodeficiency virus [and] to have consented to the release of such test results to the person who was exposed." The law assigns to health care providers the responsibility to inform patients of this provision of deemed consent prior to the provision of health care services, in other than emergency circumstances. Presumably, the patient's acceptance of health care following disclosure of this statutory provision counts as consent (deemed consent). Even if the consent is valid, the fairness of imposing this condition is still an important question.

Because consent is so important an implication of the principle of respect for personal autonomy, we often resort to fictions such as deemed consent or one of the other varieties of "consent" even when they do not appear to constitute valid consent. We extend the meaning of rules of consent and the principle of respect for personal autonomy in order to avoid conflicts with our other moral principles. But such fictions may obscure important moral conflicts. It may be more defensible to indicate that the society believes it can justifiably override a patient's autonomy, liberty, privacy, and confidentiality in order to obtain and provide information about an individual's HIV-antibody status to a health care provider who has been exposed to the risk of infection in the provision of care. The most attractive argument in favor of deemed consent is that it incorporates the patient into a larger moral community of shared concern, but this does not negate the cost of the fiction.

There is evidence that hospitals sometimes test patients for HIV antibodies without their consent (and without providing information about actions to reduce risks) (see Henry, Maki and Crossley 1988; Sherer 1988). In general, hospitals are not justified in testing patients for HIV antibodies without their specific consent, either to benefit the patients themselves or to warn caregivers to take additional precautions. Information that a patient is seronegative may create a false sense of security on the part of professionals, in view of the long time that may elapse between exposure to HIV and the development of antibodies. Thus, the best protection, though not an inexpensive or perfect one, is offered by universal precautions. In one recent study there was no evidence "that preoperative testing for HIV infection would reduce the frequency of accidental exposures to blood" (Gerberding et al. 1990:1788).

Where exposure has already occurred, and the blood is not available for testing, it is very difficult to justify forcible extraction of the patient's blood to test for HIV antibodies to reduce the caregiver's anxieties. Where the blood is already available, it is easier to justify testing after exposure, even against the patient's wishes. However, the analogy with the hepatitis B virus argues against mandatory testing, whether before or after exposure (Field 1990:104). One ethically acceptable possibility would be to obtain patients' advance express consent—not merely deemed consent—to testing if accidental exposure occurs. (I discuss testing health care professionals below.)

Premarital Screening

State-mandated premarital screening for HIV antibodies is another mix of voluntary choices and compulsory screening; individuals choose to apply for marriage licenses, but the test is required as a condition of application. Historical analogies play an important role in debates about this public health policy. For example, Gary Bauer, former assistant to President Reagan for policy development, uses mandatory premarital screening as an example of the "routine testing" that is similar to measures taken in the past to deal with threatening epidemics. He argues that mandatory premarital screening for syphilis contributed to a "sharp reduction in the infant mortality rate from syphilis" (Bauer 1987:1). However, Larry Gostin contends that "statutes for syphilis screening were largely regarded as a failed experiment" (1987:16) and notes they have been repealed by most states.

The analogy with screening for syphilis is interesting in part because, in contrast to HIV infection, syphilis is treatable and infected individuals can be rendered noninfectious. Many argue that it is even more imperative to require premarital HIV tests as a condition for marriage licenses because there is no cure for AIDS, a fatal disease. By contrast, opponents contend that the absence of effective treatment is a good reason not to require the tests. Because antibiotics can cure syphilis, it is justifiable to withhold a marriage license until there is proof of a cure, but "it would be contrary to public policy to bar marriage to seropositive individuals," who cannot now be cured (Gostin 1987:17).

The legislatures (Illinois and Louisiana) that passed statutes mandating premarital screening subsequently rescinded those statutes, largely on grounds that they were not cost effective. A report (Turnock and Kelly 1989) on the first six months of experience in Illinois indicated that only 8 of 70,846 applicants for marriage licenses were found to be seropositive, while the cost of the testing program for that period was estimated at $2.5 million, or $312,000 for each seropositive individual identified. Furthermore, half of those identified as seropositive admitted having engaged in risky behavior and could probably have been identified more efficiently through voluntary programs aimed at populations with a higher seroprevalence rate. Illinois also experienced a 22.5 percent decrease (a total of approximately 10,300) in the number of marriage licenses, while neighboring states granted licenses to a significantly larger number of Illinois residents than usual. Since the applicants had to cover the costs of the tests, the state of Illinois did not have to determine the most cost-effective ways to spend public money and make trade-offs (Field 1990). Illinois did, however, lose the revenue from marriage licenses, estimated at $77,250 for six months. The authors conclude what policy analysts had predicted prior to the experiment: "The Illinois experience with premarital testing provides a strong argument against widespread or publicly supported HIV antibody screening of low prevalence populations" (Turnock and Kelly 1989; see also Cleary et al. 1987).

While many of the proposed policies of compulsory selective screening fail the test of necessity, because there are viable alternatives, the policy of mandatory premarital screening also fails the prior conditions of effectiveness and proportionality. There is no evidence that the screening program prevented any additional illnesses and that it was a "rational or effective public health policy" (Belongia, Vergeront, and Davis 1989:2198). It mistakenly assumed that sex begins only after the marriage, and it may even have been counterproductive in driving some away from the institution of marriage. Furthermore, the costs may have kept some low-income people from applying for marriage licenses. Finally, the important public health objective of protecting spouses (and future offspring) can be pursued in other ways that will not compromise respect for personal autonomy and yet will probably be more effective and cost effective—provision of information about HIV risks and provision of voluntary testing with counseling, perhaps free of charge, to all applicants for marriage licenses. It appears that the marriage license setting is an appropriate one "for promoting individual HIV risk assessment with educational materials" (Joseph 1989:3456).

Screening Pregnant Women and Newborns

One major goal of premarital screening is to prevent infected offspring of the marriage. Because mandatory premarital screening programs are failures, voluntary premarital screening is limited, and HIV infections may occur after marriage, there has been interest in screening pregnant women and newborns at least in selected settings. Since all fifty states and the District of Columbia mandate neonatal screening for several diseases, the question arises, Why not treat HIV "just like any other disease?" However, as Kathleen Nolan (1989:55) notes, even if HIV infection were strictly analogous to these other medical conditions, such as phenylketonuria (PKU), it would be difficult to determine what it would mean to treat HIV infection "just like any other disease," because the states have various laws—for example, there is no condition for which all states mandate screening, and many states allow parental refusal. Furthermore, HIV infection differs from other diseases because of its social risks. For example, there are "boarder babies" who cannot leave the hospital because no one will take these HIV-infected babies. Hence, HIV infection, Nolan (1989:56) argues, is best viewed as a "separate case."

Still affirming the importance of analogical reasoning, Nolan (1989) identifies three criteria for justifying neonatal *genetic* screening: (1) the seriousness of the genetic condition, (2) availability of presymptomatic interventions that effectively prevent serious injury, and (3) an acceptable benefit-cost ratio. While HIV infection satisfies the first criterion, it does not clearly satisfy the other two in neonatal cases, except where there are specific reasons for testing, and then the parents will usually consent. (Furthermore, there is the problem that neonatal and infant screening, for over a year, will reflect maternal antibodies without specifically reflecting neonatal or infant infection.) In summary, Nolan argues, "calls for mandatory neonatal screening emerge primarily from beneficent clinical attitudes towards newborns, and they are rejected primarily on the grounds that not enough benefit accrues at present to justify overriding parental autonomy and family values" (1989:59) (see also Levine and Bayer 1989:1665).

But do similar arguments apply to *prenatal testing*? According to LeRoy Walters (1990), HIV testing in pregnancy should be handled in a way similar to the ways we have handled prenatal diagnosis for fetal genetic conditions or anatomic abnormalities. Prenatal HIV testing involves screening the pregnant woman, especially on behalf of her future offspring or the society, including the professionals involved in her care. Even though there may be some potential medical benefits to the pregnant woman, she also bears the social risks identified earlier. In view of the risk of transmission of HIV infection to her offspring— in the range of 25 to 50 percent—there are debates about whether it is morally responsible to continue or to terminate pregnancy and thus what counselors should recommend if they are directive (Nolan 1989; Walters 1990). Once a woman is pregnant, the test for HIV antibodies "can help contain HIV only if it leads to abortion" (Field 1990:95).

Even if the society could agree on the morally responsible choice, which is highly unlikely in view of the abortion controversy, there are further moral questions about the legal enforcement of moral obligations. Efforts to mandate prenatal testing would probably be ineffective and even counterproductive. For example, mandatory prenatal screening of all pregnant women who appear at clinics in high seroprevalence areas would put them at social risk if they were seropositive. Thus, there is "the very real possibility that mandated or universal testing during pregnancy could result in marked decreases in the number of disadvantaged women who seek prenatal care" (Nolan 1989:64). Thus, the most defensible policy, because the most respectful of pregnant women's autonomy and also the most productive of desirable consequences, is to offer pregnant women, in high seroprevalence areas or with risk factors, prenatal testing for HIV with adequate information so that they can make their own decisions, with appropriate pretest and posttest counseling and support services.

It is also important, as Nolan (1989) reminds us, to consider whether we are following defensible precedents (historical analogies) for genetic diseases and what precedents our policies regarding HIV testing may set for other genetic diseases that in the future can be detected in utero. Indeed, she suggests, our different responses to cystic fibrosis and HIV infection suggest that morally extraneous factors such as race and geography play significant parts in our societal and professional judgments, particularly in the movement from nondirective to directive counseling (for example, counselors appear to be more directive in urging HIV-infected women to abort).

In summary, mandatory prenatal testing to protect offspring appears relatively ineffective because nothing can be done to prevent the infection of the fetus; morally controversial because abortion is the only way to prevent another HIV-infected infant, and yet fetuses are infected in only 25 to 50 percent of the cases of HIV-infected pregnant women; and counterproductive in driving pregnant women away from settings where HIV screening is compulsory.

Prisoners and Others in State Custody

There are several institutional settings in which mandatory screening might appear to be justified. These are mainly custodial settings, such as prisons and institutions for the mentally infirm or mentally ill. I concentrate on prisoners, with brief attention to arrested prostitutes and patients in public psychiatric facilities. Many prisoners have been subjected to mandatory screening, because of the risk of rape and the frequency of consensual sexual intercourse in prisons where there is also high seroprevalence. Even if mandatory screening of prisoners, followed by quarantine or isolation, could reduce the spread of HIV infection, it is not clearly cost-effective and it imposes risks of injustice on seropositive prisoners, "ranging from unequal facilities for inmates to violations of a number of hard-won rights of prisoners" (Macklin 1986:22). Furthermore, it is not the least intrusive or restrictive alternative. Indeed, on grounds of respect for persons, as well as other moral principles, it is crucial for the society to reduce nonconsensual sexual intercourse in prisons (Gostin 1987:21; Field 1990:81–91). It is also important to educate prisoners and perhaps even to provide condoms to reduce the risk of transmission of HIV through consensual sexual activities. Even the provision of voluntary testing may be useful; in one study in Oregon, "two-thirds of all inmates, including those at highest risk for HIV, sought HIV counseling and testing when given the opportunity" (Andrus et al. 1989). Nevertheless, as Ruth Macklin argues, "it would not be unethical to subject to a blood test any prisoner who has sexually assaulted another inmate, and if he is found seropositive, to isolate him permanently from the general prison population" (1986:22).

Similarly, it would not be unethical, in terms of the principles of a liberal society, to confine a recalcitrant prostitute who puts others at serious risk, for example, by continuing to practice unsafe sex. A more difficult question is whether it is justifiable to require prostitutes to undergo HIV testing. Although prostitution is widely viewed as a major route for the spread of HIV infection among heterosexuals, Martha Field (1990) argues that the overall HIV infection rate among prostitutes does not justify targeting them for mandatory testing, that prostitutes tend to be well informed about safe sex practices, and that more than 99 percent of all prostitutes are never arrested. Thus, mandatory testing of prostitutes does not appear to satisfy the conditions identified earlier. However, if states pass laws to require prostitutes to be tested when in state custody, Field views two conditions as essential. First, testing should be required only of those who are convicted, not those who are arrested, because of the legal presumption of innocence. Second, patrons should be tested if prostitutes are tested; "although patrons are seldom arrested or convicted, both parties are guilty of criminal behavior that is capable of transmission" (1990:94).

Patients in state psychiatric institutions may be at risk of transmitting HIV infection through sexual intercourse. As in the case of prisoners, the state should attempt to prevent rape in psychiatric institutions—and not only because of the risk of HIV infection. Since many psychiatric patients are unable to benefit from efforts to educate them about HIV infection and safe sex, there may be a stronger argument for identifying and isolating HIV-infected patients. Even so it is necessary to make sure that there are no other alternatives and that the least restrictive alternative is chosen.

Immigration and International Travel

"Seeking to secure our national borders against an 'invasion' of AIDS, the United States now requires HIV-antibody testing of 500,000 immigrants, nonimmigrants, and refugees annually. In addition, in what may be the most massive use of HIV testing in this country, more than 2.5 million aliens living in the United States must be tested in order to qualify for legal residence" (Wolchok 1989:128). Historically, societies have responded to epidemics by closing their borders, but the current U.S. policy is ironic because the United States is probably a net exporter of HIV infection. Yet HIV infection was added to the list of designated diseases (now eight, including infectious leprosy, active tuberculosis, gonorrhea, and infectious syphilis) for which aliens can be excluded from the United States. In view of the precedent set by listing the other exclusionary diseases, it did not seem to many to be unreasonable to add HIV infection. Now temporary visitors to the United States have to indicate their HIV-antibody status when they apply for a visa, and the immigration officer may require a test. Applicants for permanent residence must undergo a serologic test for HIV infection (and syphilis) and if positive cannot receive permanent residence. Because the costs of the program fall on the applicants, the society does not have to face the question of trade-offs in the use of public funds.

Analogical reasoning is also critical here, not only in considering historical precedents but also in considering the implications of the mandatory screening of aliens for other groups. Margaret Somerville notes that viewing prospective immigrants who are HIV infected as "a danger to public health and safety would necessarily set a precedent that all HIV-infected people (already in the country) could be similarly characterized" (1989:891). In addition, it sets precedents for genetic screening as more and more tests become available.

Larry Gostin and his colleagues argue that "a just and efficacious travel and immigration policy would not exclude people because of their serologic status unless they posed a danger to the community through casual transmission" (Gostin, et al. 1990:1745–1746. Indeed, the list of excludable conditions should be revised because only active tuberculosis poses a threat of casual transmission. Immigrants are thus not a major threat to the public health, and screening them will have only a modest impact on the course of the epidemic in the United States, which already has more than one million HIV-infected persons. In addition, the screening program discourages travelers from being tested and "drives further underground undocumented aliens who live in the United States and reduces their incentive to seek counseling and preventative care" (Wolchok 1989:142). Finally, current U.S. policy does not contribute to efforts to control HIV infection in the international community (Gostin et al. 1990).

Since the current screening program does not contribute significantly to public health objectives, the major argument for excluding seropositive immigrants appears to be the cost to the society of providing health care. It may not be intrinsically unjust for a society to exclude immigrants on grounds of the costs of providing health care, but several commentators cogently argue that "it is inequitable . . . to use cost as a reason to exclude people infected with HIV, for there are no similar exclusionary policies for those with other costly chronic diseases, such as heart disease or cancer" (Gostin et al. 1990:1746). Their argument rests on the requirement of justice to treat similar cases in a similar way. And, as is true of each proposed screening target, screening immigrants raises larger philosophical and ethical questions about the boundaries of the moral community.

Other Areas of Selective Screening

I have concentrated on a few areas to indicate how the liberal framework of principles, rules, and justificatory conditions applies to proposed policies of mandatory HIV-antibody screening and testing. The arguments extend, *mutatis mutandis,* to other proposed policies. For example, what we know about the transmission of HIV renders mandatory screening in the workplace inappropriate, unless there is exposure to body fluids under circumstances that could transmit the virus.

Concern has been expressed about the possibility that health care professionals, particularly dentists and surgeons, might transmit the virus to their patients during invasive procedures. In July 1990, the Centers for Disease Control (CDC) reported a case of "possible transmission" of HIV to a patient during the removal of two of her teeth by a dentist who had AIDS. Although "the possibility of another source of infection cannot be entirely excluded," the CDC noted the absence of any other reported risk factors and a close relation between the viral DNA sequences from the patient and the dentist ("Possible Transmission" 1990:489). During the same week, researchers reported that there was no evidence that a Tennessee surgeon with HIV infection had infected any of his surgical patients, many of whom consented to HIV tests (Mishu et al. 1990). In view of the mode of transmission of HIV "it would be unexpected if HIV transmission" does not occur in surgical procedures (Rhame 1990:507). It is important, however, to keep the risk of such transmission in perspective. The probability is very low, perhaps between one in 100,000 to one in one million operations (Rhame 1990). While the risk is "exceedingly remote" of infection for any single patient, "the cumulative risk over a surgical career is real" (Gostin 1990b). The main risks appear to be in seriously invasive procedures, particularly vaginal hysterectomies or pelvic surgery, where there is "blind" (i.e., not directly visualized) use of sharp surgical tools (Rhame 1990). If there are grounds for restricting the activities of any surgeon—or dentist—who is known to be HIV infected, then there are probable grounds for mandatory testing to determine which ones are HIV infected. This area requires further careful attention, and the conclusions—at least for some forms of surgery—are likely to be applicable to both health care professionals and patients, since each party may put the other at risk of HIV infection.

Sometimes the goal of testing is to reduce costs rather than to prevent transmission of HIV infection. Both goals are present in some screening policies—for example, immigration and military screening. The goal of saving funds is often primary in workplace screening, and it is clearly the only concern in insurance screening. It is not unreasonable or even unjust for insurance companies to screen and for states to allow them to screen life and health insurance applicants for HIV antibodies, just as they screen for other conditions. It is, however, a failure of justice, compassion, and care for the society, through the federal and state governments, not to provide funds so that HIV-infected individuals and other sick people can obtain needed health care. In short, the fundamental problem is not the actions of insurance companies but rather the larger societal response to the health care needs of its citizens, including those with HIV infection.

Conclusion: The War Against AIDS

Not only do societies often react (and, at least in retrospect, overreact) through coercive measures to epidemics of communicable disease, they frequently do so in the name of *war* against the diseases. The metaphor of "the war against AIDS" has been very prominent in justifications of mandatory screening and testing. "Under the guise of a war against AIDS," one commentator notes, "American politics have recently become enamored of an argument over testing citizens" for HIV antibody (Wood 1987:35). Reflecting the prominence of military metaphors, Larry Gostin observes that it often appears that "the first line of defense in combatting AIDS is to identify carriers of the virus by systematic screening" (1987:21). And, in a sensitive discussion of major vocabularies of concern about AIDS, Monroe Price notes that "the crisis of epidemic is a natural substitute for the crisis of war," and "the question is whether the AIDS epidemic will become such a serious threat that, in the public's mind, it takes on the stature of war" (1989:81,84).

The metaphor of war is natural in our sociocultural context when a serious threat to a large number of human lives requires the mobilization of societal resources, especially when that threat comes from biological organisms, such as viruses, that attack the human body. For example, the military metaphor is one way to galvanize the society and to marshal its resources for an effective counterattack, and AIDS activists may even appeal to it for this purpose (Kramer 1990). The metaphor has, however, other entailments that need to be questioned and perhaps even opposed, especially in our sociocultural context. (On the war metaphor, see Childress 1982a; Ross 1989a and 1989b; Sontag 1990.)

From the beginning of the war against AIDS, identification of the enemy has been a major goal. Once the virus was identified as the primary enemy, it became possible to develop technologies to identify human beings who carry or harbor the virus. This led to what Ronald Bayer calls the "politics of identification" (1989). How are antibody-positive individuals to be viewed? As carriers of HIV, are they enemies to be fought? Should the society try to identify them? And how should it act on the information that a particular individual carries or harbors the virus? The line between the virus and the carrier becomes very tenuous, and the carrier tends to become an enemy just as the virus he or she carries. However much Surgeon General Everett Koop could argue that this war is against the virus, not against the people, that distinction is too subtle for many in the community. Furthermore, because the society does not consider many actions that lead to exposure to HIV as "innocent" and even views the associated life-styles as a threat to dominant social values, it is not surprising that this metaphor of war often coexists with metaphors of AIDS as punishment and as otherness (Price 1989; Ross 1989a and 1989b).

The military metaphor tends to justify coercive measures, such as quarantine and isolation of internal threats. In World War II the United

States sent Japanese-Americans to internment camps, without due process, and with the approval of the U.S. Supreme Court in *Korematsu v. United States* in 1944. These coercive policies were later discredited, and Congress even approved reparations to those who were interned. However, the coercive policy of identification and internment "demonstrates how, in times of war, like times of public health crisis, the actions of government become clothed with an unusual inviolability" (Price 1989:82). And it is even worse when the public health crisis is itself construed as warfare, because of the disjunction between "peacetime procedures" and "wartime needs" (Justice Douglas, quoted in Price 1989:84).

The metaphor of war against AIDS would not be so dangerous if our society had a better appreciation of the moral constraints on resort to and conduct of warfare, represented in the just war tradition (Childress 1982b). The justification and limitation of war, including the means employed, follow the pattern of the prima facie principles and conditions for justified infringements identified earlier. In general, like a dinosaur, the United States has been slow to engage in war but then hard to control once it starts to act. After AIDS appeared, the early societal response was limited in part because the disease was viewed as a threat mainly to those on the margins of society, especially gays, but then when AIDS was viewed as a threat to the larger society, the response was conceived in terms of war. In general, the United States has tended to engage in total war, with unlimited objectives and unlimited means, as expressed in our willingness to destroy cities in Vietnam in order to save them. In the war against AIDS it is important to recognize both limited objectives and limited means. In contrast to Susan Sontag (1990), I do not believe that the metaphor of war should be retired, but its logic must be carefully explored and its application limited by "just war" criteria and supplemented by other metaphors.

In discussions of the war against disease, caring has often been viewed as an alternative metaphor. If the military metaphor tends to conflate the virus and the carriers of the virus, the caring metaphor tends to focus on concern for individuals who carry the virus. Even a liberal society need not be a society of mere strangers; it can at least be a society of "friendly strangers." This friendliness can be expressed in care, compassion, and empathy. If the metaphor of war against AIDS tends to divide the community insofar as HIV-infected individuals are viewed as enemies, it thereby undermines some of the conditions that could make voluntaristic policies work. Trust is indispensable, and it presupposes communal commitments to provide funds for health care and to enforce rules against discrimination, breaches of confidentiality, etc.

These communal efforts are critically important, because the groups most affected by AIDS—gay men and intravenous drug users—exist on the "margins" of the community (Price 1989). Thus, they tend to view coercive policies of identification of antibody-positive individuals as analogous to the Nazi efforts to identify Jews and others for nefarious purposes (Collins 1987:10). When the "politics of identification" appeals to the sociocultural metaphor of war, it is easy to understand the fears of HIV-infected individuals, especially when they live in marginalized subcommunities. The war metaphor tends to exclude HIV-infected individuals as enemies from the larger community, while the metaphor of care tends to include them in the community. Compulsory measures, such as mandatory screening, appear to impose community, but, without the expression of community—for example, through the allocation of funds for health care and the protection of individual rights and liberties—they largely exclude coerced individuals from the community. If the society expresses solidarity with HIV-infected individuals, it is less likely to need coercive policies to replace voluntaristic ones. If the society denies solidarity, coercive policies are likely to be ineffective and even counterproductive, because they too presuppose voluntary cooperation at many points, often to enter situations where testing is encouraged or required, and generally to carry out measures to protect others.

Mandatory HIV screening, in most settings, would set a precedent of overriding rights in a crisis—in a war against disease—even when it produces no benefits, or the burdens outweigh the benefits, or there are alternative ways to protect the public health. We need to respond out of metaphors other than (or at least in addition to) war, with careful attention to the moral commitments of a liberal society and the justificatory conditions for overriding prima facie principles and rules. How we respond will shape and express our "identity and community in a democracy under siege" (Price 1989:5).

REFERENCES

Andrus, Jon K., David W. Fleming, Catherine Knox et al. 1989. HIV Testing in Prisons: Is Mandatory Testing Mandatory? *American Journal of Public Health* (July), 79(7):840–842.
Bauer, Gary L. 1987. AIDS Testing. *AIDS & Public Policy Journal* (Fall–Winter), 2(4):1–2.
Bayer, Ronald. 1989. *Private Acts, Social Consequences: AIDS and the Politics of Public Health.* New York: Free Press.

Bayer, Ronald, Carol Levine, and Susan M. Wolf. 1986. HIV Antibody Screening: An Ethical Framework for Evaluating Proposed Programs. *JAMA* (October 3), 256(3):1768–1774.

Beauchamp, Tom L. and James F. Childress. 1989. *Principles of Biomedical Ethics*, 3d ed. New York: Oxford University Press.

Becker, Marshall H. and Jill G. Joseph. 1988. AIDS and Behavioral Change to Reduce Risk: A Review. *American Journal of Public Health*, (April), 78(4):394–410.

Belongia, Edward A., James M. Vergeront, and Jeffrey P. Davis. 1989. Premarital HIV Screening (Letter to Editor), *Journal of the American Medical Association* (April 21), 261(15):2198.

Bok, Sissela. 1978. *Lying: Moral Choice in Public and Private Life*. New York: Pantheon Books.

Cates, Willard, Jr. and H. Hunter Handsfield. 1988. HIV Counseling and Testing: Does It Work? *American Journal of Public Health* (December), 78(12):1533–1534.

Childress, James F. 1982a. *Who Should Decide? Paternalism in Health Care*. New York: Oxford University Press.

Childress, James F. 1982b. *Moral Responsibility in Conflicts*. Baton Rouge, La: Louisiana State University Press.

Childress, James F. 1987. An Ethical Framework for Assessing Policies to Screen for Antibodies to HIV. *AIDS & Public Policy Journal* (Winter), 2(1):28–31.

Childress, James F. 1990. The Place of Autonomy in Bioethics. *Hastings Center Report* (January/February), 20:12–17.

Cleary, Paul D., et al. 1987. Compulsory Premarital Screening for the Human Immunodeficiency Virus: Technical and Public Health Considerations. *JAMA* (October 2), 258(13):1757–1762.

Collins, Christopher J. 1987. The Case Against AIDS Testing. *AIDS & Public Policy Journal* (Fall–Winter), 2(4):8–11.

Committee for the Study of the Future of Public Health, Division of Health Care Services, Institute of Medicine. 1988. *The Future of Public Health*. Washington, D.C.: National Academy Press.

Field, Martha A. 1990. Testing for AIDS: Uses and Abuses. *American Journal of Law & Medicine* 16(2):33–106.

Fletcher, John C. 1987. AIDS Screening: A Response to Gary Bauer. *AIDS & Public Policy Journal* (Fall–Winter), 2(4):5–7.

Gerberding, Julie Louise et al. 1990. Risk of Exposure of Surgical Personnel to Patients' Blood During Surgery at San Francisco General Hospital. *New England Journal of Medicine* (June 21), 322(25):1788–1793.

Gostin, Larry. 1987. Screening for AIDs: Efficacy, Cost, and Consequences. *AIDS & Public Policy Journal* (Fall–Winter), 2(4):14–24.

Gostin, Larry. 1990a. A Decade of a Maturing Epidemic: An Assessment and Directions for Future Public Policy. *American Journal of Law and Medicine (16)* (1 and 2):1–32.

Gostin, Larry. 1990b. Letter to Editor. *JAMA* (July 25), 264:452–453.

Gostin, Larry O. et al. 1990. Screening Immigrants and International Travelers for the Human Immunodeficiency Virus. *New England Journal of Medicine* (June 4), 322 (24):1743–1746.

Henry, Keith, Myra Maki, and Kent Crossley. 1988. Analysis of the Use of HIV Antibody Testing in a Minnesota Hospital. *JAMA* (Jan. 8), 259(2):229–232.

Joseph, Stephen C. 1989. Premarital AIDS Testing: Public Policy Abandoned at the Altar. JAMA (June 16), 261(23):3456.

Kramer, Larry. 1990. A 'Manhattan Project' for AIDS. *New York Times* (July 16).

Levine, Carol and Ronald Bayer. 1989. The Ethics of Screening for Early Intervention in HIV Disease. *American Journal of Public Health* (December), 79(12):1661–1667.

Lo, Bernard, Robert L. Steinbrook, Molly Cooke et al. 1989. Voluntary Screening for Human Immunodeficiency Virus (HIV) Infection: Weighing the Benefits and Harms. *Annals of Internal Medicine* (May), 110(9):727–733.

Macklin, Ruth. 1986. Predicting Dangerousness and the Public Health Response to AIDS. *Hastings Center Report* (December) 16:16–23.

Marzuk, Peter M. Helen Tierney, Kenneth Tardiff et al. 1988. Increased Risk of Suicide in Persons with AIDS. *JAMA* 259:1333–1337.

McCusker, Jane, Anne M. Stoddard, Kenneth H. Mayer, et al. 1988. Effects of HIV Antibody Test Knowledge on Subsequent Sexual Behaviors in a Cohort of Homosexually Active Men. *American Journal of Public Health* (April), 78(4):462–467.

Mishu, Ban, William Schaffner, John M. Horan et al. 1990. A Surgeon with AIDS: Lack of Evidence of Transmission to Patients. *JAMA* (July 25), 264:467–470.

Nolan, Kathleen. 1989. Ethical Issues in Caring for Pregnant Women and Newborns at Risk for Human Immunodeficiency Virus Infection. *Seminars in Perinatology* (February), 13(1):55–65.

Nozick, Robert. 1968. Moral Complications and Moral Structures. *Natural Low Forum* 13:1–50.

O'Brien, Maura. 1989. Mandatory HIV Antibody Testing Policies: An Ethical Analysis. *Bioethics* 3(4):273–300.

Osborn, June E. 1987. Widespread Testing for AIDS: What is the Question? *AIDS and Public Policy Journal* (Fall–Winter), 2(4):2–4.

Possible Transmission of Human Immunodeficiency Virus to a Patient During an Invasive Dental Procedure. 1990. *Morbidity and Mortality Weekly Report* (July 27), 39(29):489–493.

Price, Monroe E. 1989. *Shattered Mirrors: Our Search for Identity and Community in the AIDS Era.* Cambridge, Mass.: Harvard University Press.

Rhame, Frank S. 1990. The HIV-Infected Surgeon. *JAMA* (July 25), 264:507–508.

Rhame, Frank S. and Dennis G. Maki. 1989. The Case for Wider Use of Testing for HIV Infection. *New England Journal of Medicine* (May 11), 320(19):1248–1253.

Ross, Judith Wilson. 1989a. Ethics and the Language of AIDS. In Eric T. Juengst and Barbara A. Koenig, ed., *The Meaning of AIDS: Implications for Medical Science, Clinical Practice, and Public Health Policy.* New York: Praeger.

Ross, Judith Wilson. 1989b. The Militarization of Disease: Do We Really Want a War on AIDS? *Soundings* (Spring), 72:39–58.

Sherer, Renslow. 1988. Physician Use of the HIV Antibody Test. *JAMA* (Jan. 8), 259(2):264–265.

Simmons, A. John. 1976. Tacit Consent and Political Obligation. *Philosophy and Public Affairs* (Spring), 5:274–291.

Somerville, Margaret A. 1989. The Case Against HIV Antibody Testing of Refugees and Immigrants. *Canadian Medical Association Journal* (Nov. 1), 141:889–894.

Sontag, Susan. 1990. *Illness as Metaphor and AIDS and Its Metaphors.* New York: Anchor Books.

Swartz, Martha S. 1988. AIDS Testing and Informed Consent. *Journal of Health Politics, Policy, and Law* (Winter) 3(4):607–621.

Turnock, Bernard J. and Chester J. Kelly. 1989. Mandatory Premarital Testing for Human Immunodeficiency Virus: The Illinois Experience. *JAMA* (June 16), 261(23):3415–3418.

Walters, LeRoy. 1988. Ethical Issues in the Prevention and Treatment of HIV Infection and AIDS. *Science* (Feb. 5), pp. 597–603.

Walters, LeRoy. 1990. Ethical Issues in HIV Testing During Pregnancy. Unpublished manuscript.
Wertheimer, Alan. 1987. *Coercion.* Princeton, N.J.: Princeton University Press.
Wolchok, Carol Leslie. 1989. AIDS at the Frontier: United States Immigration Policy. *The Journal of Legal Medicine* 10:128–142.
Wood, Gary James. 1987. The Politics of AIDS Testing. *AIDS and Public Policy Journal* (Fall–Winter) 2(4):35–49.

4. AIDS and the Ethics of Human Subjects Research

CAROL LEVINE

UNDER WHAT CONDITIONS and for what purposes is it ethically justifiable for scientists to involve human beings in biomedical and behavioral research? This question, in all its many nuanced forms, has been high on the agenda of biomedical ethics for fifty years. And just when the answers seemed to be at least tentatively in place, the new disease of AIDS challenged many of the assumptions, rules, and practices that have evolved in the post-World War II era. The process of review, analysis, and change is still underway.

After a brief introduction to the evolution of ethical standards for research involving human subjects beginning in the late 1940s, this essay surveys the main ethical issues that have arisen around the new disease of AIDS. Each new stage of scientific knowledge has been accompanied by challenges to the accepted processes of ethical review. The initial epidemiological studies raised questions about protecting the confidentiality of study participants who would be interviewed about stigmatized and in some cases illegal behavior. Beginning in 1985, the use of the human immunodeficiency virus (HIV)-antibody test in epidemiological screening programs and research prompted a new range of concerns, particularly about informed consent, the justifications for anonymous seroprevalence studies, and the subject's right not to know the test results.

The relatively recent development of clinical trials to test investigational drugs or approved drugs for new uses has opened some of the most complex issues, such as the ethical dimensions of research design, the balance between protection from risk and increased access to possibly beneficial but incompletely tested agents, the duties of research subjects and physicians involved in clinical trials, equitable selection of subjects (especially vulnerable ones such as prisoners and pregnant women), and informed consent in situations where primary medical care is available only in the research setting. Finally, the goal of preventing HIV infection through a vaccine raises some additional questions, particularly about the design and implementation of international trials and protection of subjects from the social risks of vaccine-induced HIV seropositivity.

Some of these ethical issues (such as the need for special protections for confidentiality) have been largely resolved, whereas others (such as the participation of pregnant women in clinical trials) are still vigorously debated. In the future, an even broader agenda of research issues may evolve.

The Evolution of Ethical Standards for Research

The trials of the Nazi doctors at Nuremberg in 1945 mark a turning point in the modern concern about the ethics of research. The cruel experiments carried out on unconsenting prisoners for the benefit of the military of the Third Reich have now been shown to be scientifically worthless, as well as inhumane (Berger 1990). The Nuremberg Code and subsequent international codes of ethics concerning scientific research stressed that participation of subjects must be voluntary and informed and that they must be protected against unjustifiable risk.

In 1966 Henry Knowles Beecher, a highly respected Harvard anesthesiologist, charged in a now-classic article that "many of the patients [in clinical trials in the U.S.] . . . never had the risks explained to them and . . . hundreds had not known that they were the subjects of an experiment although grave consequences have been suffered as a result" (Beecher 1966). Several highly publicized studies also contributed to the raising of professional and public consciousness. Two of the most influential were the Tuskegee syphilis study (Brandt 1978) and the Willowbrook hepatitis studies (Katz 1972).

The Tuskegee syphilis study was initiated in 1932 by the U.S. Public Health Service (PHS) and continued for forty years; its stated purpose was to study the natural history of untreated syphilis. The subjects with the disease—poor black men from Alabama—were told that they had "bad blood" and that research procedures such as spinal taps were "free treatment." They were not given the standard treatment for the disease when the study began or penicillin when it became available in the 1940s. Many died needlessly. Although periodic reports appeared in the professional literature throughout the study, no concerns were raised until 1972, when press reports led to the creation of a special advisory panel of the Department of Health, Education, and Welfare.

The Willowbrook studies involved the deliberate infection with hepatitis of mentally retarded children who were residents of the Willowbrook State Hospital in Staten Island, New York. The purpose of the studies was first to study the natural history of infectious hepatitis and later to test the effects of gamma globulin in treating the disease. The major ethical criticisms concerned the deliberate infection of children (defended by the researchers because children were likely to get the disease in the institution anyway) and the inducement to parents to enroll their child in the study to gain admittance to the hospital, which was refusing new residents because of lack of space.

In 1966 Surgeon General William Stewart promulgated the first U.S. Public Health Service directive on human experimentation, stating that the PHS would not support research unless the institution receiving the grant had specified how it intended to provide assurances, through prior independent ethical review, "(1) of the rights and welfare [of the research subject], (2) of the appropriateness of the methods used to assure informed consent, and (3) of the risks and medical benefits of the investigation" (Katz 1987).

During the same period the rules surrounding the approval of new drugs were also changing. As a result of the thalidomide disaster in Europe and Australia, thousands of women who took this drug in early pregnancy gave birth to severely deformed infants. Thalidomide was never approved in the United States, although the drug was distributed on an "investigational" basis. In 1962, in response to publicity about thalidomide, Food and Drug Administration (FDA) regulations governing the introduction of new drugs were strengthened. More stringent premarketing approval requirements for evidence of safety and efficacy were established.

Thus, the basic approach to human subjects research was born in scandal and reared in protectionism. Individuals perceived as vulnerable, either because of personal characteristics suggesting a lack of autonomy or because of membership in groups lacking social power, were considered to need special protections. Over the last twenty-five years a system of federal regulations and research review by institutional review boards (IRBs) has been put in place. Most of the current federal regulations date from 1983; the regulations on fetal research, which affect research involving pregnant women, date from 1975. Research is governed by two parallel, albeit slightly different, sets of rules. One set applies to research conducted by or funded by the

Department of Health and Human Services (DHHS); the other applies to drug studies that will result in submissions for marketing approval to the FDA.

The Belmont Report, a product of the National Commission for the Protection of Human Subjects of Biomedical and Behavioral Research, sets forth the ethical principles underlying the regulations and IRB deliberations of protocols (National Commission 1978). The three ethical principles of respect for persons, beneficence, and justice are implemented through rules and practices regarding informed consent, protection of confidentiality, and selection of subjects, among other factors (R. J. Levine, 1988).

By the early 1980s, then, it seemed that the ethics of human subjects research was, if not a closed book, then at least a nearly finished chapter. The major emphases were on protecting subjects from risk, informed consent as a mechanism to ensure voluntary participation, exclusion of subjects perceived to be particularly vulnerable, and prior ethical review by a committee including some nonscientists.

After the federal regulations were finally published and discussed in 1983, a colleague asked me, in my capacity as managing editor of *IRB: A Review of Human Subjects Research,* "What will you find to publish now that all the big questions have been answered?" AIDS has mooted his query.

The basic principles underlying human subjects research have proved equal to the challenge of AIDS. Nevertheless, there are differences in emphasis and in research and regulatory practice, especially in the area of clinical drug trials. First, there is a move away from emphasizing nonmaleficence (the prevention of harm by protecting subjects from risks) toward beneficence (actively promoting patients' welfare). Second, there is an emphasis on a different aspect of patient autonomy from those that have traditionally been raised in ethical reviews. IRBs are concerned with enhancing patient autonomy by making sure that potential trial participants are free from subtle or overt coercion in making their decision whether to participate in a research protocol. Another concern is protecting autonomy by ensuring the trial participant's right to full information about risks and benefits in order to make that decision an informed one. The sense of autonomy now in ascendance stresses personal control, including the right to take risks, even serious risks, and to have access to the experimental drug one prefers for whatever reason. The physician typically talks about a drug of choice; the trial participant wants the drug preference.

Third, there is a change that brings to full equality the third principle of the Belmont Report, that is, the principle of justice—fairness and equity in the selection of subjects to receive the benefits, as well as bear the burdens, of trials of experimental drugs.

Fourth, AIDS has contributed to a reexamination of the concept of paternalism in health care. Already weakened by challenges from the patient's rights movements of the 1960s and 1970s, the idea that "the doctor knows best" has been further challenged by medicine's initial inability to treat and still to cure the disease and by the development of strong information and activist networks among patients and their advocates. It is not uncommon for doctors to turn to patients for information about or even access to the latest drugs or therapies. The concept of "patient empowerment" is a formidable challenge to the tendency of some clinicians to further the goal of beneficence by protecting patients from themselves.

Some of these changes are illustrated in the remaining sections of this essay.

Studying a New Disease: Confidentiality of Research Data

The initial research studies concerning AIDS tried to determine the etiology of what was then a largely unexplained disease. There was no question of therapeutic benefit to the subjects, who were mostly gay men, along with some drug users and recent Haitian immigrants. Because their behavior was stigmatized and in some cases illegal, people with AIDS were reluctant to divulge information about their sexual activities, drug use, or entry into this country. The potential consequences of breaches of confidentiality were severe: loss of housing, income, social and health care services, insurance, and relationships with family and friends, and all at a time of serious, usually rapidly fatal, illness.

Epidemiologists knew that they needed to be able to protect their subjects' confidentiality in order to obtain honest and accurate responses. While protection of the confidentiality of medical records and participation in research had been an important part of the development of IRB rules and procedures, in few instances had the need been so strong and the consequences of failing to win the trust of subjects so potentially disastrous to research.

To further the goals of sound epidemiological research and subjects' welfare, a research group organized at The Hastings Center developed a set of guidelines on confidentiality in research (Bayer, Levine, and

Murray 1984). These guidelines were intended to strengthen existing practices of protecting confidentiality, point out the gaps in legal protection, and establish some procedures whereby both the interests of investigators in tracking the disease and of subjects in protecting their privacy were balanced. The special problems of confidentiality in psychological and behavioral research have also been identified by many others (APA 1986; Perry 1987; Melton and Gray 1988).

One of the gaps in legal protection—the vulnerability of researchers to subpoena for research data that may contain information on identifiable individuals—has recently been addressed (Mason 1989). Congress has given the U.S. Public Health Service the authority to grant certificates of confidentiality to protect the identities of research subjects involved in research of a "sensitive nature where the protection is judged necessary to achieve the research objective." This authority, previously granted only for research on mental health, including the use and effect of alcohol and other psychoactive drugs, applies to projects whether or not they are federally funded. Investigators who receive certificates of confidentiality "may not be compelled in any Federal, State, or local civil, criminal, administrative, legislative, or other proceedings to identify [subjects]." The confidentiality certificates apply to research broadly but were clearly designed to encompass AIDS and HIV research; they have not been tested in any court.

Screening: To Blind or Unblind

The first Human Immunodeficiency Virus (HIV)-antibody test kits (then known under their original designation of HTLV-III test kits) were licensed in 1985 by the FDA for screening donated blood. Other research and nonresearch uses of the HIV-antibody test were quickly proposed. The Hastings Center confidentiality guidelines (of which I was a co-author) pointed out that "identifiers" (coded or uncoded pieces of information that enable a researcher to link data to a specific individual or to recognize that different sets of data have come from the same individual) are not always necessary to conduct research. In cases where they are essential, the guidelines stated, "Informed consent should be obtained from the human subjects of any research protocol that involves interviews with patients or family, friends, or sexual conacts; or any collection of data that results in identifiable information."

A subsequent Hastings Center research group that examined ethical issues related to screening concluded that "individuals must be notified that screening will take place," so that they can make an informed choice about whether to consent to the screening or to avoid participating in such activities as donating blood or semen or volunteering for military service (Bayer, Levine, and Wolf 1986). However, at the suggestion of one of the public health officials in this research group, the guidelines commented: "This prerequisite does not preclude the use, without notification, of blood or other samples unlinked to personal identifiers in Institutional Review Board-approved research." There was little discussion and no dissent on this point.

The "family of HIV seroprevalence surveys," conducted by the Centers for Disease Control (CDC), are precisely that type of research. Designed to determine the level of HIV seroprevalence in a nationwide sample of patients in hospitals, drug treatment centers, sexually transmitted disease clinics, family planning centers, and other settings, these studies use a random selection of leftover blood drawn for other purposes. No identifiers are kept; the only information is age, sex, and race (Pappaioanou et al. 1990).

The ethical justification for this type of research rests on the importance of the knowledge to society, the difficulty of obtaining unbiased population samples if consent were to be required, the lack of physical risk to the subjects since no extra blood is drawn, the lack of social risk since they cannot be identified in any way, and the availability of HIV-antibody testing in other anonymous or confidential settings for those who want to know their HIV status for clinical or public health reasons.

Here is one instance in which the benefits to society have appeared, in the widely held American view, to outweigh the general requirement for informed consent. Interestingly, however, this conclusion does not prevail in the United Kingdom or in the Netherlands, where similar proposals have been vigorously opposed (Bayer, Lumey, and Wan 1990). The objections are twofold: first, that consent is ethically preferable to anonymity and can be obtained without biasing the results; and second, that the lack of identifiers makes it impossible to inform those who test positive and encourage them to prevent further spread of the virus. The first objection has so far been most vigorously presented. After considerable debate within the medical and public health communities, the British Department of Health announced in November 1989 plans for anonymous screening of several patient groups in England and Wales. The plans include widespread publicity about the screening and the right of "spontaneous refusal." In the Netherlands, opposition to any compulsory public health measure is so strong that even professional and popular support for blinded studies is unlikely to overcome the barriers.

The American consensus on the ethical justifications for blinded seroprevalence studies may weaken because of increasing expressions of the second objection: the inability to notify infected individuals and offer them treatment and counseling on prevention of HIV transmission. Now that there are grounds for advising those who may be infected with HIV to seek testing and early therapeutic intervention, the pressure is building to unblind seroprevalence studies for this purpose.

In June 1989 the New York State Department of Health issued a press release in which it proposed to "modify its on-going blind newborn HIV antibody testing program to permit voluntary notification of mothers whose infants test positive." Under the proposal, new mothers would have been given the option of learning their baby's test results. (Positive antibody test results in asymptomatic newborns indicate maternal infection but are not a reliable indicator of true infection in the infant.) Community-based health care providers objected to the proposals largely on the grounds that women who have just given birth are particularly vulnerable, both to the traumatic impact of a positive test result and to potential coercion. They also stressed the lack of services for infected women and their babies who would be identified in this way. The proposal was withdrawn in favor of a more aggressive program of voluntary testing linked to concrete services.

Concerned about the potential effect on the validity of blinded anonymous seroprevalence studies if unblinding were to occur, I convened an ad hoc group of attorneys, ethicists, and epidemiologists in New York City to develop a position statement on the issue. We concluded:

> Blinded anonymous seroprevalence studies serve a vital scientific function; they offer the opportunity to sample in an unbiased and nonpoliticized way the level of infection in selected settings, with no risk to participants. These studies cannot also serve the equally important but distinct public health and clinical functions of providing individuals with the opportunity to learn their serostatus so that they can modify their behavior to prevent transmission to others and obtain appropriate care for themselves and their children (C. Levine et al. 1989)

The group submitted the statement to Charles McCarthy, director of the Office for Protection from Research Risks, who supported the conclusions and commented in a letter: "Any linkable, 'unblinded' HIV testing should be done separately from the standard, unlinkable and 'blinded' research surveys for HIV seroprevalence" (McCarthy 1989). While many members of the research and bioethics communities may hold firmly to this view, pressure from public health officials and clinicians will increase to unblind seroprevalence studies as an expedient way to identify those who fail to identify themselves.

To Know or Not to Know; to Tell or Not to Tell

When the HIV-antibody test became available as a research tool, another controversial aspect concerned the subject's right not to know the test results. While the canon of research ethics (and of medical ethics in general) stresses the subject's right to be informed of any relevant information that is developed in the course of research or therapy, the subject's right *not* to know this information has been less well examined. Many people might agree to be tested, in the interests of advancing scientific knowledge, but they may not wish to bear the psychological burden that might result from learning that they are seropositive. Although the benefits of being tested are growing, some individuals may feel that the risks are still too high, particularly when those benefits (e.g., medical care or access to drugs) may not be available. They may feel especially reluctant when the study is epidemiological or behavioral, rather than clinical.

In 1986, when this issue surfaced, Alvin Novick, a physician and AIDS activist, argued that burdensome knowledge need not be imposed, because "no ethical tradition or principle *requires* that a patient be informed of a particular laboratory test result unless he or she wishes to be informed" (Novick 1986). Furthermore, he said, "Knowledge of antibody status is not necessary for responsible behavior." Nancy Neveloff Dubler, an attorney and ethicist, argued in response that imposing this knowledge would discriminate against research subjects. Not to permit patients to refuse to learn such information, at any point along the continuum of the research, "places patients in a protocol in the position of having *fewer* rights than the general population, rather than greater rights as envisioned by the regulations" (Dubler 1986). In this debate Sheldon Landesman, another physician, took the opposite view, declaring that a research protocol that gives subjects the option of not being informed is "unethical because it shifts the moral dilemma inherent in knowing one's antibody status [and informing current, future, and perhaps past sexual partners, thereby risking the loss of valued relationships] from the subject to the researcher" (Landesman 1986). Since participation in research is voluntary, Landesman says, "if a person does not want to know his serological status he can freely choose not to participate."

The federal regulatory position is that:

. . . when HIV testing is conducted or supported by PHS, individuals whose test results are associated with personal identifiers must be

informed of their own test results and provided with the opportunity to
receive appropriate counseling (Windom 1988).

The policy allows for individual exceptions when there are "compelling and immediate" reasons to justify not informing a particular person, such as an indication that the person would commit suicide, or
exceptions pertaining to protocol design, where extremely valuable
knowledge might be gained from research subjects who would be
expected to refuse to learn their test results. In either case, the IRB
and the investigator must document the rationales for the exceptions.
Although the federal policy is now clear-cut, and in practice most IRBs
require notification of subjects with positive test results, IRBs still have
to struggle with individual protocols to determine whether specific
exceptions are justifiable and to decide how many steps researchers
must take to find and notify participants who agree to be tested but fail
to return for their test results. In general, subjects who are fully informed and counseled will, I believe, want to get their test results;
however, they should not be harassed or badgered endlessly if they
truly change their minds and are unable to cope with the prospect of a
positive result. There should always be an opportunity for such a
subject to recontact the investigator or to be retested under different
circumstances.

Another conflict concerns researchers' traditional obligation to protect the confidentiality of subjects and their obligations to society, more
specifically, to third parties who may be placed at risk by their subjects'
behavior. While the principle of confidentiality is highly valued in
professional relationships, it is not absolute. Well-known exceptions
such as the duty to report gunshot wounds and suspected cases of
child abuse have been made legal, as well as ethical, obligations. The
Tarasoff case established for psychotherapists in California a "duty to
protect" potential victims of violent behavior by their patients (*Tarasoff
v. Regents of the University of California* 1976). These examples
support a professional's decision to breach confidentiality to protect
others.

In these cases, however, the relationship between the patient and
the professional (whether a physician, social worker, psychologist, or
other) includes the professional's continuing obligation to provide care
or services to the patient or client. In most research settings the investigator has only a limited relationship with the subject; for example,
unless it is specifically prohibited, an investigator can drop a subject
from a study for any of a number of reasons and have no further
obligations to that individual, whereas a physician who wishes to ter-

minate a relationship with a patient has an ethical obligation to arrange for an alternative caregiver. Investigators who also act as primary care-givers take on dual responsibilities.

There is widespread agreement (albeit with heated opposition) that physicians have at least the discretion, if not the obligation, to inform sexual or drug-using partners of an individual's HIV status if all at-tempts to have the infected person do the notification have failed and if there is reason to believe that the third person does not know that he or she is at serious risk of becoming infected.

Does the same principle apply in the research setting? If it does, researchers may be torn between their promises of confidentiality, made even more explicit to research subjects through the consent process than to patients in medical practice, and their obligations to prevent harm. In this case, the primary conflict may be, not between the individual's interests and society's, but between two competing social claims—the advancement of knowledge and the protection of third parties at risk.

While it is essential that sensitive, effective systems of partner noti-fication be available to assist HIV-infected individuals who are unwill-ing to inform their partners themselves, the research setting seems to me to be a poor fit for that task. Most researchers, as already noted, do not have a physician-patient relationship with study participants; fur-thermore, they are generally specialists in their own fields and have no particular training in counseling skills. Most would be ill equipped and uncomfortable with the complex issues involved in partner notification and follow-up counseling.

Moreover, if partner notification were to be a standard part of re-search protocols, it might deter volunteers, especially for epidemiologi-cal or behavioral studies where individual benefit is less likely. Such a policy would have to be detailed in the informed consent process. An accurate description of the risks of participation in a research study that described the consequences of failing to inform others at risk, or of the unforeseeable consequences if the third party then disclosed the individuals' status to a wider group, would probably deter many poten-tial subjects.

The U.S. Public Health Service policy on partner notification states:

> To the extent possible, known partners of a person with HIV infection shall be notified that they may have been exposed to HIV and should be encouraged to be counseled and tested. Under usual circumstances, this process is preferably carried out in collaboration with HIV preven-tion activities of local public health departments (Mason 1990).

Does this policy apply to research? The statement is unclear. It says that the policy is applicable to "clinical activities at PHS facilities carried out by PHS personnel, where there is a physician-patient relationship or health care is otherwise provided," including the National Institutes of Health (NIH) Clinical Center. By specifically placing the ethical obligation in the context of clinical care, the policy avoids the question of whether it also applies to the research setting. In practice, however, patients admitted to the NIH Clinical Center are informed of the overall policy of the institution. In addition, consent documents for research protocols contain the same language. This system may be appropriate for the special setting of the NIH Clinical Center, where patients are admitted from all over the country and receive a wide range of clinical services in addition to participating in research protocols. It could not easily be transferred to the more typical research institution that does not automatically provide clinical care.

Imposing public health or clinical responsibilities on researchers who have not established a physician-patient relationship threatens to undermine their primary role and obligations; instead, research institutions should have procedures to refer subjects identified as HIV positive to experienced counseling services to address the issues of partner notification.

Studying a New Disease: Research Design

Most of the ethical issues that have arisen around epidemiological and behavioral studies have concerned the traditional research review questions of protecting subjects from risk (in this case, social or psychological risk) through breaches of confidentiality. The context of a highly stigmatized, new, and still ultimately fatal infectious disease has made these issues more compelling. In the case of clinical trials and other mechanisms of access to investigational drugs, however, the traditional protectionist stance has been challenged, and it is here that the ethics of research and the processes of drug development are changing most profoundly (Macklin and Friedland 1986; Grodin, Kaminow, and Sassower 1988; Freedman et al. 1989).

In an effort to make the process of drug development more flexible and responsive to patient needs, questions of research design (which have always had ethical dimensions) have taken on new significance. Some IRBs do not automatically review research design, especially when a scientific review committee has already done so. But in the case of HIV/AIDS, research design, especially when placebo arms and/

or randomization are contemplated, is an essential element of the ethical evaluation.

Since the 1950s the "gold standard" of research has been the randomized controlled trial (RCT). The RCT is considered more reliable than other research designs because random allocation to one or another drug, therapy, dosage, or placebo counteracts potential bias in assignment if the investigator were to make the choice. Furthermore, variables such as patient characteristics that might affect the outcome tend to be evenly distributed if patients are randomized. An RCT must have a control group, that is, a group of patients who do not receive the test drug or therapy but are in all other respects as similar as possible to the patients who do receive the drug or therapy. In order for an RCT to be ethically justifiable, there must be legitimate dispute or uncertainty about which arm of the trial is superior. Depriving a patient of a therapy known to be superior to the one offered in the trial is unethical.

Although the RCT's reliability makes it especially valuable, other research designs are also acceptable, even to the FDA, and in some situations may be preferable. Other trial designs may use historical controls, dose-response controls, or another therapy as control or may be open-label studies. A research proposal must be justified on grounds other than social beneficence (efficiency and reliability); an ethical justification must include considerations of justice, respect for persons, and beneficence. Just as it is unethical to place subjects at any risk in a study whose design is so flawed it cannot yield valid data, it is unethical to ignore subjects' welfare and rights to conduct a flawlessly designed study (Levine, Dubler, Levine 1990).

On the highly contentious points of placebos and randomization, a working group convened to discuss clinical research ethics concluded: "Placebo controls are especially difficult to justify in RCTs having death or serious disability as their endpoints" (Levine, Dubler, and Levine 1990). They may, however, be justified in certain circumstances, such as true scarcity of the experimental drug or in trials of short duration where participation in a placebo arm will not impair the subject's long-range prognosis if the treatment should prove effective.

Certainly the study design should not preclude the use of well-established therapies; that is, it would be unethical to deprive a subject of a therapy that will successfully treat an opportunistic infection if one should occur during the trial. But it does not seem unreasonable to ask subjects to forgo nonvalidated remedies for the duration of the trial if these drugs can be predicted to interact with the study drug in ways that would either jeopardize the subject's safety or counteract the effect of the study drug. There are alternatives to medications—many forms of spiritual, psychosocial, nutritional, and other kinds of activities that enhance self-control and a sense of well-being. If trial participants are determined to take concomitant medications, they should be encouraged to report this practice without prejudicing their participation in the trial so that this factor can be evaluated as part of the data analysis.

Access to Experimental Drugs

The FDA's emphasis on protecting consumers from unsafe and inefficacious therapies began to shift several years ago toward expediting the approval of new drugs. Budget cutbacks and other problems have, however, hindered the agency's effort to speed what is still (and many argue ought to remain) a lengthy process. AIDS has become a catalyst for more rapid change. Patients and their physicians, as well as political leaders, are pressing hard for more rapid testing and approval of a broader range of drugs. The Presidential Commission on the HIV Epidemic identified several obstacles to achieving this goal, including insufficient funding, lack of reviewers for new drug applications, and duplication of efforts in reviewing these applications (Presidential Commission 1988). The AIDS Coalition to Unleash Power (ACT UP), the primary advocacy group focused on drug development, charges that the priorities of the National Institutes of Health, "set by a closed committee, result in their failure to test promising drugs against AIDS and opportunistic infections." ACT UP is demanding "tests of thirty or more new AIDS drugs each year in small, rapid Phase I/II studies," as well as access to all scientific meetings for journalists and people with AIDS and their advocates, broadened trial inclusion criteria, and immediate release of all treatment information (ACT UP 1990). The particular target of ACT UP's protests is the AIDS Clinical Trial Group (ACTG), a network of more than forty federally funded research centers (Harrington 1990).

Much of the controversy over access to experimental drugs derives from conflicting views of the purpose of clinical trials. Investigators see them as *research* (an activity designed to produce generalizable knowledge). Patients (and some clinicians) see them as *therapy* (medical practice designed to benefit individuals). These divergent views are not unique to AIDS; Paul Appelbaum and his colleagues have written about the "therapeutic misconception" in studies with patients with diseases other than AIDS (Appelbaum et al. 1987). The "therapeutic-misconception" is the patient's belief—unwarranted but difficult to counter—that all aspects of a clinical trial are designed to benefit him or her directly. Patients want to believe that this is so, and surely investigators hope that they will benefit, but this is not the purpose of the trial.

The absence of proven therapeutic alternatives for AIDS and the belief that trials are in and of themselves beneficial have led to the claim that people have a right to be a research subject. This is the exact opposite of the tradition starting with Nuremberg—that people have a right *not* to be a research subject.

A few years ago Arthur Caplan, a philosopher, argued that people who are treated at major medical centers and derive the benefits of the most sophisticated medical care have a duty to be a research subject (Caplan 1984). If that is so, and it is arguable, the duty surely does not extend to each and every possible trial. That is, one may have a general duty to contribute to scientific knowledge but not a specific duty to enter a particular trial.

Similarly, if there is a right to be a research subject, and again that is arguable, it is not a general right to enter whatever trial one may choose but the right to be offered an equal opportunity to be considered for all trials that are appropriate, given one's medical condition and other scientifically relevant characteristics. To be more concrete, scientific eligibility criteria for trials should be broadened wherever possible to reflect the diversity of the affected patient populations; this enhances the generalizability of the knowledge gained in the trial. The criteria should not maintain unwarranted exclusions (such as excluding all current or former IV drug users on the grounds that they will not be cooperative or excluding women of childbearing age). The criteria cannot, however, be infinitely elastic or validity will suffer.

There is clearly a need for more trials, and for more decentralized trials, and for widely disseminated information about ongoing trials so that investigators can utilize this important resource of volunteers in their shared quest for better therapies. But a poorly designed trial is worse than no trial at all, because it uses scarce resources for no valid purpose. Its results may mislead others to believe that a drug has efficacy when it does not or that one is ineffective when this may not be the case.

In the past three years, in response to continued pressure, three major new mechanisms of access to investigational drugs beyond the traditional clinical trial system have been introduced: two of them, the Treatment IND and the "parallel track," operate outside the standard research setting but intersect with it. The third—community-based research—is a variation on traditional research-center-based studies but gives more power to primary care physicians and patients (Mayer 1990; Merton 1990).

The FDA's rule on the treatment use and sale of investigational new drugs (IND)—the so-called "Treatment IND" rule—went into effect in June 1987. Its goal was to facilitate the availability of promising new drugs to patients outside clinical trials. After a very slow start, eighteen drugs, including six AIDS drugs (three of them already marketed for other indications), have been approved for distribution. The Treatment IND has evolved into a mechanism that typically serves as a bridge between the late phases of clinical trials and FDA marketing approval.

"Parallel track" is a system designed to expand access to investigational drugs much earlier in the clinical trials process. The main purpose of parallel track is to make experimental drugs available to people for whom there is no therapeutic alternative while the formal clinical trial process is underway. Ideally, recruitment for clinical trials will not be adversely affected. The population eligible for parallel-track distribution includes those who are not candidates for clinical trials because they do not meet the inclusion criteria (many because they are already too ill) or because they live in areas where access to trials is limited. The National AIDS Program Office (1990) has proposed guidelines for parallel track. Even before official approval of the guidelines, one drug —dideoxyinosine or ddI—is already being distributed under parallel-track conditions. This drug is distributed by the manufacturer, Bristol Myers Squibb, to physicians who request it and document a patient's eligibility. Although the goal is not research, some basic data, especially about side effects, are being collected.

The community-based research movement grew out of dissatisfaction with the fragmentation, pace, and focus on antiviral therapies in the ACTG clinical trials. Community-based groups use community physicians as investigators and are more receptive than the ACTG to novel therapies. Because of their community connections, they may be able to recruit and retain participants more easily.

At the same time as the NIH is being pressed to develop more drugs more rapidly, and the FDA is being pressed to distribute and approve them equally expeditiously, both agencies will undoubtedly be held accountable for any serious side effects that occur when drugs are used without extensive prior testing. And there is a growing concern that the standards of clinical trials, and FDA's approval process, will be lowered to the detriment of all (Mitchell and Steingrub 1988). George

Annas, an attorney and advocate of patients' rights, sees the current trend as a threat to patients;

> The AIDS epidemic has frightened us into believing that medicine will find a cure soon, and this misplaced faith in science has helped erode the distinction between experimentation and therapy; has threatened to transform [the FDA] from a consumer protection agency into a medical technology promotion agency; and has put AIDS patients, already suffering from an incurable disease, at further risk of psychological, physical, and financial exploitation by those who would sell them useless drugs (Annas 1990).

Annas' warning is sobering to those, like me, who are advocating expanded (but not unlimited) access to promising drugs. The FDA, as a consumer protection agency, should clearly protect the public from quackery and fraudulent claims; people with AIDS, like those with cancer and other life-threatening illnesses, are particularly vulnerable to claims of "cures" or "miracle drugs." There is, however, a difference between false claims of efficacy and levels of unknown risk. Expanded access to unproven therapies undeniably involves risk-taking. The central questions are: Is the potential benefit worth the risk and who should decide? Here regulators, investigators, physicians, and patients must tread a very fine line between preventing harm and promoting well-being. The answers will depend on the particular properties of the drug, the likelihood of benefit, the level and probability of risk, and the alternatives (if any) available to the patient. While judgments will vary, and specific criteria are difficult to specify, in general the presumption should be in favor of patient participation in a carefully delineated and informed choice.

Duties of Research Subjects and Physicians

The traditional research ethic focuses on the rights of research subjects, not on their duties. Do research subjects have an obligation to abide by the terms of the protocol, when that may mean giving up unproven, but psychologically (and perhaps even physically) beneficial, medications or regimens? Once again the critical factor is one's perception of the purpose of the trial. If it is seen as research, then the burden of giving up alternative medications is one factor to be weighed in the subject's decision whether to participate. If the trial is seen as therapy, then it will seem unreasonable to the subject to be forced to forgo something that he or she perceives as beneficial. Many potential trial participants from the gay community and communities of color have a deep sense of alienation and suspicion of the health care system in general and the research enterprise in particular. They may feel that they are justified in doing whatever seems necessary to enhance their own welfare, even if that means lying to be enrolled in a protocol or failing to comply with its regimen.

Physicians may feel that it is justifiable to alter patients' records or otherwise manipulate data in order to enter them in a clinical trial. This problem is not unique to AIDS (Vanderpool and Weiss 1987). In manipulating data, physicians place their obligation to maximize their patients' interests above their professional and social obligations to advance knowledge and to benefit future patients. Expanded access to clinical trials or investigational drugs off protocol may reduce the likelihood of this undesirable behavior.

John Arras, a philosopher, has argued persuasively that subjects do have an ethical obligation to abide by the terms of the protocol. He asserts that noncompliant behavior violates ethical rules against lying, harms the interests of other potential subjects who might have participated and the interests of future patients whose treatment may be inadequate because the study is flawed, and violates the moral relationship of trust between participant and researcher (Arras 1990). In the real world, however, the assertion of moral claims must be accompanied by honest and effective efforts to redress the inequities that encourage dishonest behavior.

In order to build a partnership based on trust and mutual respect, researchers, primary care physicians, and potential trial participants will have to work together, through ongoing community consultation, to develop mutually acceptable protocols. There are several mechanisms to develop these partnerships (Melton et al. 1988; Valdisseri, Tama, and Ho 1988). One is the creation of a standing community advisory committee, which discusses with the researchers and administrators not only specific protocols as an IRB does but also more general problems of recruiting and retaining subjects, research design, and noncompliance. Another possibility is to include a person with AIDS or an AIDS activist as a full voting member on an IRB that regularly reviews AIDS research. The primary responsibility for initiating and maintaining community consultation lies with the investigator, but the system should provide ways for individuals within the affected communities to raise issues of concern.

Including the Excluded: New Problems in Subject Selection

IRBs have been charged with ensuring equitable selection of subjects, but they have implemented this responsibility largely by protecting individuals or groups from inclusion in trials simply because they are easily accessible (prisoners or poor people treated in public hospitals) or because they are vulnerable because of social, medical, or other characteristics.

AIDS and HIV have forced a reexamination of the traditional emphasis on homogeneity in subject selection and of whether restrictive criteria have been justified on scientific grounds that stressed the comparability of data gathered from homogeneous groups, on ethical grounds of protecting vulnerable people, on risk-avoidance grounds of potential liability, or on pragmatic grounds of the difficulties of outreach to nontraditional subjects. Many people who were previously considered too vulnerable to be research subjects stand to benefit most from a loosening of rules or practices on who can participate in clinical trials. Pregnant women or women of childbearing age, infants and children, prisoners, current or former drug users, members of racial or ethnic minorities—all are hard hit by HIV. They will be taking the drugs approved for use by the FDA, yet under current practice the drugs will have not been tested on subjects who are like them in scientifically relevant ways. None of these groups should be categorically excluded from research, but all of them present special problems in research review.

For example, IRBs are traditionally concerned with protecting the privacy of trial participants, as already noted. But expanding the pool of potential volunteers to nontraditional settings raises new issues of confidentiality. How can confidentiality be maintained in a prison for inmates who might benefit from an experimental drug but who might be subjected to serious harm if their HIV status becomes known? And how can their consent be "voluntary" if, as most agree, prisons are inherntly coercive institutions? In their review of the status of HIV research in prisons, Dubler and Sidel conclude that there are clear imperatives to

1. Improve medical treatment for prisoners with AIDS or HIV infection and, if medical resources are inadequate, find alternative sources for them;
2. Devise ways to improve the confidentiality of the trials, although in a prison setting this is likely to prove extraordinarily difficult or impossible;

3. Ensure that no inducements extraneous to the protocol are added (Dubler and Sidel 1989).

The involvement of women in research raises equally complex questions. A recent General Accounting Office report has substantiated the claim that women have been systematically underrepresented in drug trials funded by the NIH (Nadel 1990), despite agency policies to the contrary. Most of the women with HIV/AIDS are of childbearing age; some are pregnant or may become pregnant during a trial. On that basis alone women have been excluded from HIV/AIDS drug trials.

Does a pregnant woman's interest in participating in drug trials always override potential harm to her future child? (I use the term *future child* rather than *fetus* because this discussion applies to those fetuses that will be born either because their mothers have chosen to continue pregnancies or because they lacked timely access to abortion services). A logical conclusion of an argument in favor of a shift in policy and practice toward redressing the injustice caused by excluding women from research might be that it is *never* justified to exclude women, regardless of their childbearing potential or state of pregnancy. I am reluctant to take that absolutist position.

The ethical obligation not to do harm carried particular force when the recipient of the potential harm is an unconsenting future child, whose health and welfare may be unalterably affected. On grounds of beneficence and the harm principle, parents have moral obligations to enhance, insofar as is reasonably possible, the health and welfare of children they have conceived and that will be born to live independent existences. (Society too has obligations to provide the education, medical care, and support that is necessary for parents to fulfill their responsibilities.) Although both parents have this obligation, and there are limits to what either parent can be expected to do or forgo, mothers have particular obligations because of their biological connection.

The vast majority of women see their own primary interests as identical with those of their future children. Women do not lightly undertake any medical intervention that might have an adverse outcome on their infants; many women in fact may deny themselves optimal medical care in order to avoid risk. Some, however, may exercise their right to choose validated medical treatments despite known or unknown risks to the future child.

Research, unlike treatment, has as its primary goal the acquisition of knowledge. Approval by an IRB of a protocol is not an ethically neutral stance: it is an affirmative statement that the choices to be offered to potential subjects, while perhaps difficult to make, are ethically justifiable. Exposing a future child to known serious risk when there are alternatives or when the potential benefits to the mother are modest is not, in my view, an ethically justifiable choice.

Most HIV/AIDS protocols do not present any known or foreseeable risks to future children; for these protocols, there are, as has already been pointed out, no reasons to exclude women, especially those who are not pregnant or do not plan to become pregnant. Some HIV/AIDS protocols may carry the possibility of minimal or even moderate risk to future children but also offer the possibility of great benefit to the woman. An obvious example would be a life-saving drug or cure. Another example might be a study involving a drug to treat a debilitating opportunistic infection for which there are no acceptable alternative therapies. In these cases women should not be excluded automatically but should be given the opportunity to make that calculus for themselves, with careful explanation of the risks and benefits to themselves and their future children.

There remains, however, the small but worrisome category of studies involving drugs that present known high risk to future children and minimal or unknown benefit to women. Some would argue that risks to future children, as unconsenting participants, must always outweigh considerations of the woman's autonomy. Others would argue that there are never any grounds to override a woman's autonomy and to deny her the choice of whether to participate. In this view, valuing a future child's welfare more highly than a woman's autonomy is objectionable in principle and is yet another example, like forced caesareans and arrests of drug-using pregnant women, of treating women solely as "fetal containers."

Is there a middle ground? Protocols in other diseases may fail to gain approval on grounds of excessive risk to subjects, even when there are potential benefits. Risk to future children cannot simply be dismissed as irrelevant, even if one does not grant them "rights." But what would constitute "serious" or "excessive" risk? Opinions differ. The administration of zidovudine to pregnant women to see whether it reduces HIV transmission might strike some as posing serious risk to the more than two thirds of future children who will receive a toxic substance in utero but who will be uninfected. Yet such a study has been approved and federally funded. (Although the pregnant woman might benefit from receiving the drug, that is not the purpose of the study. In fact, according to the protocol, zidovudine will be discontinued after delivery. Of course the woman may receive it under different auspices.)

Consider this hypothetical scenario. Thalidomide, already described as a drug that causes devastating birth defects when taken early in pregnancy, is a good treatment for a serious complication of Hansen's disease (leprosy) known as erythema nodosom leprosum (ENL). Thalidomide prevents permanent damage from the fever, nerve inflammation, and eye and skin problems of ENL. Studies of cancer patients suggest that thalidomide can prevent many of the side effects, such as the sometimes fatal graft-host reaction, of radiation therapy given to bone marrow transplant recipients. The drug may also be useful in treating patients with autoimmune disease who cannot tolerate corticosteroids or who are unresponsive to these drugs (Randall 1990).

Suppose an investigator wished to study the effect of thalidomide on immunosuppression in HIV/AIDS. The benefits would primarily be the acquisition of knowledge, although if the hypothesis is correct, subjects' immune status might be enhanced. Should women of childbearing capacity be excluded? In such a case I would argue that sexually active, fertile women should be excluded because the potential harm to future children is well known, severe, and permanent and the knowledge is attainable through other means. Because no contraceptive is foolproof, the harm would occur at a point when the woman might not even know that she is pregnant. Moreover, even under the best of circumstances, informed consent is not perfect. Any subject's understanding of risks may be colored by the common misperception that research is designed for individual benefit rather than to gain generalizable knowledge. Furthermore, concern about risks may diminish over time. A woman who has no intention of becoming pregnant at the beginning of a study may fail to appreciate the risks or remember the warnings if her life situation changes.

A woman who was enrolled in such a study and became pregnant would be faced with the option of abortion (which she might find morally unacceptable) or carrying the potentially severely damaged future child to term. If the results of early studies showed that thalidomide or an experimental drug with known similar teratogenic properties had a good chance of providing substantial benefits for the woman and there were no alternatives, the drug might be offered off protocol through any one of a number of mechanisms. In this way the decision can be made on a case-by-case basis, with treatment of the individual as the primary goal, rather than as part of a research study.

Fortunately, most protocols do not present such stark choices. In the vast majority of cases women can be offered the same options as men, with full explanation of the risks and benefits to themselves, as well as to their future children.

Access to Medical Care and Informed Consent

Perhaps the greatest challenge to accepted standards of ethical review and informed consent arises, however, not from the research setting itself, but from the inadequacies of the health care system. Quite simply, there are many researchers looking for trial participants; there are very few doctors looking for HIV/AIDS patients. In a setting in which access to primary care is totally inadequate, as it is in New York City and Northern New Jersey—the epicenter of the HIV/AIDS epidemic—and in most major urban settings, entering a research trial may be the only way to obtain basic health care. How then can a decision to enter a trial be truly voluntary? And how can a decision to withdraw from a trial—one basic right of any trial participant—be truly voluntary when that decision may mean the loss of access to health care? What are the responsibilities of investigators, IRBs, and health care institutions to ensure appropriate referrals at the end of a trial?

The working group on consensus ethics in research review concluded on this point: "Institutions in which members of the medical staff serve as physician-investigators in clinical trials should assure that primary medical care is provided for patient-subjects who withdraw from clinical trials" (Levine, Dubler, and Levine 1990). Some, but not all, trials provide medical care; institutions that conduct research, as centers of economic, political, and social power, should be staunch advocates for the provision of primary care for the communities they serve if they cannot provide it themselves.

Preventing Disease: Vaccine Trials

An effective vaccine to prevent HIV infection would be a major public health advance. The lack of an animal model and a model of natural or induced immunity—essential to determining efficacy of a candidate vaccine—have been major scientific obstacles. Promising results with vaccinated chimpanzees who developed immunity to a particular HIV strain need to be confirmed and studied further.

Despite the technical hurdles, Phase I trials of candidate vaccines are under way in the United States, and it is possible that broader trials will be planned and implemented within the next few years. The candidate populations for these trials may well include those in developing nations, where HIV transmission is spreading rapidly. It will be important scientifically to know whether a vaccine works in different target populations where it is most needed.

Given the uncertainties about short- and long-term risks and benefits in these trials, and the different standards of informed consent that may prevail in various countries, as well as the history of international trials that did not give full weight to the rights of subjects, vaccine trials should proceed cautiously and with a full prior discussion of the ethical questions.

The NIH addressed the social risks of vaccine-induced seroconversion (difficulties in obtaining insurance, donating blood, joining the military, traveling abroad, for example). In trials sponsored by the National Institute of Allergy and Infectious Diseases (NIAID), participants receive documentation to certify that their HIV status resulted from participation in a research protocol (Porter, Glass, and Koff 1989). Whatever its utility in the United States, such a mechanism would undoubtedly prove unwieldy and unenforceable in a developing country.

Part of the standard of justice in research involves distributing to those who bore the risks the benefits of research. Yet in countries that have no health care system rich enough or sophisticated enough to distribute an effective vaccine (if one were to be developed) and to monitor the population for efficacy or unknown side effects, how would the subject populations who tested the vaccine benefit from its development?

Christakis suggests a reasonable set of minimum ethical standards for vaccine trials regardless of the setting: (1) suitable design and scientific merit; (2) free and, where possible, informed consent of the participants; (3) proper counseling regarding avoidance of risky behaviors; (4) the highest standards of risk/benefit analysis; and (5) fair access to any vaccine arising from the research to the populations that participated in its development (Christakis 1988).

Future Challenges

In 1974 Congress passed the National Research Act, which established the National Commission for the Protection of Biomedical and Behavioral Research. The seminal work of this commission was supplemented in the 1980s by the exemplary reports of the President's Commission for the Study of Ethical Problems in Biomedical and Behavioral Research. Today we are at another important juncture in research ethics; a new national group of committed and knowledgeable individuals should be convened to address the special issues raised by HIV/AIDS. Similar proposals have been made before (Bayer, Levine, and Murray, 1984; Levine and Caplan 1986). The proposed federal regulations on "parallel track" include the formation of a national human subjects review panel for that system and would be a good, although limited, first step.

A broadly based, thoughtful, and experienced group could provide direction and leadership when both are greatly needed. The resolutions to the questions raised by HIV/AIDS research will affect research in many other contexts. While the basic principles of research ethics have proven their value in the context of HIV/AIDS, their implementation has already been profoundly altered.

Looking to the future, some issues will clearly be on the agenda. As the number of women infected with HIV increases, there will be more pressure to include them in drug trials. Yet, as already noted, there is no consensus about the inclusion of women of childbearing age, much less pregnant women, in drug trials. The encouraging news on vaccine development from the Sixth International Conference on AIDS in San Francisco in June 1990 makes it more likely that large-scale efficacy trials will be proposed, raising to more than hypothetical status the ethical issues inherent in their design and implementation. Widespread access to investigational drugs is a major social experiment; beyond data collection on individual drugs, the process should be evaluated, especially in terms of its impact on clinical trials and on patients' well-being and autonomy.

In the coming years, debates about research ethics will focus more broadly on the economic, social, and political links between the research enterprise, the rest of the health care system, and society in general. The challenge is to uphold ethical research standards in the current health care system while at the same time trying to redress its inequities.

ACKNOWLEDGMENTS

Work on this chapter was supported in part by a grant from the American Foundation for AIDS Research. Some of the material in this article appeared in different form in my articles, "Has AIDS Changed the Ethics of Human Subjects Research?" *Law, Medicine and Health Care* (Winter 1988) and "Women and HIV/AIDS Research: The Barriers to Equity," *Evaluation Review* (October 1990). I would like to thank two groups for their contributions to my appreciation of the many values at stake in HIV/AIDS Research: the participants of the American Foundation for AIDS Research Clinical Ethics Consensus Working Group (particularly my coprincipal investigators, Nancy Dubler and Robert J.

Levine) and the past and present members of the Institutional Review Board of the Community Research Initiative in New York City. I want to pay particular tribute to the late Nathaniel Pier, M.D., a member of the IRB who was an extraordinary clinician, investigator, and advocate, while he was also a patient. Of course I alone am responsible for the views expressed in this chapter.

REFERENCES

ACT UP, 1990. Massive AIDS Demonstration to Descend on National Institutes of Health. Press release (April 16).

Ad Hoc Working Group on Unblinding Seroprevalence Surveys. 1989. Unpublished statement (September), New York City.

Annas, George J. 1990. Faith (Healing), Hope, and Charity at the FDA: The Politics of AIDS Drug Trials. In Lawrence O. Gostin, ed., *AIDS and the Health Care System*, pp. 183–194. New Haven: Yale University Press.

APA (American Psychological Association) Committee for the Protection of Human Participants in Psychological Research on AIDS. 1986. Ethical Issues in Psychological Research on AIDS. *IRB: A Review of Human Subjects Research* (July/August), 8(4):8–10.

Appelbaum, Paul S., Loren H. Roth, Charles W. Lidz. 1987. False Hopes and Best Data—Consent to Research and the Therapeutic Misconception. *Hastings Center Report* (April), 17(2):20–24.

Arras, John. 1990. Noncompliance in AIDS Research. *Hastings Center Report* (September/October), 20(5):24–32.

Bayer, Ronald, Carol Levine, and Thomas H. Murray. 1984. Guidelines for Confidentiality in Research on AIDS. *IRB: A Review of Human Subjects Research* (November/December), 6(6):1–7.

Bayer, Ronald, Carol Levine, and Susan M. Wolf. 1986. HIV Antibody Screening: An Ethical Framework for Evaluating Proposed Programs. *JAMA* (October 2), 256(13):1768–1774.

Bayer, Ronald, L. H. Lumey, and Lourdes Wan. 1990. The American, British, and Dutch Responses to Unlinked Anonymous HIV Seroprevalence Studies: An International Comparison. *AIDS* 4:283–290.

Beecher, Henry Knowles. 1966. Ethics and Clinical Research. *New England Journal of Medicine* 274:1354–1360.

Berger, Robert L. 1990. Nazi Science—The Dachau Hypothermia Experiments. *New England Journal of Medicine* (May 17), 322(20):1435–1440.

Brandt, Alan M. 1978. Racism and Research: The Case of the Tuskegee Syphilis Study. *Hastings Center Report* (December), 8(6):21–29.

Caplan, Arthur. 1984. Is There a Duty to Serve as a Subject in Biomedical Research? *IRB: A Review of Human Subjects Research* (September/October), 6(5):1–5.

Christakis, Nicholas A. 1988. The Ethical Design of an AIDS Vaccine Trial in Africa. *Hastings Center Report* (June/July), 18(3):31–37.

Dubler, Nancy Neveloff. 1986. Do Research Subjects Have the Right Not to Know Their HIV Antibody Test Results? Treating Research Subjects Fairly. *IRB: A Review of Human Subjects Research* (September/October), 8(5):7–9.

Dubler, Nancy Neveloff and Victor W. Sidel. 1989. On Research on HIV Infection and AIDS in Correctional Institutions. *The Milbank Quarterly* 67(2):171–207.

Dubler, Nancy Neveloff, Carol Levine, and Robert J. Levine. 1990. Consensus Report on Clinical Research Ethics. Unpublished manuscript.

Freedman, Benjamin and the McGill/Boston Research Group. 1989. Nonvalidated Therapies and HIV Disease. *Hastings Center Report* (May/June), 19(3):14–20.

Grodin, Michael A., Paula V. Kaminow, and Raphael Sassower. 1988. Ethical Issues in AIDS Research. *New England Journal of Public Policy* (Winter/Spring), 4(1):215–225.

Harrington, Mark. 1990. A Critique of the AIDS Clinical Trial Group (May 1). New York. Unpublished.

Katz, Jay. 1972. *Experimentation with Human Beings.* New York: Russell Sage Foundation.

Katz, Jay. 1987. The Regulation of Human Experimentation in the United States— A Personal Odyssey. *IRB: A Review of Human Subjects Research* (January/February), 9(1):1–6.

Landesman, Sheldon. 1986. Do Research Subjects Have the Right Not to Know Their HIV Antibody Test Results? The Ethical Obligations of Research Subjects to Be Informed of Their HIV Status. *IRB: A Review of Human Subjects Research* (September/October), 8(5):9.

Levine, Carol and Arthur L. Caplan. 1986. Beyond Localism: A Proposal for a National Research Review Board. *IRB: A Review of Human Subjects Research* (March/April), 8(6):7–9.

Levine, Carol, Nancy Neveloff Dubler, and Robert J. Levine. 1991. Building a New Consensus: Ethical Principles and Policies for Clinical Research on HIV/AIDS. *IRB: A Review of Human Subjects Research* (January/April), 13(1–2):1–17.

Levine, Robert J. 1988. *Ethics and Regulation of Clinical Research.* 2d ed. New Haven: Yale University Press.

Macklin, Ruth and Gerald Friedland. 1986. AIDS Research: The Ethics of Clinical Trials. *Law, Medicine and Health Care* (December), 14(5–6):273–280.

Mason, James. 1989. Research Confidentiality Protection—Certificate of Confidentiality—Interim Guidance (June 8), Washington, D.C.: Office of the Assistant Secretary for Health.

Mason, James. 1990. PHS Policy on Partner Notification (May 3). Washington, D.C.: Office of the Assistant Secretary for Health.

Mayer, Kenneth H. 1990. Progress Notes. In *AIDS/HIV Experimental Treatment Directory.* New York: American Foundation for AIDS Research (March), 3(4):46–50.

McCarthy, Charles. 1989. Personal communication.

Melton, Gary B., Robert J. Levine, Gerald P. Koocher, et al. 1988. Community Consultation in Socially Sensitive Research: Lessons from Clinical Trials of Treatments for AIDS. *American Psychologist* (July), 43(7):573–581.

Melton, Gary B. and Joni N. Gray. 1988. Ethical Dilemmas in AIDS Research: Individual Privacy and Public Health. *American Psychologist* (January), 43(1):60–64.

Merton, Vanessa. 1990. Community-based AIDS Research. *Evaluation Review* (October), in press.

Mitchell, Sheila C. and Jay Steingrub. 1988. The Changing Clinical Trials Scene: The Role of the IRB. *IRB: A Review of Human Subjects Research* (July/August), 10:(4):1–5.

Nadel, Mark V. 1990. National Institutes of Health: Problems in Implementing Policy on Women in Study Populations. Testimony Before the Subcommittee on Health and the Environment, Committee on Energy and Commerce, U.S. House of Representatives (June 18).

National AIDS Program Office. 1990. *Federal Register* (May 21), 55(96):20856–20860.

National Commission for the Protection of Human Subjects of Biomedical and Behavioral Research. 1978. *The Belmont Report: Ethical Principles and Guidelines for the Protection of Human Subjects of Research*. Washington, D.C.

Novick, Alvin. 1986. Do Research Subjects Have the Right Not to Know Their HIV Antibody Test Results? Why the Burdensome Knowledge Need Not Be Imposed. *IRB: A Review of Human Subjects Research* (September/October), 8(5):6–7.

Pappaioanou, Marguerite, Timothy J. Dondero, Jr., Lyle R. Petersen, et al. 1990. The Family of HIV Seroprevalence Surveys: Objectives, Methods, and Uses of Sentinel Surveillance for HIV in the United States. *Public Health Reports* (March–April), 105(2):113–119.

Perry, Samuel W. 1987. Pharmacological and Psychological Research on AIDS: Some Ethical Considerations. *IRB: A Review of Human Subjects Research* (September/October), 9(5):8–10.

Porter, Joan P., Marta J. Glass, and Wayne C. Koff. 1989. Ethical Considerations in AIDS Vaccine Testing. *IRB: A Review of Human Subjects Research* (May/June), 11(3):1–4.

Presidential Commission on the HIV Epidemic. 1988. Final Report (June). Washington, D.C., pp. 50–53.

Randall, Teri. 1990. Thalidomide's Back in the News, but in More Favorable Circumstances. *JAMA* (March 16), 263(11):1467–1468.

Tarasoff v. Regents of the University of California. 1976. 131 *California Reporter* 14.

Valdiserri, Ronald O., Geraldine Maiatico Tama, and Monto Ho. 1988. The Role of Community Advisory Committees in Anti-HIV Agents. *IRB: A Review of Human Subjects Research* (July/August), 10(4):5–7.

Vanderpool, Harold Y. and Gary B. Weiss. 1987. False Data and Last Hopes: Enrolling Ineligible Patients in Clinical Trials. *Hastings Center Report* (April), 17(2):16–19.

Windom, Robert E. 1988. Policy on Informing Those Tested About HIV Status. Letter to PHS agency heads (May 9).

5. AIDS and The Crisis of Health Insurance

GERALD M. OPPENHEIMER &
ROBERT A. PADGUG

> The American Medical Association has made a series of propos-
> als whose implementation would not only increase access to
> health care but also go a long way toward providing appropriate,
> effective care in the proper setting. . . . The undergirding prem-
> ise is to each according to his or her need and from each
> according to his or her means. When did this become undemo-
> cratic? (Todd 1989:46)

IN THE MID-1980s and the years thereafter, many argued that AIDS
portended catastrophe for the U.S. health insurance industry. This
assertion was, to some degree, based on early estimates that lifetime
hospital costs for an individual with AIDS were as high as $147,000
(Hardy et al. 1986:209–211). Only recently have we come to realize
that the epidemic is a manageable problem for health insurance carriers, with a lifetime cost one third to one half the original estimate
(Scitovsky 1989:319; Padgug and Eisenhandler 1990).

Whereas the original prediction has proved false, its converse has
occurred: our health care reimbursement system has profoundly and
negatively affected persons with AIDS and those perceived to be at risk
for it. More specifically, the characteristics and practices of our health
insurance industry and the serious crisis that marked its history in the
years directly preceding the epidemic have posed a substantial threat,
particularly to our ability as a society to handle AIDS in an efficient,
compassionate, and equitable manner.

Comprehension of that threat starts from the fact that the United
States, unlike most other industrialized nations, primarily uses private

The opinions expressed in this essay are those of the authors and do not necessarily
represent the views of the institutions with which they are associated.

enterprise to meet a social welfare need, namely, payment for health care. In addition, for most of the population covered by private carriers, entitlement to private insurance derives directly or indirectly from employment in an organization willing to pay the requisite premiums. Under these circumstances, the pool of those with insurance coverage has always been narrower than the general community, all of whose members are at risk of illness.

Because private means have proven inadequate, our society has developed public programs, Medicare and Medicaid, that grant entitlement to medical care to persons who meet eligibility criteria of poverty, disability, age, or—in the single instance of end-stage renal disease— diagnosis. Nonetheless, many remain excluded from the privately or publicly supported categories of entitlement. Unfortunately, the number and proportion of those in the United States who are bereft of any coverage have been growing over the last decade. Whereas roughly twenty-five million Americans were without insurance in 1977, that number rose to perhaps as many as thirty-one to thirty-seven million ten years later (Walden, Wilensky, and Kasper 1985:3; Monheit and Short 1989:35).

In part, this state of affairs derives from the competitive or market demands of the insurance industry, demands that have, over the years, forced it to include in its pools only the most economically attractive participants. Paradoxically, excluded increasingly from the pools are those with the greatest need to be covered: the very ill and those most likely to become so (Oppenheimer and Padgug 1986:19). In effect, the industry's drive for profitability (efficiency) has made it difficult, if not impossible, to offer insurance, and thus an appropriate level of health care, to all who require it in the community (equity).

The ordinary manner in which the health insurance industry operates threatens those with AIDS (along with others who are "economically unattractive") with decreased access to medical care. Unfortunately, the situation is substantially complicated by the fact that this "crisis of community"—the exclusion of many in the community by insurers—is intensified by the social characteristics of those infected by the human immunodeficiency virus (HIV). They have, to date, mainly been gay men and intravenous (IV) drug users, who were, even before the epidemic, considered outside the boundaries of the normative American community.

The normative community has tended to perceive IV drug users and gay men as outsiders who are reservoirs of a terrifying and fatal virus, as well as victims of a disease they in some degree brought on themselves. As such, they are less deserving of sympathy and aid than other groups might be. Moralism of this kind has intensified the discrimination that gays and drug users experienced even before the epidemic. Insurers share in these prejudices. Thus, gay men, for example, became for insurers both economically and socially unattractive, a double determination that makes gays more vulnerable than others to exclusion from the narrowing risk pools.

Ironically, the HIV epidemic, followed by the exclusionary tactics of the insurers, occurred at a time when lesbians and gay men, at least, had organized themselves into cohesive communities within major U.S. cities and had crafted sophisticated means to lobby for political ends. Sensitive to exclusion and discrimination, the gay community responded to insurers by questioning the validity and legitimacy of their actions. In this they were joined by others who expressed alarm at the attempts by the insurance industry to shift the costs of the epidemic and of catastrophic illness in general outside the market sector. As a consequence, the structure and practice of the insurance industry, which had for a long time faced little public scrutiny, became the object of careful examination by policy analysts and the daily press.

The perceived threat of AIDS to insurance and the threat of insurance to AIDS have, consequently, raised significant policy questions that transcend the HIV epidemic and affect all of American society. For example: is there an unresolvable contradiction between society's need to establish equity in the provision of health care and the insurance industry's need to safeguard its economic profitability? Can the United States meet the challenge of equity for patients with AIDS and for others with catastrophic chronic disease within the parameters of the current system of health care financing? Specifically, can the current system develop mechanisms for including our whole community within its domain?

Insurance: From Inclusion to Exclusion

In the 1930s, when the Blue Cross and Blue Shield Plans created the policies that served as prototypes for our current health insurance system, insurance premiums were based on what is known as community rating. That is, the costs of health care were spread among the entire population—or community—that was covered by a particular type of policy, and premiums were set at the same level for everyone (Eilers 1963:88–89). This system represented a broad spreading of the risks, and thus of the costs, of health care utilization over a relatively large population.

The original principle of community rating was substantially replaced over the next few decades by what came to be known as experience rating. Impressed with the success of Blue Cross, commercial insurers entered the market. They provided employers with health policies whose rates were based upon the actual claims experience of their specific employee groups, normally made up of younger and healthier persons than the community-at-large (Stevens 1989:260–262). Eventually, in order to survive, most Blue Cross and Blue Shield Plans were forced to follow suit for the majority of their business. As a consequence, insurance risks were spread less widely than previously and were defined by a relatively narrow, employment-related base.

Many small groups and all individuals (with the exception of those covered by a few Blue Cross and Blue Shield Plans, mainly in the Northeast) became subject to significant underwriting. Through underwriting, insurers determine "whether and on what basis insurance can be issued at 'standard rates,' offered at higher premium rates or with other limitations (such as the exclusion of a specified medical condition from coverage), or whether insurance should be refused (declined) altogether" (U.S. Congress, OTA 1988:5). For small groups and individuals, which continued to be lumped together to some degree, underwriters determined premium rates and extent of coverage by assaying such variables as age, current and future health status, and type of occupation and geographical location, all of them factors believed to be correlated closely with projected health care utilization.

Once evaluated and accepted, the insured are grouped into pools of relatively homogeneous risk and premium levels. As a consequence of underwriting, as well as of experience rating, the universe of the privately insured is atomized into a multitude of self-contained, self-supporting units rather than a broad, mutually supportive community-at-risk.

The result of basing the private insurance system on employee groups and on underwriting was, paradoxically, the exclusion of precisely those risk groups most in need of health care. The elderly, the disabled, those with serious chronic diseases, and the poor were essentially excluded from coverage either directly or through unaffordably high premiums. Access to the health care system was provided through a succession of governmental acts—most notably Medicaid and Medicare—that included many of those the private insurance system rejected. Nonetheless, only those who met the categorical requirements of these programs were covered by them. Consequently, large numbers of persons remaining outside public or private entitlements were forced to rely on what personal resources they possessed for access to health care or to depend on charity care.

By the 1970s, the trend toward atomization of the community-at-risk into narrow, self-inclusionary units proceeded to the next logical step: in order to reduce costs further and to escape from state legislation and regulation, large employers instituted what is called self-funding or self-insurance, paying the health care costs of their employees directly from their own funds (Rublee 1986:787–789). As a result of this trend, which has now been extended to more than 60 percent of large firms in the United States (McDonnell et al. 1986:1), the costs of health care, which under experience rating were at least shared between employer and insurer, now rest squarely on the employer, unless the latter has purchased relatively expensive "stop-loss" insurance. An employer lacking reinsurance and with any significant number of sick employees will be in danger of serious fiscal hemorrhaging and perhaps insolvency. As a consequence, employers might safeguard themselves by truncating benefits or by reducing the number of those previously covered, thereby further excluding individuals from health insurance.

Starting in the late 1970s, insurers and self-funded employers were confronted with substantial, spiraling increases in the costs of health care. Faced with a massive rise in costs, insurers and employers added to their plans a variety of "cost containment" measures aimed at reducing expenditures for employee health care. Thus, in addition to pooling and other underwriting techniques, insurers now developed mechanisms to constrain both provider behavior (the introduction of "second opinion" for elective surgery or preauthorization of inpatient hospitalization, for example) and patient demand. Of the procedures to reduce demand, one of the most important was "cost-shifting" (euphemistically known as "cost-sharing") to those who use health care services.

Unacceptably large increases in the cost of health coverage have led some firms, mainly smaller employers, to drop health insurance entirely (Freudenheim 1990:A1), or, more commonly among larger employers, to place a growing portion of their costs onto the members of the group. Fewer firms, for example, now pay the entire premium for individual or family coverage, and the majority of employer plans have ceased to reimburse the full costs of even inpatient care, as they did earlier (U.S. Congress, Library of Congress 1988b:36–38). In addition, employers who are self-funded, and therefore no longer under the jurisdiction of state insurance laws, can truncate their insurance packages to suit their needs, increasing employees' deductibles and coinsurance and decreasing the benefits offered (McDonnell et al. 1986:11–12; Taravella 1990:52).

This trend, in which the cost of illness is increasingly shifted to the individual or family, is in many ways merely the logical conclusion of the movement from community rating to ever narrower insurance pools. Community rating assumed that insurance benefits should be distributed according to need. Experience rating and underwriting allocate the costs of insurance to those who generate them (Stone 1990:65); at least theoretically, no group or individual pays for anyone else. In the last analysis, each pays for himself or herself. Ultimately, health insurance becomes only a savings plan against future need on the part of those clients accepted by insurance carriers (Stone 1990:65).

The cost spiral and more stringent use of underwriting have had an especially deleterious effect on smaller employers. A survey carried out by the Small Business Administration in 1987, for example, found that 60 percent of the respondents reported that insurance costs precluded offering health insurance to employees (U.S. Congress, Library of Congress 1988b:25–26). Another government study found that as carriers introduced more aggressive underwriting techniques, smaller employers were being progressively excluded from the health insurance market (U.S. Congress, Library of Congress 1988a:37–38). Many small groups and individuals were forced to drop coverage entirely during the 1980s. Some who had never before been without health insurance —small entrepreneurs or professionals and their families—were pushed into the "uninsured pool" (Kosterlitz 1990:272).

Unfortunately, competitive strategies (efficiency) prevented any insurer from softening its underwriting rules for fear of adverse selection, that is, of attracting the worst risks and thus being forced to raise premiums to uncompetitive and unprofitable levels. The only viable alternatives were for insurers to leave the small business market entirely, as some did (Kosterlitz 1990:272), or to develop new mechanisms that force all insurers to liberalize their rules simultaneously, mechanisms that are increasingly under discussion both within and outside the industry (Freudenheim 1990:A1).

Thus, the private insurance system had, by the early 1980s, reached a serious impasse. Its viability depended in part on crafting ever more inclusive risk pools that atomized the "community of insured" while continually enlarging the number of those without coverage. Unfortunately, this occurred at a time when government was itself retrenching, trying to cut costs associated with medical and disability reimbursement and characterizing health care more as a commodity than as a social need or entitlement (Fox 1986:16–17; Fox and Thomas 1990:199).

For example, during the first term of the Reagan administration, Congress passed the Omnibus Reconciliation Act of 1981 (OBRA), which, in the spirit of cost containment, set new limits on Medicaid eligibility while reducing the federal financial share in the program (Holahan and Cohen 1986:1, 33–37). At the same time, the average state ceiling for Medicaid eligibility (measured as a percentage of the official poverty level) fell substantially (Beauchamp 1988:44). As a consequence, compared with the years before OBRA, the number of Medicaid recipients decreased each year between 1981 and 1984. In the same period, the number of nonelderly living in poverty in the United States grew substantially faster than the number of nonelderly enrolled in Medicaid programs (Holahan and Cohen 1986:5–32). Under such circumstances, public entitlement programs were unable to extend their protection to those who were pushed out of the private insurance system. The crisis of health care costs had adversely affected both the private and public foundations of the U.S. health care financing system, exacerbating previous contradictions.

Insurance: Excluding the Risk of AIDS

The AIDS epidemic could not have emerged at a worse time. It came to public notice precisely as the crisis of health insurance intensified. At first, the disease was perceived as ominous: of unknown origin and trajectory, uniformly fatal, difficult and probably expensive to treat. When early estimates, particularly by the Centers for Disease Control (CDC), suggested that the per case costs of AIDS were exceptionally high, the cataclysmic nature of the new disease made these very inaccurate estimates credible. At the same time, the perceived credibility of those data, coming as they did from the respected CDC, reinforced the sense that AIDS was potentially an economic catastrophe (Green, Oppenheimer, and Leigh 1989). Insurers held they had good reason, indeed the necessity, to guard against persons with AIDS and those believed most likely to contract it.

The insurers responded by invoking sound underwriting policy, as they had in other cases when current conditions or risk factors were thought to be predictive of high medical utilization. As a result, insurers refused to cover individuals with AIDS or AIDS related complex (ARC) at all, while asymptomatic, HIV-infected persons seeking nongroup policies were virtually uninsurable.

A 1987 survey by the Health Insurance Association of America, for example, found that of the insurers responding, 100 percent considered as uninsurable applicants with AIDS, 99 percent applicants with ARC, and 91 percent applicants with asymptomatic HIV infection (Intergovernmental Health Policy Project 1990:6). That same year, a survey carried out by the Congressional Office of Technology Assessment (OTA) revealed that many insurers had already begun or planned to screen both individual and group applicants for HIV infection (U.S. Congress, OTA 1988:80, 85). According to the OTA, 77 percent of commercial or Blue Cross carriers who insure small groups and more than 50 percent of those who cover large ones either already screened for HIV infection or would do so. In short, the specter of high costs appears to have generated an expansion of medical screening, particularly within the group market.

The underwriting methods insurers utilize—especially those aimed at ascertaining health status and demographic characteristics—allow carriers to differentiate between individuals with varying risks of incurring losses. According to insurers, such discrimination is "fair," where "fair" means measuring, to the extent possible, the potential loss shifted to the insurer by the policy holder and then charging a corresponding premium (Stone 1990:64).

However, in the case of AIDS, when the insurers applied underwriting rules, it was (and is) often difficult to distinguish between "fair" and "unfair" discrimination. That difficulty is particularly acute when gay men are the target population. From an early stage in the epidemic, the insurance industry, following most clinical, epidemiological, and popular attitudes, identified all gay men as a risk group, indeed *the* risk group, for AIDS and, therefore, for incurring far higher than normal costs of health care. As a risk group in both the epidemiological and underwriting sense, gay men became a group of potential, and in many cases actual, uninsurables, a development assisted by significant prejudices against gay persons that have for long existed within American society and that were reinforced by the AIDS epidemic itself.

Consequently, large numbers of insurers use sexual orientation in underwriting policies, despite the efforts of the National Association of Insurance Commissioners to ban the practice. The OTA survey, for example, reveals that 30 percent of the commercial carriers responding considered sexual orientation as a factor in underwriting insurance (U.S. Congress, OTA 1988:64).

Some insurers determine the sexual orientation of an applicant by hiring investigative agencies or through other means (U.S. Congress, OTA 1988:64). However, the sexual orientation of individual or group applicants is less often ascertained than inferred, based on supposedly correlative variables. Insurers have excluded individuals living in areas with a high proportion of gay men or cases of AIDS. One insurer, for example, rejected all single male applicants from San Francisco (Lambert 1989:A1). Some carriers hold ineligible for insurance individuals or groups engaged in occupations that popular prejudice has identified as associated with gay men: beauty parlors, florists, entertainment and arts groups, hair stylists, and interior decorators (Minkowitz 1989:19; Anderson 1990:42). Similarly, one commercial insurer warned its agents against unmarried men working in occupations that demanded no physical exertion (Lambert 1989:A10). In this fashion, an unspecified number of insurers have incrementally shifted from "fair" discrimination against those with risk factors for serious illness to "unfair" discrimination against a whole class of people, many of whom may never have engaged in high-risk behavior, and only a minority of whom were HIV positive (ACLU AIDS Project 1990:24–26, 74–78).

More frequently, carriers screen some or all persons by asking AIDS-related questions on the insurance application or by requiring HIV-antibody tests—the enzyme-linked immunosorbent assay (ELISA) and the Western blot series. Use of these tests as a screening mechanism appears more rational than the inferential methods described earlier, for the tests will eliminate only individuals with positive results. Nevertheless, they engendered opposition. Gay community groups fought the introduction of HIV testing; they argued, presciently, that the antibody test would be used to identify, and to discriminate against, gays and that it would be used successfully to foreclose access for many to insurance and the health care system (Bayler and Oppenheimer 1986:31; Bayer 1989:101–123). In addition, after the ELISA was licensed in 1985, California, Wisconsin, a number of other states, and the District of Columbia prohibited insurers from requiring HIV tests of applicants for health insurance. These states acted, in part, out of concern for gays but also out of fear that an increasing proportion of AIDS-related costs would be shifted to the public sector.

Insurers successfully fought the state curbs on their underwriting powers. To justify its actions, the industry argued that without testing, adverse selection and the unusually high cost per case of AIDS portended economic disaster for carriers. In addition, it claimed that eliminating a viable screening device would constitute "unfair" discrimination against those at low risks for HIV infection, who would be forced to bear higher premiums (to "cross-subsidize") as a consequence. Finally, the HIV-antibody test was unexceptionable, consistent with the industry's history of medical testing—using blood profiles and urine analysis, for example. Today only one state, California, fully prohibits carriers from requiring HIV tests for health insurance, a sign of the strength of the insurers' drive to maintain control over their underwriting powers.

The battle over HIV testing has, however, had some significant consequences. One of them was a study by the OTA that examined current and possible future medical tests in the light of their actual and potential adverse effects on access to health insurance and employment. Would advances in predictive and diagnostic tests operate, like the HIV antibody test, to "make private health insurance unavailable or too costly even to a number of presently insured persons and their dependents if analysis of their risks improved" (U.S. Congress, OTA 1988:3)? Would insurance pools of individuals and groups consequently become even narrower? Would the number and proportion of the uninsured and underinsured subsequently increase, placing a growing burden on the public sector? These questions have also been posed by the lay press, including the mainstream news magazine, *Newsweek* (Quinn 1987:55) and the liberal journal of opinion, *The American Prospect* (Stone 1990:62–73).

The insurers' arguments, made in an effort to counter their critics, have subsequently "politicized" underwriting. When insurers protest that they treat AIDS like any other disease, their wider practices become precisely the problem. As insurers claim that sound underwriting requires them to identify and to eliminate risk groups with high patterns of utilization, it becomes clear they are shifting the highest utilizers from the health insurance market to government programs or private charity. When insurers argue that without underwriting, people with average patterns of utilization would unfairly be subsidizing those with higher ones, they beg the question. Their rejection of cross-subsidies among pools is neither an actuarial nor a natural law but a policy choice of their own making that can be reopened and debated. That debate, if taken to its logical conclusion, would go to the very heart of the nature and limitations of the present private health insurance system in the United States. That is, the debate should center on whether the costs of health care should be shared by the entire community or be prorated on the basis of actual need for health care.

Unfortunately, insurers were not alone in differentiating and sometimes discriminating against those with AIDS. A minority of self-insured employers, fearing the financial consequences of HIV infection in their workforce, have imposed lifetime limits on what they will reimburse for AIDS, limits substantially below those set for other disorders (Taravella 1990:52). Often these caps on AIDS expenditures are far lower than the $50,000-60,000 currently estimated as the lifetime cost of that disease (Scitovsky 1989:319); in some instances the maximum has been set as low at $5,000 or $10,000 (Taravella 1990:52). Because self-funded firms are free of state insurance regulations, including those for minimum benefits, but fall instead under weak federal statutes, successful court challenges to these actions may prove difficult. Currently, only a few groups have limited benefits in the fashion described. They have, however, set a precedent, dangerous in an environment of medical cost crises, cost containment through exclusion, and general prejudice against gays and IV drug users.

As a result of such prejudice, employed and insured gay men may face a tragic paradox with respect to their coverage. To use health insurance for AIDS or related conditions identifies one not only as a potentially expensive employee and, therefore, a threat to the pool, but also as a member of a group that some employers might wish to exclude from coverage on moral grounds. In such circumstances, although insured, HIV-infected gay men may choose to pay their own costs for medical care at the onset of their illness and, in some cases, even later, when the burden of illness and expense have become far greater.

Even for employees with health care coverage who have not suffered from discrimination, AIDS has nonetheless clearly demonstrated the structural limitations of the present health insurance system. First, almost all existing policies require copayments and deductibles, which, even in the presence of "stop-loss provisions" in the insurance contract, can prove prohibitive. The necessity, in many instances, to pay for expensive services at the time they are rendered and wait for reimbursement adds substantially to the burden of cost as well. In addition, many policies, including some provided by large employers, contain preexisting conditions clauses, which limit payment for illnesses considered to have started before the effective date of the insurance contract; in most instances, mere evidence of antibodies to HIV, not to speak of an actual diagnosis of AIDS, is considered sufficient to invoke a preexisting condition clause.

Finally, and significantly, few policies cover all the care a person with AIDS or related illness is likely to require. For example, Americans must still pay out-of-pocket for 74 percent of pharmaceutical-related expenses (HCFA 1987:1–36). Yet prescription drugs currently play an unusually important role in AIDS-related treatment, a role that will only increase as medicine learns to intervene earlier in the natural history of the disease (Pascal et al. 1989:37–38). In addition, experimental therapies are almost universally excluded from insurance reimbursement (Antman, Schnipper, and Frei 1988:46), but it is precisely such therapies that are, of course, particularly common in AIDS treatment because of the relative novelty of the syndrome.

Also of importance are those exclusions that affect nonacute care. Because most health insurance has been based on employment, it has tended to focus on acute care designed to return to the workplace members of a relatively healthy workforce. Such insurance has omitted coverage for long-term care, in particular nursing homes and home health care. Since AIDS is rapidly becoming a chronic condition, parallel to the illnesses traditionally associated with the nonworking elderly, the tendency to exclude coverage for long-term care is particularly onerous to persons with AIDS.

AIDS has also made it difficult for many to continue to work, thereby eliminating their insurance coverage entirely. The vast majority of those in this position lack continued access to coverage through the family policies of their spouses. Most people with AIDS are gay, and gay relationships are rarely recognized as falling within the category of the family.

Legislative and regulatory initiatives that extend insurance through mandated conversion to individual policies or through time-limited continuation of employer coverage at individual expense (the so-called COBRA provisions at the federal level) have mitigated this problem somewhat. These initiatives are, however, seriously weakened by problems of inadequate benefits, in the instance of individual policies, and higher premiums than most can afford, in the extension of membership in employee groups. In addition, the COBRA provisions do not apply to groups with fewer than twenty workers, a type of employer group common in New York City, San Francisco, and some other urban areas most affected by AIDS.

As a consequence of all these developments, persons with AIDS have seen their access to health insurance, and therefore health care itself, seriously threatened during the epidemic. The threat has been reduced for many with AIDS by Medicaid and other public programs. Medicaid has, however, substantial disadvantages. These include the need to be categorically eligible (although persons with AIDS are "presumptively eligible," those with HIV are not and may have to wait some time for coverage); the need to meet poverty criteria that may force the patient to first "spend down," that is, divest himself or herself of assets; the lack of uniformity across states in either eligibility or benefit levels; and the refusal of large numbers of health care providers to accept Medicaid because of its generally low level of reimbursement (Holahan and Cohen 1986:99–110; Perloff, Kletke, and Neckerman 1987:222). Some states, including New York where the policy was pioneered, use Medicaid funds to pay the premiums of those clients with catastrophically expensive diseases who retain eligibility for private health insurance, but only a small number of persons with AIDS are covered by such programs (New York State 1982; Taravella 1989:9; Tarini 1989:13, 15).

Insurance: The Social Response to Exclusion

The U.S. private health insurance system both poses a danger to the health and financial well-being of individuals and shifts the social burden of those most in need of health care outside the insurance marketplace. Where public programs are absent, the social costs fall on the patient and his or her social network.

In the instance of AIDS, the private insurance system has shifted considerable costs onto the communities most affected by the epidemic, in particular the gay community and, increasingly, the poor and minority communities. The gay community, for example, has had to make an enormous financial commitment in order to ensure that those of its members without health insurance or with inadequate coverage receive proper medical and other treatment. Because of this financial commitment, there has almost certainly been a sizable, albeit impossible to measure, transfer of wealth, especially from the gay community, to institutions and individuals in the majority community, most notably to health care providers and pharmaceutical companies (Hansell 1990).

Many middle-class gay men and some IV drug users with AIDS do have health and other forms of insurance to draw upon to offset the costs of the disease (Taravella 1989:9). But others are not so fortunate. The gay community, in particular, has had to compensate for the lack of such financing or for the shortfall of social service and long-term care benefits in most private insurance policies by establishing elaborate care-giving institutions of its own. Among these are the Gay Men's Health Crisis in New York, the Shanti Project in San Francisco, and hundreds of similar organizations in many other cities (Altman 1986:82–109). In recent years, these institutions have served as models for analogous organizations in the black and latino communities. All these organizations require large amounts of voluntary contributions and labor, drawn mainly from within the communities themselves (Arno and Feidan 1986; Arno 1987; Griggs 1989).

The burdens of the epidemic on the gay and minority communities result not only from a lack of insurance or from the disproportionate number of community members with HIV infection. The burdens are due as well to prejudice against those with the new disease. This prejudice has led to a significant breakdown of the communal principle that hardships of this type should be shared by the entirety of American society (analogous to the aid provided to whole groups of people after flood, hurricane, or earthquake disasters).

This breakdown has had, in turn, an adverse effect on those areas of the country in which gay people and IV drug users form substantial minorities of the population. The lack of a true communal (a national) approach to AIDS has meant that the State and City of New York, for example, have had to spend immense sums directly or indirectly (in the form of Medicaid) for the provision of health care. Nor have the health care systems of these localities fared any better: the absence of health insurance for an unusually large number of persons with one particular disease has added to the financial and other problems of already overburdened hospitals and other health care institutions (Bigel Institute 1988; Andrulis, Weslowski, and Gage 1989:784–794).

In summary, the character and techniques of the U.S. health care system have posed a profound threat to our ability as a society to handle in an equitable and compassionate manner the current HIV epidemic. At the heart of this threat is a contradiction: instead of a community pool that spreads risks across the population, so that the many well cover the costs of the sick few, our private system creates discrete pools of the relatively well that do best when they exclude the costs of the sick. That the insurance system is employment based reinforces its fragmented and cost-benefit nature. To compensate for the inadequacies of the private system, our society has supplemented it with publicly sponsored programs; the supplementary system is itself, however, clearly an inadequate safety net. Consequently, the number of Americans without any coverage has grown significantly over the past decade to perhaps thirty-seven million individuals (Monheit and Short 1989:22). The U.S. health care financing system may be creating, as it were, "a growing army of the uninsured."

In large measure, the health insurance industry has not treated AIDS differently from other expensive diseases. To the degree that this is so, AIDS has served as a sort of prism to make manifest much that was invisible in health insurance. But AIDS has served in that capacity largely because HIV infection appeared first as, and seemed uniquely, a disease of gay men. Consequently, when the normative community reacted to AIDS with indifference, gays responded to it as a matter of personal and communal survival (Padgug 1989). As a result, the gay community, well organized, politically sophisticated, and highly sensitive to discrimination, fought vigorously for its share of the resources held by the larger American community. As part of that struggle, the gay community, including those already infected, clashed dramatically with insurers over their policies and procedures: the HIV test; redlining on the basis of geographic area, occupation, or sexual orientation; limitations on benefits or coverage maxima. For the first time, a segment of the uninsured (and soon-to-be uninsured), because they had a political base and awareness, sought to confront the insurance industry (Padgug 1989:307–308). To do so, they had to learn the insurance system thoroughly, much as persons with AIDS learned about therapeutics so that they could lobby providers and the federal bureaucracies.

The gay community has been able to battle employers and insurers over the terms in which health insurance is offered or refused, as well as, and with rather more success, over direct discrimination within the insurance industry, owing to its own organizational sophistication and the efforts of many nongays. It is not clear that the lesbian and gay community and, even less, any of the other affected groups, has the resources to continue to fight forever. Nor should they have to: it is time that the rest of American society—the normative community—takes on the contradictions of health insurance.

Restoration of Community

It is clear that the American health care financing system, centered around private health insurance, has not served persons with AIDS well. It has, in fact, placed additional burdens on both individuals and groups rather than contributed to an easing of the already serious problems the epidemic has caused. It has proved to be a divisive force in the community rather than a unifying one.

All of this has consequences. As Michael Walzer has observed:

> Membership [in the democratic community] is important because of what the members of a political community owe to one another and to no one else, or to no one else in the same degree. And the first thing they owe is the communal provision of security and welfare. This claim might be reversed: communal provision is important because it teaches us the value of membership. If we did not provide for one another, if we recognized no distinction between members and strangers, we have no reason to form and maintain political communities (Walzer 1983:64).

The financing system's inability to generate "communal provision of security and welfare" has rendered even more fragile whatever sense of mutual assistance exists on a quotidian basis in the United States.

AIDS, in turn, demonstrates the serious flaws of our current health care financing system. Most significantly, it reveals the contradiction inherent in meeting a basic social need through a private insurance system whose nature and internal development is determined by profitability and cost issues, narrowly construed as the interests of insurance companies and employers rather than of those of society as a whole. The most striking aspect of this contradiction is the need of the system to build in socially undesirable exclusions of economically unattractive people and groups. Such a system can scarcely be expected to serve as an efficient mechanism for the inclusion of the entire community of Americans within an equitable system of access to necessary health care.

A significant portion of the problems of the system derives directly from its basis in employment. Placing employer-provided insurance at the heart of health care financing has had the effect of vitiating universality and uniformity of coverage. It has supported and reinforced a network of fragmented insurance pools that are too vulnerable to high medical costs. Finally, it places in the hands of employers and insurers an unusual degree of power to decide issues of fundamental importance to the entire society and to their employees: who will be covered, what benefits will be offered, how much reimbursement will be made. Instead of public bodies, private organizations are making decisions concerning matters of social welfare.

If we are to solve the major problems of health care financing that exist for persons with AIDS and other major health problems, our health care financing system must move away from its current dependence on market principles. We must, instead, taking note of the system's original organization and the issues raised by its fragmentation, attempt to reconstitute "a community of insured." This can best be achieved through a type of system that offers universal and uniform coverage to all Americans, regardless of location within the employment system or familial relationship to other citizens. In this system, "illness is the relevant reason for distributing medical care and health protections" and for reimbursing the providers of such care (Beauchamp 1988:3).

How can we construct a system of universal and uniform coverage? There are many possible approaches, each with its strengths and its problems; we can only discuss them schematically here.

The most obvious and, at least conceptually, simple approach is some version of government-sponsored and government-provided national health insurance, which would replace the current system entirely. In a system of this sort, the community of insured and society-at-large should closely coincide. With such a system, access to health care might also strengthen the fragile communal ties that remain to us. As Dan Beauchamp has argued:

The common system stabilizes the politics of equality, setting up an alternative source of attraction for citizens' loyalty beyond the market, forging an enduring majority of the middle and lower income groups, and strengthening the ties of a common justice and community (Beauchamp 1988:40).

National health insurance in one form or another has, over the years, appealed to at least a large minority of Americans. Its implication raises, however, a number of serious issues that must be taken into account in any debate over the future of health care financing in this country. At present, the most important issues of national health insurance involve cost and program design.

With respect to costs, the major concern is that a system of national health insurance would simply be too expensive and, given our current federal and state budget deficits, unaffordable (Kinzer 1990:468). Some analysts have estimated, however, that the United States would save a large proportion (at least 8–10 percent) of its current total health spending if it adopted national health insurance, because it could dismantle most of the bureaucratic complexes required to sell, administer, and regulate our private reimbursement system (Himmelstein and Woolhandler 1986:442–443). In addition, analysis of health care spending across nations with different health care systems has shown that countries with strong national health insurance or health care systems, such as those found in Canada, Great Britain, and West Germany, were better able than the United States to control over time the proportion of their gross domestic product dedicated to health expenditures (Pfaff 1990:21–23). Evidently, "the more universal the coverage, the greater the scope of the public sector to act as a consumers' cooperative [which] . . . permits the community to hold down the share of its income which it must take over to providers" (Pfaff 1990:22).

One might argue that national health insurance, although expensive, would potentially allow the United States to gain control over its health care expenditures and achieve savings over time, as compared with projected costs under the present system. This might lead to beneficial results for all persons with serious illness, including persons with AIDS. In addition, a less fragmented system subject to community input through democratic institutions would be more likely to have a greater interest than the major protagonists of the present system in the more efficient and equitable handling of major epidemics and health crises.

The second significant issue raised by the implication of a national health insurance system is that of program "design" (Kinzer 1990:468–470). What form should a national health insurance system take?

Which of the present "players"—providers, insurers, employers, manufacturers, administrators—should be included? How should all the pieces fit together? What financing and quality and cost control mechanisms should be used? These questions, beyond the scope of this essay, will be debated if and when national health insurance again becomes part of a truly public debate.

However, in what appears to be the absence of a viable movement to create a national health insurance system at present, we will almost certainly have to accept something less than a thoroughgoing replacement of the current system, at least in the near term. A less dramatic, but still largely acceptable, approach would build on the strengths of the present system and attempt to mitigate its weaknesses through significant systemic reforms. Such an approach is unlikely to be successful unless it involves the participation of government (both as the voice of the citizenry and as a major purchaser of medical services), as well as employers and insurers. To achieve reform, government must lead the way through sweeping legislative and regulatory initiatives.

Some promising proposals have already appeared and some measures have already been promulgated. At the state level, both Massachusetts and Hawaii have implemented insurance programs that lay the foundation for universal health care coverage, the Health Security Act and the State Health Insurance Program respectively. The legislatures of many other states, including New York and California, either are discussing proposed legislation that would implement some type of universal coverage plan or have initiated official studies of the possibilities of such plans (New York State Department of Health et al. 1990). In March 1990 the Pepper Commission, a bipartisan congressional panel charged with studying the problems of the uninsured, recommended a program of universal health care coverage through a combined employment-based and public system (U.S. Bipartisan Commission 1990). The Kennedy-Waxman bill, the "Basic Health Benefits for All Americans Act," now before Congress (Senate S. 768, House H. R. 1845), contains a similar proposal.

The best of these proposals are based on a set of interconnected elements. First, they mandate employer-provided insurance, with small employers sometimes allowed the option of paying into a public program instead; all employees and usually their dependents receive at least a minimum package of benefits, with limited patient premium and copayment responsibilities. Second, they offer a publicly funded program designed in particular for those, like the working poor, who lack access to either private or categorical public (Medicare, Medicaid) coverage. Third, they expand Medicaid eligibility thresholds to at least the federally defined poverty level. Lastly, they alter the insurance underwriting environment, especially for smaller groups and individual applicants, to recreate some version of community rating, including open enrollment, acceptance of all who apply, and uniform premiums (albeit sometimes adjusted for acceptable demographic factors) for identical coverage.

Programs constructed using these elements, although they do not necessarily create a theoretically ideal health care financing system, should eliminate many of the worst flaws of the current system. They will provide to all (or almost all) members of the community access to a specified bundle of health services (whose adequacy varies by proposed program). They commit public funds, although the target population for those funds differs by program, ranging from the poor to the whole community. They prevent employers from eluding their responsibility in an employment-based insurance system to cover their workers. Through government participation, they foster public debate over the nature and practices of health care financing. They should, therefore, go far toward creating, or building toward, universal, uniform, and equitable health coverage and access to health care. They will at the very least eliminate many of the most serious social problems faced by those with HIV infection, as well as by all others with serious illnesses.

To ensure that programs that fall short of a complete government-sponsored national health insurance system work most efficiently and equitably, it will be necessary, especially in the case of AIDS, to combine them with other proposals that deal, directly and indirectly, with the issue of discrimination. Most importantly, we need to ensure that gay people and persons with AIDS are no longer "the other," abandoned to their own devices, beyond the boundaries of the normative community. Consequently, we must widen the struggle against fear and loathing of gays, minorities, and those with HIV infection through education campaigns headed, ideally, by our political and moral leaders. In addition, we need to pass and put into effect federal and state legislation that bans all discrimination against persons with disabilities —including AIDS—as well as discrimination against gay men and women.

Finally, we need to strengthen the ties of a common justice and of community by elaborating a national commitment to those areas of the country devastated by the epidemic. We have made a start through the approval by Congress in the spring of 1990 of the Comprehensive AIDS Resource Emergency Act, which earmarks funds for hospital, nursing home, and home care services to people with AIDS in the hardest hit cities and states (Hilts 1990:B9). Analogous legislation should be enacted to subsidize social services as well.

Like great wars, major epidemics test a society's institutions and values, its resilience and coherence as a community. In the case of health care financing and its institutions and values, we have attempted to muddle through the AIDS epidemic, changing as little as possible. As a consequence, the weakest of the "players," those who are ill or perceived to be at risk, have had to pay the consequences.

It remains to be seen whether the organized voices of the gay community, joining with others who recognize the need for "communal provision of security and welfare" for the acutely and chronically ill, will succeed in changing the status quo. Ten years into the epidemic, are we prepared to place mutual assistance above market principles? If we are not, we may lose our belief in adequate health care for all who need it in our society. In the process, we may further encourage social forces of polarization and distrust. In that case, the reality of community will continue to erode in America, with massive inequities and injustice the rule, not only for gays, IV drug users, and persons with AIDS, but also for all too many of our citizens.

REFERENCES

ACLU (American Civil Liberties Union) AIDS Project. 1990. *Epidemic of Fear. A Survey of AIDS Discrimination in the 1980s and Policy Recommendations for the 1990s*. New York: ACLU.

Altman, Dennis. 1986. *AIDS in the Mind of America*. Garden City, N.Y.: Anchor Press/Doubleday.

Anderson, Porter. 1990. Insurers Nix Arts Coverage. *American Theater* (January), pp. 42–43.

Andrulis, Dennis, Virginia Beers Weslowski, and Larry S. Gage. 1989. The 1987 U.S. Hospital AIDS Survey. *JAMA* 262:784–794.

Antman, Karen, Lowell E. Schnipper, and Emil Frei III. 1988. The Crisis in Clinical Cancer Research, Third Party Insurance and Investigational Therapy. *New England Journal of Medicine* 319:46–48.

Arno, Peter. 1987. The Contributions and Limitations of Voluntarism. In John Griggs, ed., *AIDS: Public Policy Dimensions*, pp. 188–192. New York: United Hospital Fund.

Arno, Peter and Karyn Feidan. 1986. Ignoring the Epidemic: How the Reagan Administration Failed on AIDS. *Health-PAC Bulletin* (December), 17:7–11.

Bayer, Ronald. 1989. *Private Acts, Social Consequences: AIDS and the Politics of Public Health*. New York: Free Press.

Bayer, Ronald and Gerald Oppenheimer. 1986. AIDS in the Workplace: The Ethical Ramifications. *Business and Health* (January/February), pp. 30–34.

Beauchamp, Dan E. 1988. *The Health of the Republic*. Philadelphia: Temple University Press.

Bigel Institute for Health Policy and United Hospital Fund of New York. 1988. New York City's Hospital Occupancy Crisis. New York: United Hospital Fund of New York.

Eilers, Robert D. 1963. *Regulation of Blue Cross and Blue Shield Plans*. Homewood, Ill.: Richard D. Irwin.

Fox, Daniel M. 1986. AIDS and the American Health Polity. *The Milbank Quarterly* 64 (Suppl.) 1:7–33.

Fox, Daniel M. and Emily H. Thomas. 1990. The Cost of AIDS: Exaggeration, Entitlement, and Economics. In Lawrence O. Gostin, ed., *AIDS and the Health Care System*, pp. 197–210. New Haven: Yale University Press.

Freudenheim, Milt. 1990. Insurers Seek Help for Uninsured. *New York Times* (January 11), p. A1.

Green, Jesse, Gerald Oppenheimer, and Madeline Leigh. 1989. The $147,000 Misunderstanding. In *AIDS, The Scientific and Social Challenge*. The 5th International Conference on AIDS. Montreal, Canada, p. 1030 (abstract).

Griggs, John, ed. 1989. *Simple Acts of Kindness: Volunteering in the Age of AIDS*. New York: United Hospital Fund of New York.

Hansell, David. 1990. The Impact of the Epidemic on the Financial Status of Gay Men (April 2). Testimony presented at hearings on "The Social Impact of the HIV Epidemic on the Lesbian and Gay Community in New York City," organized by the National Academy of Sciences, Panel on Monitoring the Social Impact of the AIDS Epidemic, New York Study Group.

Hardy, Ann M., Kathryn Rauch, Dean Echenberg et al. 1986. The Economic Impact of the First 10,000 Cases of Acquired Immunodeficiency Syndrome in the United States. *JAMA* 255:209–211.

HCFA (Health Care Financing Administration), Division of National Cost Estimates. 1987. National Health Expenditures, 1986–2000. *Health Care Financing Review* (Summer) 8:1–36.

Hilts, Philip J. 1990. House Approves $4 Billion in Relief for AIDS. *New York Times* (June 14), p. B9.

Himmelstein, David U. and Steffie Woolhandler. 1986. Cost Without Benefit, Administrative Waste in U.S. Health Care. *New England Journal of Medicine* 314:441–445.

Holahan, John F. and Joel W. Cohen. 1986. *Medicaid: The Trade-off Between Cost Containment and Access to Care*. Washington, D.C.: Urban Institute Press.

Intergovernmental Health Policy Project. 1990. State Financing for AIDS: Options and Trends. *Intergovernmental AIDS Reports* (March–April), 3:1–8, 12.

Kinzer, David M. 1990. Universal Entitlement to Health Care, Can We Get There from Here? *New England Journal of Medicine* 322:467–470.

Kosterlitz, Julie. 1990. Sick About Health. *National Journal* (February 3), no. 5, pp. 270–273.

Lambert, Bruce. 1989. Insurance Limits Growing to Curb AIDS Coverage. *New York Times* (August 7), pp. A1, A10.

McDonnell, Patricia, Abbie Guttenberg, Leonard Greenberg, and Ross Arnett III. et al. 1986. Self-insured Health Plans. *Health Care Financing Review* (Winter), 8:1–16.

Minkowitz, Donna. 1989. Redlining the Arts, Insurers Brand Artists AIDS-Prone. *Village Voice* (August 22), p. 19.

Monheit, Alan C. and Pamela Farley Short. 1989. Mandating Health Coverage for Working Americans. *Health Affairs* (Winter), 8:22–38.

New York State, Department of Health; State University of New York at Albany, School of Public Health; Intergovernmental Health Policy Project, The George Washington University. 1990. Universal Health Care: Voices from the States, State Initiatives (May). Proceedings of the Conference on Universal Health Care: Voices from the States, Albany, N.Y.

New York State, Department of Social Services. 1982. Administrative Directive, Payment of Health Insurance Premiums on Behalf of Public Assistance and Certain Medicaid-Only Recipients (August 10). Transmittal no. 82 ADM-48 [Medical Assistance].

Oppenheimer, Gerald M. and Robert A. Padgug. 1986. AIDS: The Risk to Insurers, The Threat to Equity, *Hastings Center Report* (October), 16:18–22.

Padgug, Robert A. 1989. Gay Villain, Gay Hero: Homosexuality and the Social Construction of AIDS. In Kathy Peiss, Christina Simmons, and Robert A. Padgug, eds., *Passion and Power: Sexuality in History,* pp. 293–313. Philadelphia: Temple University Press.

Padgug, Robert A. and Jon Eisenhandler. 1990. AIDS Costs and Utilization: Trends Among 10,438 Cases Insured by Empire Blue Cross and Blue Shield. In Sixth International Conference on AIDS, San Francisco. *AIDS in the Nineties: From Science to Policy* 3:285.

Pascal, Anthony, Charles L. Bennett, Russell L. Bennett, and Marilyn Cuitanic (1989). The Costs and Financing of Care for AIDS Patients: Results of a Cohort Study in Los Angeles. In William N. LeVee, ed., *Conference Proceedings: New Perspectives on HIV-Related Illnesses: Progress in Health Services Research,* pp. 34–41. Rockville, Md.: National Center for Health Services Research.

Pfaff, Martin. 1990. Differences in Health Care Spending Across Countries: Statistical Evidence. *Journal of Health Politics, Policy, and Law* (Spring), 15:1–67.

Perloff, Janet D., Phillip R. Kletke, and Kathryn M. Neckerman. 1987. Physicians' Decisions to Limit Medicaid Participation: Determinants and Policy Implications. *Journal of Health Politics, Policy, and Law* (Summer), 12:221–235.

Quinn, Jane Bryant. 1987. AIDS: Testing Insurance. *Newsweek* (June 8), p. 55.

Rublee, Dale A. 1986. Self-funded Health Benefit Plans. *JAMA* 255:787–789.

Scitovsky, Anne A. 1989. Studying the Cost of HIV-related Illnesses: Reflections on the Moving Target. *The Milbank Quarterly* 67:318–344.

Stevens, Rosemary. 1989. *In Sickness and in Wealth.* New York: Basic Books.

Stone, Deborah A. 1990. AIDS and the Moral Economy of Insurance. *The American Prospect* (Spring), pp. 62–73.

Taravella, Steve. 1989. Programs Help Low-Income AIDS Patients Pay for Insurance. *Modern Healthcare* (June), 19:9.

Taravella, Steve. 1990. Self-insured Employers Limit AIDS Benefits. *Modern Healthcare* (February 19), 20:52.

Tarini, Paul. 1989. Mich. Tries Paying Premiums for Private AIDS Insurance. *American Medical News* (November 10), pp. 13, 15.

Todd, James S. 1989. It Is Time for Universal Access, Not Universal Insurance. *New England Journal of Medicine* 321:46–47.

U.S. Bipartisan Commission on Comprehensive Health Care. 1990. *Recommendations to the Congress by the Pepper Commission: Access to Health Care and Long-Term Care for All Americans.* Washington, D.C.: U.S. Government Printing Office.

U.S. Congress, Library of Congress, Congressional Research Service. 1988a. *Insuring the Uninsured: Options and Analysis.* Prepared for the Subcommittee on Labor Management Relations and the Subcommittee on Labor Standards of Committee on Education and Labor, and the Subcommittee on Health and the

Environment of the Committee on Energy and Commerce, House of Representatives, and the Special Subcommittee on Aging, U.S. Senate, Part I (May).

U.S. Congress, Library of Congress, Congressional Research Service. 1988b. *Insuring the Uninsured: Options and Analysis.* Prepared for Subcommittee on Labor Management Relations and the Subcommittee on Labor Standards of the Committee on Education and Labor, and the Subcommittee on Health and the Environment of the Committee on Energy and Commerce, House of Representatives, and the Special Subcommittee on Aging, U.S. Senate, Part II (October).

U.S. Congress, OTA (Office of Technology Assessment). 1988. *Medical Testing and Health Insurance,* OTA-H-384, Washington, D.C.: U.S. Government Printing Office.

Walden, Daniel C., Gail R. Wilensky, and Judith A. Kasper. 1985. *Changes in Health Insurance Status: Full-Year and Part-Year Coverage.* Washington, D.C.: National Center for Health Services Research (DHHS Publication no. PHS 85–3377).

Walzer, Michael. 1983. *Spheres of Justice: A Defense of Pluralism and Equality.* New York: Basic Books. Cited in Dan E. Beauchamp. 1988. *The Health of the Republic.* Philadephia: Temple University Press.

6. Ethical Issues in AIDS Education

NORA KIZER BELL

> From our limited knowledge of the subject, we are, therefore, to conclude that for the solution of the problem of venereal diseases there is but one recourse, and that is education. Not altogether that education which is to begin at the change of fourteen years or older, but that education which shall begin with the earliest lisp of the little child when it begins to ask the question of the origin of its being and the uses of its external sexual organs . . .
>
> —G. W. Goller, in "AIDS and Public Health,"
> by A. Yankauer

ALTHOUGH WRITTEN IN 1916 by Dr. G. W. Goller, Health Officer of Rochester, New York, these words capture equally well what has been the prevailing sentiment in recommendations for public health approaches to acquired immune deficiency syndrome (AIDS) prevention. Today, as then, persons are urging that education is our best hope against the human immunodeficiency virus (HIV).

What has emerged in the moral debate, however, is strong disagreement over the substance of, and rationale for, such programs. There is no clear consensus on how early education should begin, to which groups it should be directed, who should do it, how long it should be continued, or what kinds of information it should include. Furthermore, there is no clear consensus on the role it should play in an overall public health strategy. Currently, the moral climate within which public health policy is being developed is still one of fear, distrust of medical information, and intolerance. The current climate is also still characterized by efforts to identify and isolate (literally and figuratively) those succumbing to infection and illness. These facts are mirrored in public demands for renewed efforts to institute compulsory or coercive public health interventions to halt spread of HIV. As a consequence, policymakers have suggested a range of compulsory measures (adapted from communicable disease models) to halt spread of HIV, from premarital testing or other forms of compulsory exclusionary screening, to mandatory reporting of positive test results, to incarceration or quarantine of the recalcitrant infected.

Unfortunately, there has been no clear statement of what moral principles might motivate one to choose education as against choosing compulsion. And there is still heated debate over how effective educational programs have been to date in accomplishing public health objectives. In short, a great many issues in AIDS education call for careful examination.

Few health care issues in recent years have captured public attention to the extent that AIDS has. Much about AIDS has thrown it into the spotlight—its modes of transmission; the life-styles associated with behaviors that place one at highest risk; the public image of wasted, suffering human beings at the edge of death; media reports of "AIDS orphans" abandoned in developing countries and likely to be abandoned in urban areas in this country; burgeoning health care costs associated with clinical care of persons with AIDS; and further challenges to civil liberties. As a consequence, discussions about which public health measures will effectively break the chain of transmission are overlaid with social and value questions. And in the absence of a national plan or policy for halting its spread, response to AIDS has been haphazard. Predictably, many policymakers have responded to the emotional and political effects of AIDS rather than to the medical realities of the disease.

Those who urge that we have a duty to society to control and eradicate this horrible disease sometimes also urge that individual rights and needs will have to be compromised in the effort. In fact, a survey of public attitudes toward those infected with HIV revealed that an overwhelming 81 percent of the respondents felt that individual rights would have to give way to the goal of controlling further spread of disease, while 74 percent of those in the survey believed that the necessity of identifying those who are HIV infected would require compromising privacy rights (Blendon and Donelan 1988). Many persons portray the moral dilemma in combating AIDS as requiring that we choose either to affirm individual rights or the good of society. The moral maxim that we seek to promote good and to prevent harm, they argue, compels us to move to protect the well-being of society, and that cannot be accomplished if we continue to champion the privacy rights or individual needs of persons with AIDS/HIV or if we continue to embrace voluntarism.

It is no surprise that AIDS policy issues have been debated publicly. Public health questions, by their very nature, are often decided in the public arena. But while most societies agree that government can override certain individual rights and needs in order to protect and promote public welfare, knowing where to draw the line in controlling spread of AIDS/HIV remains a delicate balancing act—especially in a society that embraces the principles of a liberal democracy.

This difficulty goes right to the heart of the controversy surrounding strategies proposed for breaking the chain of HIV transmission, and it forces an examination both of the moral appropriateness and the efficacy of a variety of AIDS prevention proposals. Such as undertaking is especially important *at this point* in the unfolding of the AIDS epidemic.

It is clear now that we are entering a new phase in our understanding of this disease. Since it was first clinically identified in 1981, AIDS has moved from being viewed as a disease causing a series of acute care crises requiring inpatient treatment of varying intensity and duration to a chronic disease—a continuum of infection requiring ongoing outpatient treatment and monitoring. In addition, new medical and demographic profiles of AIDS suggest that, while the numbers of persons infected with HIV remain greatest in homosexual and bisexual men (largely because of the infection rate in that population in the early days of AIDS), new cases of HIV infection are more frequently appearing in other populations. Notably, those newly infected are increasingly heterosexual men, women, and youth who are drug addicted, black and Hispanic, rural and urban poor, or the offspring or sexual partners of any and all of these groups.

In other words, we now have a reasonable grasp of the magnitude of the public health threat, the modes of transmission of HIV, the change in the "AIDS profile," and AIDS/HIV treatment options/benefits. As a consequence, we are at a point in AIDS policy development where we will be forced to make difficult choices about the proper role of education, compulsion, and voluntarism. Public health efforts to control the spread of HIV represent some of the most controversial aspects of the debate over individual rights versus protection of the public. Nowhere is this more obvious that in current deliberations about the form, the substance, and the soundness of AIDS education programs.

In what follows I want to examine some of the theoretical presuppositions underlying public health education, judgments made of the efficacy of AIDS education programs, what those judgments presuppose about people who live in a liberal democracy, and what the implications of different conceptions of education hold not just for controlling AIDS but also for many other public health issues.

A recurring problem in discussions of AIDS education is that education keeps getting run together with many other AIDS issues. In particular, education has been recommended over and against the adoption of compulsory public health strategies; the claim has been that, from a moral perspective, the two approaches are incompatible. Part of what I must do, therefore, is to spend some time examining that claim.

The Efficacy of Education

Many persons arguing for the use of compulsion in the control of HIV believe that education and the ready availability of current and accurate information on HIV transmission and prevention simply are not enough, that they have not been successful in changing behaviors, and that they cannot be expected to be successful. Hence, they argue, education should be supplemented by—or, better yet, abandoned in favor of—mandatory and coercive strategies.

It is here that they are fond of pointing to the history of syphilis as a counterexample to the efficacy of education. Thus, those early educational efforts bear brief examination.

As Alfred Yankauer reminds us, public health officials in the early part of this century viewed education as a panacea (Yankauer 1988). Social reformers believed that forthright education would end the problem of sexually transmitted infection (Brandt 1988). The commitment to education was so complete that allowing sex education to be taught in the schools was a relatively uncontroversial solution to halting venereal disease (VD). For example, it was agreed during that time that "[i]f parents failed to perform their social responsibilities and inform their children, then the schools should include sex education" (Brandt 1988:368).

Sex education during the first half of this century took, however, the form of instruction in sex hygiene. Many, if not most, of the courses emphasized teaching cleanliness, the avoidance of "polluted sources" of sexual gratification, the loathesomeness (and disfiguring aspects) of venereal disease, and the dangers of sexual activity, namely, disease and unwanted pregnancy. In short, most of these educational programs were strongly antisex (Cleaves, in Brandt 1988). Such programs unrealistically hoped to *end* sexual activity outside of marriage—by teaching *fear* of the activity.

As Brandt argues, however, such educational efforts may actually have contributed to the stigma that attached to disease because of the fears generated by the possibility of infection. More importantly from the perspective of those in public health, they did not seem to have any appreciable effect on reducing rates of infection.

Educational programs whose goal was to modify behaviors—that is, make them "safer" rather than to eradicate them—had slightly more "success." One such precedent is found in a military education program undertaken during World War II. Operating with a different underlying assumption, namely, that sexual activity was *going to continue* to occur, military officials sought to discover how, given their assumption, soldiers could best be kept fit and healthy. Their program emphasized prevention of transmission of VD through condom use, and condoms were widely distributed (Brandt 1988). A concerted effort was made to separate the task of education and prevention from the moral debate about promiscuous or adulterous sex.

From criticisms of these early health education programs, however, it is clear that there was strong consensus that they were *unsuccessful* —albeit to varying degrees. It is also clear from commentaries on what counted as success in those early venereal disease efforts that education was intended to effect behavior change. Neither the critics nor the proponents of these early education programs distinguished the educational goal of dispensing information to persons likely to be sexually active from the goal of restructuring the risky behaviors of those persons.

AIDS educational efforts have fallen prey to the same confusion of goals. As I discuss later in this essay, measuring the success of AIDS education programs will require that we have a clearer understanding of what should count as the criteria of success. Behavior change may be only one of those criteria.

Models of Behavior Change

An article by Marshall Becker and Jill Joseph reviewed much of the literature on education/behavior change to reduce risk for AIDS/HIV. Contrary to what some have tried to argue, they found that the bulk of the data supported the contention that significant changes in behavior have occurred as more information about AIDS has become available. Changes in behavior among homosexual/bisexual men in large city AIDS epicenters have been called the "most rapid and profound response to a health threat which has ever been documented" (Becker and Joseph 1988:407; McCusker et al. 1988).

Perhaps the most powerful data came from San Francisco, in studies undertaken in three separate cohorts from 1982 to 1986, which suggested an almost 90 percent reduction in unprotected anal intercourse during that four-year period (Becker and Joseph 1988). Data from New York City that compared behaviors during the interview year with behaviors recalled for the previous year indicated that the number of reported receptive anal sex episodes declined by 75 percent and that the use of condoms during anal intercourse increased from 2 percent to 19 percent of the episodes. In fact, 40 percent of study participants decreased their overall level of risk between the two time periods (Becker and Joseph 1988).

Becker and Joseph also documented substantial behavior change in intravenous (IV) drug users. In New York City, for example, a variety of behavior changes was elected by 59 percent of methadone maintenance patients as early in the epidemic as 1984. A further study noted that "novel behaviors" such as purchasing new needles and syringes or disinfecting used needles and syringes increased eightfold during a two-year period and were reported by almost half of a cohort of IV drug users interviewed in 1987 (Becker and Joseph 1988).

Studies of behaviors among hemophiliacs, heterosexuals who are not IV drug users, heterosexual women who are partners of IV drug users, prostitutes and their clients, and adolescents and young adults were also reviewed in the Becker and Joseph article. While some evidence of behavioral risk reduction was found in all of these groups, additional data also indicated that there was very little behavior change among potentially vulnerable adolescent and young adult populations (Kegeles, Adler, and Irwin 1988) or among urban blacks and Hispanics (Becker and Joseph 1988). In addition, research in smaller urban and rural areas revealed that rates of high-risk sexual behaviors in those locales are much higher than rates of risky behavior in most large AIDS epicenters (Fleming et al. 1987; Jones et al. 1987; St. Lawrence et al. 1989).

Other data are also important to evaluate in an examination of models of behavior change. For example, many of the studies indicated worrisome rates of instability in behavior change (Becker and Joseph 1988). While backsliding is a common phenomenon with many health behaviors, in the case of HIV this phenomenon is ominous and may provide an argument *against* attempts to eliminate rather than to modify those behaviors that can transmit disease. Furthermore, such behavioral instability can be attributed both to recidivism and to the introduction of newcomers into previously high-risk populations, another fact that suggests the importance of ensuring that interventions are ongoing and repetitive (Recent Reports 1990).

Finally, equally worrisome data on behavior change were reported in a study that examined sexual practices and attitudes of sexually active adolescents in San Francisco—a city where information about AIDS prevention has been abundantly available on television, bill-boards, buses, and in newspapers (Kegeles et al. 1988). In spite of media and school attention to AIDS prevention information, 40 percent of the females and 69 percent of the males continued to have multiple sex partners and only 2 percent of the females and 8 percent of the males reported using condoms every time they had intercourse.

In other words, behavior change has been widespread, but it has not been complete.

Criteria for Success

Many different hypotheses have been offered in explanation of the dramatic behavior change, as well as the absence of behavior change, noted above. Social norms within these special populations are said to be one factor. The fact that gay men in New York and San Francisco were able to construct new norms for governing their interpersonal relationships, norms of self-respect and mutual protection, is said to have helped lead to changes in their sexual interrelationships. As AIDS became clearly *their* concern, the gay communities in large city epi-centers worked to improve their network of social supports and through them to encourage behavior change. Owing perhaps to an absence of "gay community," this has not been seen to occur to the same extent in many smaller urban and rural areas.

Social norms can also have a negative impact on behavior change. When social norms fail to encourage condom use or the use of nonox-ynol-9, when most persons believe that suggesting condom use implies that one already has HIV infection or AIDS, when talk about safer sexual practices is taken to imply a distrust of one's partner, or when persons deny being among those at risk, sexual behavior is likely to reflect those norms.

Social norms in many places not only discourage talk about condom use and safer sex but also stand squarely opposed to the dispensing of condoms (in schools, in prisons, in residential care facilities such as group homes or halfway houses, in rest areas or rest rooms, and so on) —the argument being that the ready availability of condoms encour-ages sexual promiscuity. Social norms in many areas, particularly in smaller urban and rural areas, have also been traditionally antigay. Unlike larger urban areas, there has been little acceptance of, or oppor-tunity for, a gay network and/or gay community or social organizations.

The stigma attached to being gay still persists. Gays in most areas of the country still suffer isolation, lack of familial and social supports, the absence of role models, and the absence of legal recognition of "bonded" relationships they may have formed with another gay individual. Black gays, in virtue of their double minority status, suffer double the stigma.

Religious conservatism and the intolerance of homosexuality it fosters have both served as impediments to the development of social norms that would be conducive to risk reduction in homosexual/bisexual behavior. This conservatism has also had a profoundly troubling effect on sexual behavior in the heterosexual community. The denial of heterosexual transmission of AIDS and the general cultural denial of sexuality, coupled with religious instruction opposed to contraception, are responsible for norms of heterosexual behavior that are also unsafe.

The same conservatism that has been a barrier to many risk reduction programs in the gay community has been an especially serious impediment to risk reduction programs in the IV-drug-using community. Because of language and literacy problems (and socioeconomic differences), communication with the drug subculture is far more difficult to accomplish.[1] Yet, data from users potentially at greatest risk (i.e., those not in treatment programs) show that from 1985 to 1987, 47 percent of users who shared needles reported that they usually or always disinfected them with bleach. This was an increase from 6 percent who reported such practices in 1985. Similarly, the proportion of users reporting that they never used bleach fell from 76 percent to 36 percent in the same two groups (Becker and Joseph 1988). At the same time, in a study that sought to determine whether needles were still being reused in the face of the AIDS epidemic, increased demand for new needles was also noted. Brief ethnographic data even suggested that the illicit market for sterile needles in New York City had increased significantly and that some drug dealers were dispensing "free" needles or syringes (Becker and Joseph 1988).

In spite of reports of data like these in numerous studies, many in public health have worried that AIDS education and primary prevention programs are *not* reaching those at risk (Kelly et al. 1990). In fact, as I mentioned earlier, for some the claim that education is not working —that behavior change has not been adequate to break the chain of transmission—has been used as a reason for recommending a move toward adopting more coercive strategies for intervention in this phase of the epidemic, toward revisiting policy proposals rejected early in the epidemic as antithetical to public health goals.[2] Several states, for example, are considering requiring mandatory testing of all newborns. Some states are reconsidering mandatory testing in a variety of other populations, notably in prisons, extended care facilities, and some workplace settings. Legislation that would require premarital screening for HIV is now pending in thirty-five states (Brandt 1988). Several states have already mandated partner notification. And in some states, an infected person who engages in behaviors that could transmit HIV risks criminal prosecution.

Yet, the fact that significant behavior change has not been noted in adolescents or in smaller urban and rural gay or minority populations may be less an argument against the effectiveness of AIDS education programs than it is a comment on how those programs are designed and made available to persons in special at-risk populations or how such populations should be expected to respond to AIDS information.

Clearly, development of public health policy rests on assumptions about what prevention measures should accomplish. These assumptions obviously shape recommendations for new public health policy. What, then, are the presuppositions that underlie the claim that current prevention strategies are not working? What are the criteria for success in AIDS educational programs?

The message in reports that evaluate risk reduction data is unmistakable: that "only" 8 percent of males and 2 percent of females are reporting using condoms following exposure to AIDS education messages, that 60 percent of adolescent females and 31 percent of adolescent males are "still" engaging in promiscuous sex, and that the use of condoms by homosexual/bisexual men during anal intercourse increased "only" from 2 to 19 percent. It is also unmistakable that many of the reports conclude that AIDS education programs have failed for those reasons.

The standard is clearly behavior change. Furthermore, it seems equally clear that the bottom line for those in AIDS prevention, the public health goal in AIDS education, is elimination of disease—zero transmission, 100 percent risk reduction. Short of that, public health efforts are said to have failed.

This seems an impoverished notion of education. With AIDS/HIV, serious public health and social consequences can flow from a failure to appreciate how likely it is that most educational programs in a democratic society will not bring about complete behavior change— and perhaps equally serious consequences can flow from an expectation that they would.

Democratic Education

Many ethical issues in AIDS education arise because we take the notion of democratic education very seriously. In other words, we do not easily entertain a conception of education that has complete mind or behavior control as its mission.

By its very nature democratic education—that is, education that occurs in the context of a liberal democracy—will eventuate in something less than complete compliance with, or complete assimilation to, its instructional mission. A truly democratic society is willing to give up some degree of control over citizens' (mis)behavior in order to encourage the responsible exercise of individual freedom. A commitment to democratic education means, therefore, accepting compromise in its results. This is especially true in a culture that is pluralistic. Pluralism provides for the kind of social diversity that "enriches our lives by expanding our understanding of differing ways of life" (Gutmann 1987:33).

Education understood in such a context (and by extrapolation, AIDS education) must, therefore, accommodate all different kinds of cultural perspectives and individual variations, handicaps, strengths, and proclivities. Surely, part of what it means to accept the concept of democratic education is to accept that education should not advance any particular cultural perspective any more than education can *solve* the myriad of problems confronting those whom it seeks to educate. AIDS is only one of a number of social problems (such as teen pregnancy, inadequate parenting, delinquency, and substance abuse) for which this claim has relevance. Rather than recommend more draconian measures of behavior control, the concept of democratic education seems to suggest offering people information about a range of options, all of which can have better or worse impact on their lives. Such a conception of education relies heavily on the conviction that not everyone will be attracted to the same options and that, even if they are, they will be able to achieve them to greater or lesser degrees. Furthermore, such a concept of education underscores the value of voluntary choice.

Thus, even if we were to agree that completely eliminating risky behaviors is desirable in combating HIV and should be advocated in AIDS education programs, our commitment to the desirability of democratic education ensures that AIDS education programs will not accomplish that end.

If education cannot accomplish *eliminating* behaviors that transmit

HIV, what is there about education as a strategy to recommend it? Here we must return to what should count as criteria for success.

For a democratic society that places a high value on pluralism, the principle of respect for persons has important moral force. Respecting persons requires a presumption in favor of individual responsibility, just as it leads us to "embrace certain values, such as mutual respect among persons, that make social diversity both possible and desirable" (Gutmann 1987:33). The principle of respecting persons requires not only that we accept all persons as equally possessing moral status and moral agency but also that we *treat* them with such respect, that we affirm their moral right to be treated equitably, and that we affirm their moral right to be different.[3] Ensuring respect for persons, in Gutmann's language, is accomplished by the principles of nonrepression and nondiscrimination. The authority of democratic education must be so limited (Gutmann 1987:95).

The criteria for a successful AIDS educational program in such a context might be vastly different from the way public health educators conceive it. Under such a conception, strategies for reducing transmission of HIV must rely heavily on moral persuasion, rational deliberation, and, hence, on the availability of current and accurate information on HIV transmission and prevention.

Under such a conception of education, success is achieved if persons and societies are enabled to govern themselves. Success is achieved if persons can be participants in their own learning and if they can differentiate and accept responsibility for moral choices. AIDS education has been successful if persons are enabled, for example, to establish norms of mutual protection and self-respect that would allow them to change behaviors and preserve their social identification. Proponents of such a conception of education have confidence that people *will* learn, albeit at different rates and in different ways. Their learning will be conditioned by their various perspectives. Measuring success under such a conception of education means something vastly different than merely determining whether particular percentages of persons change their behaviors.

One of the principles that is said to provide the philosophical underpinnings for a liberal democracy derives from a principle articulated by John Stuart Mill and typically identified as the "harm principle": one is free to do as one chooses so long as one's actions harm no one else. This principle, while often used to justify paternalistic interventions designed to prevent harm to others, does not justify limiting one's freedom for one's own good. A commitment to the concept of democratic education, then, suggests not only that we cannot eliminate all risky behaviors that threaten *others* in society but also that it is inappropriate to seek to prevent voluntarily chosen *self-destructive* behaviors (such as unprotected sex).

Such a conception of education obviously involves certain risks or liabilities—namely, that some people *will* learn but will not change their behaviors, that they will forget, that they will make mistakes, that disease will not be entirely eliminated. Education may make some persons more willing to take risks with themselves and others than they were before—say, because they learn that the risk of infection with HIV from one act of intercourse with an infected person without using a condom is considerably smaller than they had believed. Education may even make some people *less* responsible citizens than they were before. These are all risks inherent in an AIDS education program understood as democratic. These are also risks that those who are determining public health policy seem unwilling to accept.[4]

Alternatives to Education

For many in public health, the undesirability of such risks has suggested that society should pursue prevention alternatives other than education.

Throughout the first four decades of the twentieth century, the search for an effective treatment for venereal disease was a major objective of those in public health. In 1943, Dr. John S. Mahoney of the United States Public Health Service announced his finding that penicillin was effective in treating rabbits with syphilis. After these findings were replicated in human subjects, it seemed clear that a treatment for syphilis really had been found. With a single shot of penicillin—a "magic bullet"—syphilis could be cured. By 1949, Mahoney and others were able to say that antibiotic therapy had virtually eradicated gonorrhea and syphilis (Brandt 1988).

History also teaches us, of course, that the decline in the rates of venereal disease infection was short-lived. By the late 1950s, many of the other public health strategies that had been in place for combating spread of venereal disease (such as public education) were no longer being funded or implemented. In the early 1960s, rates of infection began to climb again and have climbed steadily since.

Clearly, the lesson to be learned from this experience is that even the discovery of a "cure" is unlikely to achieve the goal of zero transmission.

What then? Are we led, as so many others seem to have been led, to recommending a strategy of coercion?

As I indicated earlier in the essay, people often talk as if our choices in adopting AIDS prevention measures lead us to choose either education or coercion. In fact, they are really quite separate issues. It is one thing to try to determine whether we should have AIDS education and what that education should include. In a democratic society there is really no choice whether or not to educate persons about a disease as potentially devastating as AIDS. We have a responsibility to provide that education, whether or not it eventuates in behavior change. The fact that we as a society have a responsibility to provide AIDS education does not, however, address the question of whose responsibility it is to provide such education—merely that education ought to be provided.

Only if we think that education must necessarily eventuate in specific behaviors are we pushed to think that we must choose between it and coercion. So, for example, while we might agree that AIDS education should include telling people what their responsibilities to others are, it is a very different project to determine what will happen to persons who fail to heed that educational message. Unfortunately, one reason coercion or compulsion appeals to so many persons is that it provides an outlet for the anger and resentment felt toward those who are already infected or are at risk for AIDS. The preference for compulsion seems to be correlated with the belief that persons who contract HIV are deficient in moral character and self control—that they have *chosen* immoral behavior and are, therefore, morally culpable rather than victims (Reamer 1983).

The issues involved in sorting out how to think about AIDS education should not, however, be conflated with whether we will or will not make appeal to coercive measures in containing HIV transmission.

Distinguishing Features of HIV

Having addressed the question of what counts as success in AIDS education or prevention programs, I now turn to an examination of the content of AIDS educational efforts. But first, I want to identify several features of AIDS and HIV infection that are idiosyncratic and are thus a factor in evaluating AIDS education strategies.

Most obvious of the distinguishing features of AIDS/HIV is the fact that there is not yet a magic bullet to treat AIDS or HIV infection. AIDS and its sequelae are currently incurable. Even with early diagnosis and therapeutic intervention, available treatments are able, at best, to slow one's progression along the disease continuum.

A second distinguishing characteristic of HIV is that persons at risk of infection, or already infected, are asked to undertake *lifelong* changes in their behaviors, whereas persons infected with other sexually transmitted diseases are required to alter sexual behaviors temporarily (or to be more discriminating in their choice of sexual partners) (Becker and Joseph 1988). What is more, there is little in the way of an incentive for behavior change to offer persons who are already infected. (In fact, perhaps the only incentive is a moral incentive—that is, avoiding harming someone else.) This fact stands in sharp contrast to many other risk-reducing public health recommendations.[5] Presumably, there are all sorts of incentives for those who are not yet infected to make behavior changes, but that is a different point.

Modes of transmission of HIV, in addition to calling attention to *sexual* behaviors that are problematic areas of behavior change, also call attention to *addictive* behaviors that elude clear-cut intervention/education strategies. Substance abuse addiction, for example, seems particularly resistant to educational efforts. The sharing of needles has long been a part of the subculture of drug addicts. Addicts driven by withdrawal are not likely to seek out new or disinfected "works" (Fineberg 1988). Coupled with the problem of substance abuse, the developing racial, gender, and class issues of HIV disease also create newer and more difficult barriers to developing sensible education and intervention programs.

A third distinguishing (and disquieting) feature of AIDS/HIV is that it is stigmatized more than its other infectious disease counterparts. Persons with AIDS or HIV infection have already experienced discrimination at the hands of society in a variety of forms for which there is no single analogue. A recent study reported in the *New York Times* gives even greater cause for concern about AIDS stigma. According to that study, undertaken by the American Civil Liberties Union (ACLU), acts of discrimination against people with AIDS have steadily increased, in spite of the fact that most people now know that AIDS is not spread through casual contact. In fact, approximately 30 percent of the cases of discrimination reported in the study were against persons perceived to be at risk for HIV and against those who cared for persons with AIDS—not against those already infected (Hilts 1990).

A final and important (though not distinguishing) feature of HIV is that nearly all transmission involves consensual risk-taking. Nearly every activity that spreads HIV disease is voluntary. Furthermore, most of these activities are inherently private—hence, not easily (or effectively) regulated. While coercive strategies for controlling HIV transmission might have both moral and public health warrant in isolated cases, such as in blood or organ donation, coercion, in general, is not likely to have the desired effect. Nor, on my view, is such broad use of coercion justified.[6]

Although social, cultural, and sexual norms have an undeniable effect on behavior and behavior change, there is also an undeniable link between education and the development of these norms. In my view, education must be the *centerpiece* of public health policy for managing AIDS/HIV; it is our most promising (and cost-effective) strategy. To say this is not to say that coercive measures are never appropriate. As I indicate in the paragraph above, in very limited cases coercion might be necessary and appropriate.[7] Nor is it to say that AIDS researchers should not pursue finding both a cure and a vaccine. Obviously, it is important to urge that they do. Rather, it is to say that while HIV transmission might be partially controlled by one or another of these strategies, the behaviors that place one at risk for HIV infection will not be eradicated. For that reason, a mixed strategy, one that gives the most central role to education, may be the best public health approach.

The Educational Message

Education, clearly, can take many forms. It can take place not only through the use of printed materials, lectures, presentations, videos, and so on, but also, importantly, through voluntary counseling.[8] At its best, education can enhance autonomy and help shape voluntary choices. Determining the message of AIDS education is not, however, so easily accomplished. Among other things, AIDS educational programs have to be designed to meet the needs of vastly different audiences: adults, youth, persons whose life-styles and behaviors place them at greatest risk of HIV infection. It might be helpful to look first at educational messages appropriate for adults at greatest risk.

Many public health and education experts agree that AIDS/HIV education will be most effective in altering risky behaviors if its language is explicit and nontechnical; it leaves existing values, roles, and attitudes intact (i.e., does not warn or forbid); it achieves ethnic and gender congruence with its population; it is nonjudgmental; its message actually targets the populations it is intended to reach; and it is personalized (Stone et al. 1989).

Behavior modification requires creativity, and to the extent that it can, say behavior change experts, it should be accomplished within the social milieu of the targeted population. Currently, for example, the major source of heterosexual transmission of HIV is intravenous drug use. Since many partners of IV drug abusers see the users, not themselves, at risk for HIV, and since 50–80 percent of the female sex partners of IV drug users do not themselves inject drugs (Cohen, Hauer, and Wofsy 1989), educational interventions have to be considered in at least two arenas: one, in any forum where the user/abuser accesses the system, and the other by outreach and support to those at the fringe of the drug culture (Bell 1989). Parts of this population will be especially hard to reach, and the effectiveness of educational outreach will depend on there having been clearly established a climate of trust, not of fear or retribution. Primary prevention programs among drug users may have to include instruction on sterilizing and cleaning needles and syringes with bleach. Educational outreach may have to include needle exchange opportunities and condom distribution. Finally, and crucially, interventions directed at drug abusers should stress both self-protection and altruism (the need to protect one's partners and one's children) (Stone et al. 1989).

Such educational interventions are most effective when personalized. For that reason, persons already in drug treatment programs may be those who are best able to reach into the drug-using community; women whose partners infected them without warning them may best be able to communicate with other women in similar positions. There has been some resistance to this notion, primarily because addiction counselors oppose encouraging any reestablishing of contact between persons in treatment programs and the drug culture itself. Yet, who could know better the language and the social norms of user/abusers? At the very least, these persons could be used to help develop educational materials and strategies. Expanding access to drug treatment programs is a further means of educating and counseling about risk reduction.

The message of HIV education must also adapt itself to a variety of attitudes about sex. If sex is regarded as an act of economic exchange more than of pleasure, for example, barrier contraceptives can be introduced as useful or practical and not just as something that can enhance sexual enjoyment; alternatives to vaginal or anal intercourse can be described as well. This approach has had some success in persuading prostitutes to have their customers use condoms and to engage in oral-genital sex as their predominant mode of sexual activity (Becker and Joseph 1988).

Similarly, educational materials that can teach ways to make safer sex practices more erotic are likely to have greater impact among those who place the pleasurable aspects of sex above its possible consequences. Several authors have noted that materials attempting to educate about safer sexual practices among gay men, for example, both failed to acknowledge homosexuality as a sexual orientation (Rhame 1988) and couched discussion of gay sex in the "language of AIDS" (Aiken 1987). Aiken concluded that teaching how to make gay sex safer would have been better accomplished "in the language of sex."

Critics of frank and explicit AIDS education believe, however, that educational interventions should focus on teaching abstinence and restraint—even though studies have shown that celibacy was not the preferred method of risk reduction, for example, among homosexual/ bisexual men (Becker and Joseph 1988).

Objections to the Message

Of course, AIDS education that is frank and sexually explicit or that advises how to make drug use safer creates considerable cause for controversy (Barnes 1989). Opponents of such educational efforts generally resist it on two grounds: (1) it legitimates or gives tacit approval to activities that are thought to be morally (and in some cases, legally) wrong, and (2) it is offensive and violates traditional social norms of decency.[9]

True, in some cases the activities that spread HIV are illegal. There is already considerable debate about whether all of those activities *should be* illegal (sodomy, for example)—especially if they take place between consenting adults. Regardless, it is important to distinguish between permitting an objectionable behavior to occur—or even making it easy to engage in—and acknowledging that certain behaviors are *going to continue* to occur and educating to make their occurrence less risky to all involved.

One strand of the debate over the content of AIDS education involves a factual dispute: does explicit information about decreasing one's risk in engaging in certain behaviors actually help bring about a reduction in high-risk activities? This dispute can be resolved, obviously, by studies that seek to discern just this. As Becker and Joseph argued, empirical studies that give us such factual data are an essential first step in the development of successful strategies for effecting behavior change (1988:408).

The more worrisome strand of the debate is, however, that offered by the "legal moralist." Expressed commonly in the context of discussions about homosexuality (and more recently in discussions about drug use), legal moralism is the view that society has a right to protect its existence against behaviors or life-styles that threaten its basic moral principles by enforcing those standards of behavior that constitute a common and shared morality. It is the legal moralist who often recommends sweeping punitive or coercive AIDS strategies in the name of protecting morality and common decency. It is the legal moralist who, consistent with some versions of religious conservatism, sometimes suggests seeking retribution for the "harm" posed to society by the life-styles of those infected with AIDS/HIV.

What from one point of view is protective of morality, however, from another point of view is scapegoating. While there may in fact be certain public principles governing behavior that are shared by the majority, it does not follow simply from their being shared that such principles are morally defensible. Nor does it follow that private acts of (alleged) immorality damage public morality. It is one thing to argue that persons whose activities recklessly endanger others are a public hazard and deserving of blame and punishment. It is another to know what those activities are. While I agree that recklessly endangering another is wrong, I disagree with the moralist that we can infer from persons' life-style that they will engage in those activities. Determining the moral worth of principles or behaviors that are to be advanced as worthy of promulgation or enforcement requires more than determining the level of moral indignation among members of the public. It is important to insist that such decisions be based on fact and on sound moral reasoning, not on prejudice, emotional response, or a mere report of majority feelings.[10] Having said that, however, it is important to reiterate that these are judgments that are most appropriately made at a different level—namely, when people transgress what we take to be important moral principles governing human interrelationships.

Still, the relevance of my worry about the moralist to the argument about the content of AIDS education cannot be overlooked. Until there is convincing moral argument for why public health policy should not adopt those strategies most likely to reach persons at risk—and for why public health education should be willing to write off entire segments of the population—AIDS education is an inappropriate platform for certain kinds of public moralizing.

The second objection to explicit AIDS educational messages is slightly more difficult to address. Unquestionably, the explicit nature of the materials in educational programs that are targeted to specific at-risk populations will offend some persons. Brochures and videos (and other educational media) depicting eroticized safe sex practices could surely be viewed by persons who never imagined such practices. In fact, it would be realistic to expect that they would find wider distribution. Graphic portrayals of risky sex and drug use could well cause persons to view activities they find offensive. Involuntary exposure to such materials might arguably be said to constitute an intolerable intrusion into their privacy—just as it might inform them of activities and possibilities they would not otherwise have entertained.

A solution offered to such objections is to minimize their offensiveness by selective distribution of such materials—making them available primarily in places where persons whose behaviors place them at risk are likely to be. Drug treatment facilities, VD clinics, gay bars, adult bookstores—all these come to mind as places where explicit educational messages would be least likely to offend.

In my view, however, to opt for selective distribution is to hide one's head in the sand. Many persons choose to ignore or deny the risks involved in their activities and for that reason do not seek out places where such information might be available. A study conducted recently in South Carolina, for example, revealed that interstate rest areas were a common location of risky sexual activity (unprotected anal and oral sex) between men, 85 percent of whom described themselves as bisexual or "straight." Of those in that study who reported being "rest area regulars," 80 percent reported engaging in high-risk activity (and reported an average of 7.9 such rest area sexual encounters a month). Not only did these men not self-identify as homosexual or bisexual, their denial of their sexual orientation led them to deny that their behaviors put them at risk for HIV infection. So complete is the social stigma attached to being gay that several of them explained that gay bars were the last places they wanted to be seen (Exoo 1990).

In spite of the fact that public health officials and others in the homosexual/bisexual community had long been aware of rest area sexual activity, there was considerable public (and official) resistance to placing condom machines in rest area rest rooms and to using rest areas as a locus for explicit AIDS education posters and brochures. Yet, there is good reason to believe that no other educational effort would reach this at-risk population. In a democratic society, can we expect less than such an effort?

The offensiveness debate and the arguments for limiting distribution of explicit educational materials have other consequences worth examining. Although no one would deny the effectiveness of explicit television campaigns against smoking, and although no one seems to object to the graphic content of television campaigns against drunk driving, there has been little support for such a campaign against HIV transmission. Rather, most AIDS public service announcements advise viewers to call an AIDS hotline number for information about risk factors and transmission. What is worse, the messages are aired in off-hours.

When one considers the explicit sexual content of much of television programming, and when one considers the graphic portrayals of violence on television (occurring with alarming frequency even in network news), it is hard to imagine how pictures of condoms or depictions of proper condom use could be more offensive. One standard for tolerable offense is often said to be the social utility of the offending message. Yet, claiming that campaigns against smoking and drunk driving have high social value, and for that reason can be thrust on unwilling and captive television audiences, is inadequate as a response. Surely there is equally high social utility in slowing transmission of HIV. In other words, the offensiveness of explicit media messages about AIDS is mitigated by the importance of getting that message to persons likely to be at risk and by the social value of reducing HIV transmission. The same holds true, I would argue, for the importance of explicit AIDS education in a variety of other settings: prisons, halfway houses, psychiatric hospitals, residential care facilities, and so on.

It is not difficult to believe, however, that a partial explanation for the failure to institute broad-based, aggressive, and explicit AIDS education campaigns lies less in the offensiveness of the message than in the identification of AIDS with life-styles that are considered offensive. Nonetheless, in a democratic society it is important to society as a whole to ensure that *all* possibilities for informing persons be left open and to provide fair access to information that can affect persons' choices about their futures.

AIDS Education and Youth

A final arena where both these objections to explicit AIDS educational messages have had a substantial (in this view, negative) impact is health education programs for adolescents, preadolescents, and teens. Here the ethical issues arise because youths, not adults, are the target audience.

After former Surgeon General Koop endorsed condom advertisements and explicit AIDS education, many state and local school districts established health education programs designed to allow/provide AIDS instruction—as did other institutions and organizations whose mission is primarily to serve youth. Although the prevalence of HIV among adolescents and teens is not known, there is increasing concern about their risks for developing AIDS. Some in public health even project sharp future increases in rates of HIV infection among young people (Shafer in Kegeles, Adler, and Irwin 1988). One important indicator of teens' risk is their high rate of other sexually transmitted diseases (Kegeles, Adler, and Irwin 1988). The need for sexually active adolescents to understand and engage in the use of condoms and other barrier methods of contraception is vital as a step toward reducing transmission of HIV.

Although instruction in sex hygiene in public schools has been common practice since the early days of syphilis and gonorrhea, it is widely acknowledged that such instruction usually "misses the mark." Students complain that it is simpleminded, rarely addresses the real concerns they have about their sexuality, and uses terminology alien to most teens' way of talking about sex. In its attempt to be neutral to the moral issues at stake, it avoids teaching much of anything. Parents, on the other hand, have argued against recent efforts to expand sex education curriculum, complaining that instruction about sex that attempts to deal with more than sex hygiene is likely to teach values that may conflict with the moral and religious values of individual families.

When AIDS was introduced into the equation, the debate over sex education in the schools heated up. The arguments for democratic education are complicated in this context by the fact that adolescents and teens are legally minors, and hence, rarely accorded either legal or moral autonomy. Several layers of paternalism, therefore, smother students' rights to know how to protect themselves from HIV infection. Schools may act *in loco parentis,* to be sure, and could arguably decide that explicit AIDS education is in the students' best interests. But schools are run by school superintendents, school boards, and parents —not to mention state legislatures and county and city governing boards. And parents have traditionally been allowed authority in areas considered to be religious or moral instruction.

Because of the politics of AIDS (and the politics of public education), many states have allowed school districts to determine, district by district—with the help of parents and other interested parties— what the content of AIDS educational programs will be. The consequence in many schools is, unfortunately, that the very information students need to protect themselves from transmission is the information that is not permitted to be included. Omitting some of that information can actually be very harmful; including *as information* material that teaches hatred and intolerance can be very destructive.

In school districts in areas dominated by religious conservatism, for example, health education instructors are sometimes *required* to teach abstinence and *forbidden* to mention condoms or spermicide use as methods of prevention or transmission. Suggestions have been made in some school districts that AIDS education should include instruction that homosexuality is perverted and morally wrong. Even in some more enlightened districts, AIDS educational materials can include discussion of the modes of transmission but cannot include mention of condoms or spermicides. And so on.

The situation is equally difficult for those who teach or counsel in many out-of-school settings such as the Girls or Boy Scouts, YMCA/ YWCA, athletic programs, college health clinics, social service agencies, churches/synagogues, after-school programs, social clubs, group homes, halfway houses, and so on. Many of these are settings where young people naturally congregate and where the atmosphere is relaxed and informal enough to allow for frank discussion of AIDS and HIV prevention—where questions can be asked without fear of embarrassment. Yet, teaching about AIDS in these settings often meets with more resistance than providing AIDS education in public schools because of the perception that such extracurricular settings are not purely educational, are not staffed by professional educators, and are not as carefully controlled.

These reports are frightening. Many persons in public health (and many ethicists) would argue that adolescents and teens deserve the same standard of treatment and information as any other risk group in this epidemic. Some might even argue that because of their "nonage" we have a strong obligation to give them more instruction and counseling, especially as concerns sexual relationships and the consequences of their sexuality. At least one study indicated that merely providing information to adolescents that condom use can reduce risk of AIDS and other sexually transmitted diseases may not lead to increased condom use. That study suggested that AIDS educational programs for adolescents also needed to target their perceptions of personal vulnerability (Kegeles et al. 1988).

Gutmann, in a section of her book on sex education, explains what confidence in a democratic education commits us to. She argues as follows: While it is true that sex is intimate, personal, and private (and is importantly interwoven with personal and familial values), it is not enough to say that because it is private in that sense, it should not be taught in public schools. Nor is it enough in a democratic community to say that it should be mandatory for everyone in public school because the consequences of sex affect the interests of others so profoundly. Rather, democratic education commits us to acknowledge the legitimacy of both interests—which is why we find that most schools require sex education and allow persons to opt out of it on personal moral grounds (Gutmann 1987: 108–110).

What should we say, then, about the proper *forum* for, and the *content* of, AIDS education in a democratic society? Although one cannot deny the importance of parents' interests in their children's education—and the legitimacy of that interest—the importance of adolescents and teens having access to AIDS prevention information overrides the incentive to give parents the final say in this matter. This is true even though there will be parents who profoundly object to the message of AIDS education. In a democratic society, it is important that persons have the capacity to deliberate among alternatives in their personal lives. It is unthinkable that religious, educational, and social institutions whose mission is to prepare youth to be good citizens and responsible adults, and to be informed in the exercise of their moral agency, would be permitted to deprive them of knowledge essential to that mission—and more important, knowledge that might save their lives.[11]

For these reasons, I would argue that the content of AIDS education should be uniform across school districts, that it should be provided in other extracurricular settings where young people gather and are educated and trained, that it should be reiterated often in all of these contexts, and that it should be as explicit and as nearly complete as possible.

I have argued that the mainstay of a well-integrated AIDS primary prevention program is not merely a vaccine or a drug, nor is it the use of broad-based coercion. Managing AIDS/HIV means, among other things, managing fear, hatred, and ignorance, and that is best accomplished through a concerted educational effort. Because many solutions for halting transmission of HIV will require the development of public consensus and will need significant assistance from persons inside the communities most at risk, debate in policymaking arenas is likely to be heated. Developing coherent education programs will require a tolerance or acceptance of alternative life-styles, cultural practices, and sexual orientations that is anathema to many who are in positions to decide public health policy. For these reasons, the challenges posed by AIDS will require unprecedented emotional and intellectual flexibility. They will also require a careful consideration of the real likelihood of eliminating AIDS as opposed to slowing its spread.

Coherent intervention also requires developing programs for protecting persons from discrimination. Because they fear the repercussions of coercive policies to halt HIV transmission, persons whose behaviors place them at risk for infection are likely to remain "underground" without such protections. This fact makes the obligation to provide education more compelling and is a further argument in favor of making explicit AIDS education *more widely* available.

Communicating information through education is easy; changing behaviors, especially addictive and pleasurable behaviors, is not. If one adopts the eliminative approach, one is likely to opt merely for a strategy of compulsion and coercion. In a democratic society, however, it is the process that is as important as the result.

> Public health cannot be separated from a concern for democracy and its requirements for an educated electorate, for public health in its broadest sense is public welfare and its foundations lie in social justice (Kreiger and Lashof 1988:414)

ACKNOWLEDGMENTS

I acknowledge the considerable help of Ferdinand Schoeman in the shaping of this paper. Without his invaluable criticisms and suggestions about its focus and direction, my discussion would be far less interesting or compelling. I also thank Frederic Reamer for having sufficient interest in this topic to inspire me to write this piece. His comments and suggestions were germane and truly invaluable. A final word of thanks to my colleague Jerry Wallulis for reading an early draft of the paper.

NOTES

1. As several authors point out, members of the IV drug-using community (unlike members of the gay community) are more likely to be minority, poorly educated, and of disadvantaged socioeconomic status. Furthermore, the stereotype of the IV drug user is considerably more negative than that of the homosexual/bisexual male.

2. As I discuss in my paper, "Social/Sexual Norms and AIDS in the South," Ronald Bayer and others attribute this to an erosion of the alliance between the gay and public health communities—an alliance that promoted a voluntarist approach to controlling spread of HIV. However, as the AIDS profile has changed, the populations most newly affected seem less able to form such an alliance. Whereas the gay community was predominantly white, well educated, middle class, *and* organized and politically savvy, the populations most newly affected (i.e., IV drug users and black and Hispanic women and children) are not well organized, politically well aligned, or savvy. On the contrary, they are unusually fragmented, historically disenfranchised, and hence more vulnerable to (and less able to resist) the imposition of coercive measures.

3. This poses a special challenge for American culture, given the moral stigma

generally attached to people with AIDS and those whose behaviors place them at risk for HIV infection.

4. Interestingly, to say that is *not* to say that AIDS education must be provided by those in public health. They cannot be faulted for having goals different from the goals of education.

5. As Becker and Joseph point out, smokers who successfully stop smoking can expect improved respiratory function and reduced risk of heart disease within a relatively short period of time. Changes in diet and exercise habits also provide similar incentives for behavior change.

6. Although there is not space here to address the implications of such a claim as fully as I would like, it has been demonstrated by several studies that the financial cost of the broad use of coercive AIDS strategies outstrips their success (Cleary et al. 1987; APHA/SIA 1988). In conditions of scarcity, this seems a wasteful use of health care dollars. It has also been pointed out that the anguish caused by false positives in a climate of coercion is an important additional cost to be factored (Cleary et al. 1987; Gostin and Curran 1987; Walters 1988). Other arguments are probably well known to most readers.

7. One can point to public health campaigns where coercion seems to have been effective—for example, laws that mandate the wearing of seat belts. And there are public health campaigns that we could predict would not be successful if coerced—for example, alcohol use and abuse. To say that, however, does not really address whether, effective or not, we believe that these kinds of choices available to people *should* be mandated. I must admit that I am inclined to think that they should not. Significantly, although persons advocating compulsory measures for preventing spread of HIV have reached back into the history of sexually transmitted diseases to demonstrate the precedent for mandating "turnstiles" for testing (Buckley 1986), many of these same advocates of compulsion fail to recall with any accuracy that mandatory premarital serologies never proved to be particularly effective in finding new cases of syphilis—or thus in preventing transmission to marital partners and offspring. Furthermore, although the United States Congress passed legislation during World War I to allow the incarceration of infected prostitutes, as well as the incarceration of women suspected of being infected or spreading disease, the venereal disease rates during that time continued to climb (Brandt 1988).

8. I mean to include here the professional counseling provided by nurses, psychologists, social workers, and others trained to help people who are struggling to control high-risk behaviors.

9. The same controversy surrounds school-based family planning clinics and school-based programs for teenage mothers.

10. I advance this same argument in my paper "Social/Sexual Norms and AIDS in the South." It is interesting to wonder whether the legal moralist would accept my arguments about what should count in determining whether publicly shared principles are morally defensible if the tables were turned—that is, if majority sentiment endorsed homosexuality, sexual promiscuity, or IV drug use.

11. This claim is clearly consistent with the Supreme Court's recent insistence that abortion statutes are unconstitutional unless in the best interest of the child they allow her to avoid parental control by seeking a court's permission to abort. While that does not prove that it is right to circumvent parental control on either of these issues, it does show that there is significant state interest in securing children's rights in a democratic society.

REFERENCES

Aiken, J. 1987. Education as Prevention. In H. Dalton, S. Burns, and Yale AIDS Law Project, eds., *AIDS and The Law*, pp. 90–105. New Haven: Yale University Press.

APHA (American Public Health Association): SIA (Special Initiative on AIDS). 1988. *Contact Tracing and Partner Notification* (November), APHA/SIA Report 2.

Barnes, M. 1989. Toward Ghastly Death: The Censorship of AIDS Education. *Columbia Law Review* 89:698–724.

Becker, M. and J. Joseph. 1988. AIDS and Behavioral Change to Reduce Risk: A Review. *American Journal of Public Health* 78(4):394–410.

Bell, N. 1989. Women and AIDS: Too Little, Too Late? *Hypatia* 4(3):3–22.

Blendon, R. and K. Donelan. 1988. Discrimination Against People with AIDS. *New England Journal of Medicine* 319(5):1022–1026.

Brandt, A. 1988. AIDS in Historical Perspective: Lessons from the History of Sexually Transmitted Diseases. *American Journal of Public Health* 78(4):367–371.

Buckley, W. 1986. Identify All the Carriers. *New York Times* (March 18), p. A27.

Cleary, P. et al. 1987. Compulsory Premarital Screening for the Human Immunodeficiency Virus. *JAMA* 258(13):1757–1762.

Cleaves, M. 1910. Transactions of the American Society for Social and Moral Prophylaxis. In A. Brandt, AIDS in Historical Perspective, pp. 367–371.

Cohen, J., L. Hauer, and C. Wofsy. 1989. Women and IV Drugs: Parenteral and Heterosexual Transmission of Human Immunodeficiency Virus. *Journal of Drug Issues* 19:39–56.

Exoo, G. 1990. Ladson, SC, Rest Area Interviews: Summary (April 26). A study funded by the Unitarian Universalist Social Concerns Grants Panel.

Fineberg, H. 1988. Education to Prevent AIDS: Prospects and Obstacles. *Science* 239:593–596.

Fleming, D., S. Coch, R. Steele et al. 1987. Acquired Immunodeficiency Syndrome in Low-Incidence Areas: How Safe Is Unsafe Sex? *JAMA* 258:787.

Fox, R., N. Odaka, and B.F. Polk. 1988. Effect of HIV Antibody Disclosure on Subsequent Sexual Activity in Homosexual Men. *AIDS* 1:241–246.

Gostin, L. and W. Curran. 1987. AIDS Screening, Confidentiality, and the Duty to Warn. *American Journal of Public Health* 77(3):361–365.

Gutmann, A. 1987. *Democratic Education*. Princeton: Princeton University Press.

Hilts, P. 1990. AIDS Bias Grows Faster Than Disease, Study Says. *New York Times* (June 17) p. A14.

Jones, C., H. Waskin, B. Gesety et al. 1987. Persistence of High Risk Sexual Activity Among Homosexual Men in an Area of Low Incidence of Acquired Immunodeficiency Syndrome. *Sexually Transmitted Disease* 14:79–82.

Kegeles, S., N. Adler, and C. Irwin. 1988. Sexually Active Adolescents and Condoms: Changes Over One Year in Knowledge, Attitudes, and Use. *American Journal of Public Health* 78(4):460–461.

Kelly, J., J. St. Lawrence, T. Brasfield et al. 1990. AIDS Risk Behavior Patterns Among Gay Men in Small Southern Cities. *American Journal of Public Health* 80(4):416–418.

Krieger, N. and J. Lashof. 1988. AIDS, Policy Analysis, and the Electorate: The Role of Schools of Public Health. *American Journal of Public Health* 78(4):411–414.

McCusker, J. Anne M. Stoddard, Kenneth H. Mayer et al. 1988. Effects of HIV Antibody Test Knowledge on Subsequent Sexual Behaviors in a Cohort of Homosexually Active Men. *American Journal of Public Health* 78(4):462–467.

Reamer, Frederic. 1983. The Free Will-Determinism Debate and Social Work. *Social Service Review* 57(4):626–644.

Recent Reports: Unsafe Sex and Relapse. 1990. *Focus: A Guide to AIDS Research and Counseling* 5(6):4.

Rhame, F. 1988. More on 'Safe Sex.' *New England Journal of Medicine* 318:1760–1761.

Shafer, M., C. Irwin, and S. Millstein. 1988. In S. Kegeles, N. Adler, C. Irwin (1988). Sexually Active Adolescents and Condoms, pp. 460–461.

St. Lawrence, J., H. Hood, T. Brasfield, and J. Kelly. 1989. Risk Knowledge and Risk Behavior Among Gay Men in High-Versus-Low-AIDS Prevalence Areas. *Public Health Reporter* 104:391–395.

Stone, A., D. Morisky, R. Detels, and H. Braxton. 1989. Designing Interventions to Prevent HIV-1 Infection by Promoting Use of Condoms and Spermicides Among Intravenous Drug Abusers and Their Sexual Partners. *AIDS Education and Prevention* 1(3):171–189.

Walters, L. 1988. Ethical Issues in the Prevention and Treatment of HIV Infection and AIDS. *Science* 239:598–603.

Yankauer, A. 1988. AIDS and Public Health. *American Journal of Public Health* 78(4):364–366.

7 . Ethics and Militant AIDS Activism

COURTNEY S. CAMPBELL

WE TAKE AS a defining mark of a civilized society that it is able to resolve disputes and conflicts through political or legal institutions and processes. In a democratic polity, we expect that political representatives will be accountable to the citizenry and that our fundamental values will be embedded in and expressed through the law. If such avenues do not prove responsive to particular interests, we encourage, as a constitutionally enshrined right, freedom of assembly as a means to redress grievances, and though compliance with law is an important condition for social cohesion and order, we find it a vital sign of a liberal democracy that there is social space for peaceable protests and demonstrations.

As we near the end of the first decade of an epidemic that has killed more Americans than the Vietnam War, the emergence of militant AIDS activism requires that we examine anew the limits of political and social tolerance toward protest tactics that are increasingly more confrontational, coercive, or even illegal. In a society committed in its foundational documents to freedom, due process, and justice, how should we think morally about methods to effect political or institutional changes through threats or civil disobedience? Consider the following examples:

In August 1989, in a public meeting at the Food and Drug Administration (FDA), the federal agency charged with overseeing the regulatory review and approval process for experimental drugs for acquired immune deficiency syndrome (AIDS), activist Larry Kramer promised: "If we do not get these drugs, you will see an uprising the like of which you have never seen before since the Vietnam War in this country. We will sabotage all of your Phase II studies," that is, scientifically controlled clinical trials to evaluate the effectiveness of a drug (Kolata 1990). Kramer's threat came before an agency that has already been widely criticized for relaxing some of its policy and ethical controls over the drug approval process to expedite expanded distribution of experimental AIDS drugs and that less than a year previously had been the object of a mass demonstration and civil disobedience by more than a thousand activists, nearly 180 of whom were arrested.

The issue that mobilized nearly a thousand activists in New York in late March 1990 was somewhat different—institutional inadequacies in the provision of medical and social services for persons with AIDS (PWAs)—but certainly no less charged. Responding to a call by the AIDS Coalition to Unleash Power (ACT UP) to "shut down the State Capitol in Albany" and proclaiming that "New York is a healthcare disaster area," the activists picketed the executive mansion and drowned out remarks by Governor Mario Cuomo, then converged on the Capitol building, where some doused red paint on its steps, while others proceeded inside to stage "die-ins" in legislative offices or unfurled banners rebuking state officials for their indifference to and mismanagement of the AIDS epidemic. This demonstration followed by a day the actions of some twelve activists who entered the legislative chamber, blowing air horns and shouting slogans, in the midst of a debate between lawmakers over a bill concerning benefits for volunteer firefighters.

As a result of their participation, approximately eighty activists were arrested for disorderly conduct or harassment, criminal trespass, and obstruction of governmental administration. This seemed to have minimal deterrent value on many of the protesters, however, who indicated this protest was only the beginning of a sustained attempt to draw attention to the social scope of AIDS by disrupting government activities. "There will be no peace," commented one protester, "until the funds and the attention [are] marshaled to meet the AIDS crisis. We tried talking, we tried insisting, and now it's time to escalate" (Hughes 1990; Verhovek 1990).

We may consider the rhetoric of protest and the activities of civil disobedience as little more than minor social annoyances (the Albany protest cost New York State about $10,000 for law enforcement, paint removal, and related expenses) or, alternatively, as the manifestation of political pragmatism, politics carried on by disruptive, but at least nonviolent, means. In this political frame, activists will typically draw attention to the success of their methods, such as the "dramatic results" in drug policy that activists attribute to the 1988 FDA protest: "Since then four new treatments for secondary complications of AIDS

have been approved in record time, and the FDA now permits wider
distribution of drugs still being tested" (Harrington 1990:4). Opponents of the methods (though not necessarily the goals) of militant
activism, meanwhile, may feel inclined to counter the rhetoric of "uprising" or "escalation" by raising the prospect of a "backlash" or emphasizing the counterproductive consequences, as expressed in the
reaction of one New York legislator to the Albany protest: "It hurts [the
activists] a lot. If anybody in government lets people who disrupt the
orderly process of government get their way, then you have no government. It's unfair to all the poor people who are suffering" (Hughes
1990).

Framing the problem of activism as solely a political question, whose
value resides exclusively in pragmatism and effectiveness, is, however,
inadequate in some important respects. Militant AIDS activism, whether
it takes the form of jeering public speakers, dramatic street die-ins that
disrupt vehicular traffic, rendering telephone switchboards nonfunc-
tional, legally permitted demonstrations, public threats, or civil disobedience, has been decisively shaped by a particular *history* that bears
inquiry. Before we rush too quickly to judgment, our first response
must be one of understanding.

Moreover, as the comments of both the activist and legislator suggest, there is more to militant activism than *Realpolitik*. Such actions
raise profound *ethical* questions about the moral authority of the state,
fairness, social priorities, and the saving of lives. Concerns about the
implicit anarchy attributable to the disruption of due process appear to
collide with ultimate imperatives that warrant moving beyond talking
to lawbreaking. Thus, unless we are committed to a view that political
action is inherently amoral, or an ethical perspective that the ends
justify any and all means, we need to supplement the fixation on
pragmatism and effectiveness with a richer set of ethical considerations.

In the following, therefore, I illustrate how the adoption of militant
and confrontational tactics by AIDS activists cannot be understood
apart from a perceived long-standing neglect and callousness toward
PWAs or others at risk for the disease on the part of government
officials at all levels and embedded to some extent in the scientific and
medical response to AIDS. I also contend, however, that this narrative
of neglect does not dispose the ethical issue. The moral limits of political tolerance are stretched by threats that border on manipulation and
coercion, and a moral line is crossed when an individual or a collective
body deliberately violates the law and intentionally disrupts the political
process to pursue goals and ends. AIDS activists who engage in civil

disobedience thereby bear a burden of justification for their actions, and it is important to explore whether this burden is both recognized and satisfied.

Silence and Red Tape

Why is it that AIDS activists have adopted tactics that have not been resorted to, for example, by advocates for patients with cancer or heart disease? Why is it that some organizations have moved beyond lobbying politicians or fundraising through special musical, theatrical, and artistic performances—activities that are no different in kind than those performed by any special interest group with expectations of benefits, political and medical, for their constituency and that in themselves do not present the distinctive moral questions raised by the specter of sabotage or the activism of civil disobedience?

That such issues can be posed at this point in the AIDS epidemic may at first strike us as perplexing. After all, the concerns of activists about social priorities and resources, as expressed in budgetary allocations, have increased extensively (indeed, some would say disproportionally in relation to the scope of the problem). Federal expenditures for AIDS research have risen from $7 million in 1982, the year after the first cases of what we now call AIDS were reported by the Centers for Disease Control (CDC), to more than $1.3 billion currently (The Latest Word 1990). Such outlays exceed the research investment in diseases such as cancer and heart disease that kill far more Americans each year than AIDS has over the past decade. Substantial changes have also transpired in the scientific and regulatory processes governing testing, approval, and distribution of new drugs. Although even presidential commissions have been sharply critical of the political response to AIDS as hesitant, mismanaged, and fragmented from the beginning of the epidemic, in light of recent fiscal and bureaucratic breakthroughs, is it fair to characterize the current political and medical situation regarding AIDS as constituting "passive genocide" (Spiers 1989:34)?

From the perspective of activists, several factors mitigate the significance of such developments. It is most likely the case that government outlays for research, treatments, and care would not be as high as they are currently but for the efforts of activists using various means, from letterwriting to lawbreaking, to make the issue of resource allocation unavoidable for political representatives. It is not to be forgotten, moreover, that unlike many of the diseases cited for comparative purposes,

AIDS is an infectious disease. The scope of its threat is, therefore, potentially catastrophic.

Meanwhile, not only do advocacy groups continue to express serious concerns about the adequacy of legal statutes protecting privacy and prohibiting discrimination (in employment, housing, or medical care, for example), but also, to activists, the use of appropriate funds by the scientific research community seems suspiciously inefficient. Some six years after the discovery of human immunodeficiency virus (HIV), the causative agent for AIDS, there is but one federally approved antiviral drug, azidothymidine (AZT), and only minimal research attention to secondary infections and cancers. Our economics seems to have proceeded apace of our ethics, for as one activist has commented, "People with AIDS have *different priorities*" than researchers or drug companies (Harrington 1990:4; my emphasis). Finally, AIDS remains a uniformly lethal disease, most prevalent among members of subcultures, gay men and intraveneous (IV) drug users, who have historically been marginalized in our society. Paradoxically, threats of uprisings and acts of civil disobedience are emerging as tactics to effect political and regulatory changes precisely at a period in the epidemic when scientific research is most intensive and fiscal support most extensive.

Two symbols of AIDS activism are particularly suggestive for illuminating this paradox. The first is the maxim of ACT-UP, "Silence = Death," which, while calling the members of the AIDS community to activism, expresses as well an indictment of political indifference. The second is the spectacle of activists literally binding themselves with red tape and staging die-ins in the October 1988 FDA demonstration to protest policies of regulatory review deemed to hinder the availability of drugs for AIDS.

These symbols suggest the importance of historically contextualizing the militant character of current AIDS activism, for it does represent an "escalation," as the Albany protester noted, from earlier forms of activism. In the initial years of the epidemic, the AIDS activism of the gay community, for example, was less confrontational than it was preservationist. It focused on practices to sustain the internal cohesiveness of the community in the face of threats of dissolution from either death or from calls for repression and coercion emanating from the dominant culture. Within the community, activists devoted attention to such methods as education, mobilization, the formation of health support groups, seeking financial support for the medically indigent, and provision of care and meals to the homebound and critically ill. As well, vigorous efforts were directed outward to resist increasing pressures for state coercion, stigmatization from blood donation policies, or exclusion via quarantines or isolation (Bayer 1983, 1989; Shilts 1987; Kramer 1989).

These measures of sustenance and preservation were particularly significant, given that nearly three years (1981–84) elapsed between official reports of the first AIDS cases and the discovery of what we now refer to as HIV; this prolonged period of scientific uncertainty shaped a perception that AIDS was a disease that potentially threatened all members of the most afflicted communities. Writing in 1983, for example, Larry Kramer, cofounder of the Gay Men's Health Crisis (and later of ACT UP) asserted:

> After almost two years of an epidemic, there still are no answers. After almost two years of an epidemic, the cause of AIDS remains unknown. After almost two years of an epidemic, there is no cure. . . . Our continued existence as gay men upon the face of this earth is at stake. Unless we fight for our lives, we shall die. In all the history of homosexuality, we have never before been so close to death and extinction. Many of us are dying or are already dead (Kramer 1989:33).

The interpretation activists would later ascribe to this delay in identifying the causative agent of AIDS became important, as I note subsequently, in cultivating an ethos of militant, confrontational activism.

This is not to say that confrontational tactics were not contemplated during this period. Indeed, civil disobedience was considered as an option to protest neglect by federal, state, and local political officials at least as early as March 1983. In a famous essay in the *New York Native,* Kramer disclosed that "a number of AIDS Network Members have been studying civil disobedience with one of the experts from Dr. Martin Luther King's old team." Kramer expressed a hope that such a protest method would not be necessary to evoke a comprehensive response from governmental authorities to AIDS but nevertheless concluded his essay with an appeal for "volunteers" for civil disobedience: "It is necessary that we have a pool of at least three thousand people who are prepared to participate in demonstrations of civil disobedience. Such demonstrations might include sit-ins or traffic tie-ups. All participants must be prepared to be arrested" (Kramer 1989:48–50).

Kramer has since noted that this appeal was "not successful," in that it drew only fifty persons. It is nevertheless indicative of a move, albeit premature, toward militant activism rather early in the AIDS epidemic for precisely the same rationale, pervasive governmental apathy, that prompts current demonstrations and civil disobedience. Obviously, the sheer magnitude of the epidemic in intervening years (Kramer entitled his 1983 essay, "1,112 [cases of AIDS] and Counting"; he concludes a 1989 essay with the phrase, "105,990 and Counting") and its attendant consequences, such as woefully inadequate health care services, account partly for this transformation in tactics. Yet, both unsuccessful and successful attempts to mobilize activism into confrontational protests have drawn on the same resource for motivation, political neglect in the face of a killer disease.

For many activists, politically institutionalized indifference was personified by former President Ronald Reagan; the symbol of leadership and social vision in this country, Reagan did not utter the word "AIDS," let alone make a public address on the topic, until several years into both his presidency and the epidemic. Indeed, it was not until some 25,000 persons were known dead from AIDS that Reagan authorized the Department of Health and Human Services "to determine as soon as possible the extent to which the AIDS virus has penetrated our society" (Crimp 1989:11).

AIDS activists have thus seen their foe as not merely a virus that attacks the immune system but also a government that has failed to attack directly a virus responsible for the deaths of a substantial number of its citizens. A sustained and comprehensive educational and scientific effort and aggressive, visionary leadership would, in this view, have made a significant impact on the development and the *control* of the epidemic; instead critical leaders and institutions often appeared to fail to acknowledge either the presence or the scope of AIDS, making a desperate situation border on the catastrophic. The enormous degree of culpability activists have ascribed to government at all levels, but most particularly at the federal level, is attested to in the comment of activist Herbert Spiers that "There would not be an AIDS activist movement, *perhaps not even an epidemic,* had the government originally responded to the disease forthrightly as a medical issue" (Spiers 1989:34; my emphasis).

That response, in the perspective of activists, has instead been decisively formed by the history of marginalization and disenfranchisement toward the communities most affected by AIDS. This provides the only plausible explanation for why it required three years to discover HIV when very recent threats to public health had illustrated that government and scientists could act concertedly and with some dispatch as the occasion required. Hence, "Many gay men, their friends, and political allies, concluded, rightly, that their lives were dispensable, or certainly weren't worth as much as the lives of middle-class busi-

nessmen who were struck with Legionnaires' disease some years previously [1970s], an illness that prompted much official activity to discover its cause and find its cure" (Spiers 1989:34).

The Trial of Drug Trials

If the political system in the United States is perceived as generally
unresponsive to the medical and social needs of PWAs, scientific and
regulatory processes relating to research, approval, and distribution of
drugs for AIDS are deemed no less blameworthy. The research convention of establishing scientific validity of a treatment, through reliance
on randomized control trials (RCTs) with placebo wings to generate
generalizable knowledge about the toxicity and efficacy of a prospective therapeutic agent, has seemed to activists to be beset with all the
vices of a bureaucracy encumbered by excessive red tape. Particularly
as the numbers of deaths from AIDS began climbing dramatically in
the mid-1980s, and Public Health Service estimates of those infected
with the disease ranged from 500,000 to 1,500,000 persons, activists
began to question the wisdom of adhering to protocols and policies that
had been established in the past with minimal regard for the special
problems that might arise in the face of an epidemic from an infectious
disease. Treatments were needed immediately to save identifiable lives,
and yet the extensive testing and extended approval process seemed to
promise only to add to earlier delays, culminating in either avoidable or
at least premature deaths. Reflecting the perspective of many, one
activist has pointedly observed that "the research bureaucracy lives on
a different time line than the one on which people with AIDS live"
(Harrington 1990:5).

When our society has confronted the ethical question of setting
priorities between identified and statistical lives in the past, it has
typically chosen on the side of present persons in need, and the evolving debate over research and approval of new drugs for AIDS has
proved no exception to this. That issue was at the center of the controversy over the September 1986 interruption of the RCT conducted by
Burroughs-Wellcome on AZT and over subsequent decisions by the
FDA to expand distribution of the drug and to revise its drug classification scheme to permit expedited approval for promising treatments.
The clinical convention required for thorough scientific authentication
of a drug as safe and effective may benefit future PWAs; however, it
appears to have minimal merit to present PWAs, who may well die
before regulatory review of research is completed.

It is within this context—the agonizing trajectory of a PWA toward death would not wait for science or the federal bureaucracy—that the most prominent AIDS activist organization, ACT UP, came into being. Before an audience of some two hundred and fifty people at New York's Gay and Lesbian Community Center in March 1987, Larry Kramer observed, "A new drug can easily take ten years to satisfy FDA approval. Ten years! Two-thirds of us could be dead in less than five years." The practical conclusion seemed obvious," We have to go after the FDA—fast. That means coordinated protests, pickets, arrests" (Kramer 1989:131, 136).

The FDA was, then, identified as the fundamental "brick wall" blocking access to drugs for dying persons, and three different, but related, models of activism were gradually articulated and implemented with the objective of effecting sweeping changes in the drug approval and distribution process and modifying, if not abandoning altogether, the regulatory reliance on RCTs. The "gadfly" model focused on *visible, public* protests, including civil disobedience, to bring pressure for institutional change from outside the standard avenues of political change; at the very least, this approach held out the prospect of garnering considerable media attention to dramatize the inhumane face of science and medicine. Thus, the "red tape" demonstration at the FDA, in which members of ACT UP, joined by other advocacy groups, carried tombstone placards reading "I died for the sins of the FDA," "I got the placebo," and "Dead from lack of AL-721," was fueled by a sense of frustration that the "Food and Drug Administration . . . took more time to license new drugs than many PWAs could expect to live" (Harrington 1990:5).

A second activist model relied on *invisible, internal subversion* to ensure the failure of the governing regulatory structure. In the federal policy debate over AZT distribution, some participants concluded that conducting conventional RCTs could well become an exercise in futility, because seriously ill PWAs, desperate to obtain any agent that held out the prospect of palliation and deferring death, would engage in noncompliance and deception. For example, patients might seek to determine the identity of the drug they receive in an RCT and refuse to participate further in the study if they are receiving a placebo or an unsatisfactory drug or take other unauthorized drugs as supplements. Kramer underscored and advocated this practice in his remarks that culminated in the formation of ACT UP: "Double-blind trials are also exceptionally foolish, because PWAs lie to get the drugs. I'd lie. . . . If they told me what to say to get a promising treatment, I'd say it, whether it was true of not. I have friends who have forged their medical records, who have gone to medical libraries to learn the correct terminology to fill in the blanks. So all the results from all these double-blind studies aren't going to tell anyone a thing" (Kramer 1989:132).

Noncompliance, deception, and lying are not sabotage, but in the context of clinical trials, they may well accomplish the same end, the invalidation of scientific data on drug safety and effectiveness. They reflect a refusal to play by the regulatory rules of the game, whose consequence is that its overriding objectives are compromised. AIDS activists have subsequently contended that the "ethical validity" of a clinical trial is directly correlated with the extent of patient noncompliance: "Noncompliance can be used as a surrogate marker, if you will, for the extent to which you've been able to infuse your trials with some level of ethics" (Palca 1989:20).

A third activist model has focused on *negotiation and consultation* with researchers and policymakers, although the feasibility and effectiveness of this alternative, perhaps initially, was conditioned by the existence of the protest and subversion models. That is, in the case of the FDA, the threat to its supervisory status and regulatory role had to be serious enough for members of the medical research community and the political establishment to be willing to listen to proposals by activists for a system more responsive to the need of PWAs or those who have tested HIV positive. The efficacy of this model also requires that activists become well educated about the drug-testing and regulatory process, an important result of which has been that the expertise of some ACT UP members has been drawn upon, either directly or indirectly, by researchers at the National Institutes of Health (NIH) and FDA policymakers (Crossen 1989:A7; Kramer 1989:126). In assuming advisory roles with direct policymaking implications, activists can presumably function as effective advocates for community interests and as indispensable resources for scientists concerned to tailor research to meet community needs.

The various models of public protest, internal subversion, and political persuasion are not mutually exclusive and may well be unified by the common end of achieving change in the regulatory structure. This does not mean, however, that there has not been considerable debate and disagreement between activists over *how* to bring about such changes most effectively. The various tactics employed, from protests and civil disobedience, to deception, to assuming advisory roles or engaging in conventional political lobbying, reflect not simply activist adaptability to what is expedient in a given set of circumstances but also dissent and diversity over the extent of cooperation and noncooperation with a political and health care system assessed as unjust.

Thus, while some activists have deemed confrontational methods necessary and most efficacious, others have distanced themselves from the most strident language and militant methods. Kramer's "call to riot" as part of a "massive disruption" by activists at the Sixth International Conference on AIDS in San Francisco (1990) was publicly disavowed by leading members of ACT UP and ultimately rejected by every AIDS activist organization in attendance (Kramer 1990; see also Gross 1990). Indeed, two spokesmen for ACT UP at the conference asserted: "No violence will be started, continued, or condoned by any ACT UP organization" (Specter and Gladwell 1990).

Nor is there always consensus on nonviolent disruptive action. The speech of Dr. Louis Sullivan, the Bush administration's Secretary of Health and Human Services, at the San Francisco conference prompted a large and vocal protest marked by a chorus of "shame, shame," condom and paper throwing, and whistles and air horns that together effectively rendered Sullivan's remarks inaudible; still, some activists "feared the hostile show would exhaust any remaining sympathy for activists within the administration" (Chase 1990). Similarly, the December 1989 disruption of a mass in St. Patrick's Cathedral by members of ACT UP, while condemned by civic and religious leaders, as well as by national AIDS advocacy organizations, also ignited a vigorous debate among the protesters themselves in subsequent ACT UP meetings. The focus in these dissents is not on the general objectives of activism but on the ethics and efficacy of specific confrontational tactics.

The collaborative approach likewise has not been without its critics from within activist circles. Those who have been invited to participate on various research and regulatory bodies may risk being perceived not as constructive intermediaries but rather as possessing divided loyalties. An instructive example of this tension is conveyed in the role compartmentalization proposed by a leading activist, Jim Eigo, following his nomination to the AIDS Research Advisory Committee of the National Institute of Allergies and Infectious Diseases (NIAID): "[T]o protect ACT UP and to protect me from any perceived conflict of interest, I propose that in accepting the nomination, I make it clear that *I am not accepting as an ACT UP member,* that on ARAC I will not be speaking for ACT UP, and that ACT UP and I are not responsible for each other's words and actions" (Eigo 1989; my emphasis). On these terms, one cannot be both an activist and a bureaucrat and retain integrity. Indeed, the militant critique of working to improve the drug-monitoring process from within the research or policy establishment concerns less the problem of effectiveness and instead focuses on the prospects of complicity, bureaucratic cooptation, and dirty hands in the perpetuation of injustice. It seems clear that even if activists have answered affirmatively the question whether research and regulatory change will occur, they may not be entirely of one mind on just how to accomplish the changes they seek.

Breakthroughs and Bottlenecks

The precise influence AIDS activists and their various methods of public protest, internal subversion, and political persuasion have wielded in the evolving process of balancing the needs of desperate and dying PWAs and the concerns for scientific validity is difficult to determine precisely, because a complex nexus of political, scientific, social, and fiscal factors is involved in policy decisions. Nevertheless, the general goals of activists throughout this period have been to restructure the drug regulatory process through expanded research, expedited approval, greater access, and affordable costs, and whatever their influence, it seems undeniable that the outcome of the process facilitates achieving those goals.

Indeed, despite strong ethical and policy opposition on grounds of scientific validity, patient welfare, and informed consent to risk-taking in clinical research (Annas 1990), it is indisputable that the current research and regulatory structure for AIDS drugs is substantially different than even four years ago, when AZT was approved for expanded distribution. Since that decision, the federal government has authorized more than $250 million in research projects under the auspices of the AIDS Clinical Trials Group (ACTG), a nationwide consortium of forty-six centers that have enrolled more than eight thousand patients in clinical trials. An interesting example of the increasingly significant consultative role of activists is displayed in the recent attention ACTG working groups have given to an ACT UP document entitled "A National AIDS Treatment Research Agenda," released at the Fifth International Conference on AIDS in Montreal in 1989. The document articulated criteria for conducting clinical trials, including involving PWAs in trial design, greater attention to drugs for opportunistic infections, flexible protocols, broader requirements for patient enrollment, and trial end points other than death to determine the efficacy of a drug.

While the ACTGs remain the primary testing venue for AIDS drugs, testing, distribution, and approval are in several respects no longer confined to this setting. Activists have been instrumental in the emergence of Community Research Initiatives (CRIs), semiautonomous or fully autonomous community-based treatment programs, as a second forum to conduct tests on nonvalidated drugs. Such programs have already had a significant impact: testing carried out by CRIs was responsible for the 1988 FDA approval of aerosol pentamidine, a potential preventive agent against the secondary infection *Pneumocystis carinii* pneumonia, after the ACTG program failed to conduct its own proposed studies.

Nor do PWAs have to rely on being enrolled in either an ACTG or a CRI to obtain nonvalidated drugs. The FDA revised its policies in 1988 to permit U.S. citizens to import unapproved drugs from foreign countries for personal use, and federal imprimatur has recently been given to the "parallel track" policy, which allows the release of experimental drugs to patients (via physicians) not enrolled in clinical trials, so long as certain safety standards have been satisfied. This mode of expanding access was exemplified in the widespread distribution of dideoxyinosine (ddI) in late 1989, even though long-term toxicity studies had been completed on fewer than one hundred patients. Finally, unauthorized drugs may be distributed to PWAs in unauthorized *trials,* such as the controversial "underground" study of the Chinese drug compound Q in San Francisco.

This is not to contend that these developments on several policy fronts have left activists at all content. After all, even after four years, AZT remains the only federally approved drug for AIDS, and for activists the pace of research continues to be mockingly slow. Having made rather substantial gains in the middle of the regulatory structure, activists have looked to achieve similar successes with beginning (research) and ending (cost) "bottlenecks" in the distribution of drugs for AIDS.

Indeed, "success" stories of how the protest model has been applied in the past to effect change have subsequently been invoked as a precedent for further confrontational actions. The "dramatic results" attendant to the FDA "red tape" demonstration have been cited, for example, in activist literature promoting "another assault on the AIDS bureaucracy," a demonstration and civil disobedience against the NIH on May 21, 1990, to "protest its midguided drug testing policies." NIH AIDS research is portrayed as "a fiasco, a catastrophe, a morass of red tape and incompetence which kills us daily," and the ACTGs in particular as "a massive, dysfunctional failure in its inept efforts to lengthen and improve the lives of HIV infected people." Several hundred activists presented many demands for substantial changes in research, including immediate testing of all potential treatments; research on AIDS as a whole, rather than an exclusive focus on antiviral treatments against HIV; a move from secrecy to *"glasnost"* by the NIH through opening its meetings and committees to the public, and particularly to

PWAs; immediate disclosure of test results; and an end to "medical apartheid" by broadening enrollment criteria to include present and former drug users, persons of color, and women. In this attempt to "storm the NIH," some eighty-two protesters were arrested, fined, and released for various acts of civil disobedience, including twenty-one who occupied the office of Dr. Daniel Hoth, director of the AIDS division at NIAID (Hilts 1990).[1]

All such efforts to make as many drugs available as quickly as possible, whether pursued through militancy and confrontation or consultation and negotiation, could well be hampered by economic considerations, as was exemplified with the release of AZT. Following federal approval, the annual charge for some three years for this drug ranged between $8,000 and $10,000, meaning that the *only* federally approved treatment for AIDS was beyond the financial means of most PWAs. To protest this situation and draw attention to the refusal of Burroughs-Wellcome, the pharmaceutical manufacturer of AZT, to provide subsidies for indigent patients, even though it had recouped development costs and was achieving a 50 percent profit margin on new sales, four members of ACT UP occupied the office of a corporate executive in April 1989, damaging property with chain saws and drills. The activists were subsequently arrested and charged with trespassing and destruction of private property, but the matter did not end there.

Members of ACT UP, together with representatives from fifteen other AIDS organizations, subsequently met with corporate representatives; this reliance on the model of negotiation failed to change company policy. Nor did ACT UP's call for a nationwide boycott of Burroughs-Wellcome products. Finally, in September 1989, in the role of very visible gadfly, protests were organized at the London, San Francisco, and New York stock exchanges, with activists encouraging investors to sell their stock in the pharmaceutical company. Some two weeks later, Burroughs-Wellcome cut the price of AZT by 20 percent, although the company disclaimed any causal relation (Crossen 1989:A7; Spiers 1989:34; Handelman 1990:82). In January 1990, the FDA halved the recommended dosage of AZT, based on studies that revealed the lower dose was safer and just as effective. This recommendation also meant, of course, that the cumulative cost of AZT would drop substantially.

It is likely that if ability to pay becomes a criterion for access to drugs approved and distributed in the future, the resort to models of protest, followed by attempts at negotiation and then protest, displayed in the activism against Burroughs-Wellcome, will be replicated and on a much larger scale. Alternatively, pharmaceutical companies might be compelled to take preemptive measures to avoid controversy (and unfavorable publicity) over issues of access and cost. For example, the experience of Burroughs-Wellcome has been cited by some as influential in the decision by Bristol-Meyers to release ddI free to five thousand patients who could no longer take AZT (Handelman 1990:89).

The tactics of protest with regard to access to drugs, however small in scope (the brief occupation of one research administrator's or one corporate executive's office is not on the same scale, for example, as the long-term occupation of a university president's office, as in protests against the Vietnam War), have sought to draw attention to fundamental disparities in power and moral issues of fairness. Those persons and institutions with adequate rhetorical, fiscal, and medical resources at their disposal have seemed to keep them out of the reach of those whose resources are scanty by comparison. Yet it is precisely this latter community that has borne the substantial burden and deaths from the AIDS epidemic.

The preceding narrative of indifference and inequity may render intelligible efforts by activists to disrupt political proceedings, commercial traffic, telephone services, and corporate or scientific "business as usual." Yet such tactics are not morally innocuous. Moreover, in spite of, or perhaps because of, success in effecting change attributed to the protest model, the rhetoric of AIDS activism is now advocating even more militant methods, including an "escalation" of tactics, an "uprising" reminiscent of the antiwar protests, and ongoing demonstrations. The question that now needs to be addressed directly is whether activism that crosses the boundaries of peaceable political protest can be morally justifiable. I focus this discussion by concentrating on the issue of justified civil disobedience, although the framework of evaluation I utilize would apply as well to issues of coercion and manipulation expressed, for example, in threats to sabotage clinical research.

Crossing the Line

Civil disobedience raises profound questions of political theory about the nature of political obligation; it assumes that the scope of the moral authority of the state is limited and the obligation to obey the state and its laws is not absolute. The constituent features of civil disobedience are philosophically contested; nevertheless, for purposes of this discussion, I understand civil disobedience to involve public and nonviolent violations of law to protest an actual or proposed law or practice in which the protesters are willing to submit to legal sanctions as punishment for their actions (Childress 1971:11; 1986:94). On this account,

AIDS activists are clearly correct to invoke the concept "civil disobedience" to describe many of their protests and demonstrations.[2] However, specific acts may differ depending on (1) the extent of persuasion and coercion in disobedient acts, (2) the relation of the laws violated to the injustice that is the object of the protest, and (3) the legal and translegal warrants for disobedience. I first illuminate the character of the civil disobedience of AIDS by identifying some comparisons on these points with the historical legacy of civil disobedience in our culture before proceeding to examine the arguments for justified civil disobedience.

Persuasion and Coercion

Acts of civil disobedience may be differentiated according to their reliance on elements of persuasion and education, attitudinal change in others, or coercion to bring about change. Henry David Thoreau, Martin Luther King, Jr., and Mahatma Gandhi, the classic exponents of civil disobedience, all attributed a pedagogical function to civil disobedience. In the essay that brought the term "civil disobedience" into our political and moral vocabulary, Thoreau described his refusal to pay a state poll tax to protest slavery, the Mexican war, and mistreatment of native Americans as "doing my part to educate my fellow-countrymen (Thoreau 1962:100). Similarly, King, who was deeply influenced by Thoreau's essay, acknowledged in his famous "Letter from Birmingham City Jail" that one might break an unjust law and submit to the legal penalty "to arouse the conscience of the community over its injustice . . ." (King 1969:78–79).

The aspiration to use civil disobedience as a means of educating a society that certain laws or policies are inconsistent with other important values is clearly present in the practices of AIDS activists. Indeed, the sociological presupposition of AIDS civil disobedience is that much of our culture is radically unaware of the crises in health care (inadequate treatments, exorbitant costs, restricted access to care) that PWAs confront. This educational rationale in part informs the stress activists have given to designing their disobedient actions in a way that is congenial with coverage by the mass media.

There are, however, different methods by which informing public consciousness can be accomplished, and the techniques of AIDS activists often push beyond persuasive appeals to moral sensitivity to provocative action that may offend moral sensitivity. An important difference arises in this respect from some of the classical exponents of civil disobedience, which focuses on the "civility" of protesters in their attitudes toward those they deem as oppressors. For King, for example, effective nonviolent action required of the lawbreaker a spirit of love and reconciliation toward the other. This redemptive approach was intended to elicit respect and trust that would provide the basis for constructive negotiations. Gandhi, meanwhile, affirmed that the lawbreaker should embody "courtesy" and "gentleness" and seek, if at all possible, "not to embarrass the opponent" (Childress 1971:7).

The contrast with some techniques of AIDS activists could not be more marked on this point. Their intention, not unlike antiwar protesters, is precisely to evoke shame and embarrassment and to expose institutional hypocrisy. Actions born of anger, frustration, and suspicion of government rhetoric are purposely provocative: "A basic feature of [AIDS] demonstrations is that they are *meant* to intrude, to provoke, to irritate, and to offend" (Novick 1989:36). Provocation thus becomes an unsettling, discomforting mode or technique of effecting change on AIDS issues and carries with it risks of alienation rather than reconciliation.

With the exceptions of a few instances of property destruction, for the most part AIDS civil disobedience has been constituted by acts of illegal trespass and die-ins, the AIDS version of sit-ins; as Hugo Adam Bedau has noted, "any government can accommodate this sort of civil disobedience and still survive, no matter how widespread it becomes" (Bedau 1969:22). The coercive dimensions of civil disobedience emerge when such actions seek to effect change primarily through disrupting the "as usual" operations of government or other institutions, whether scientific, business, or ecclesiastical. It is this feature of designed disruption that leads many commentators to view Thoreau's tax resistance as more laden with coercive than educational intent, for as Bedau comments, the nature of tax refusal "is to deny to government its capacity to govern, to administer and enforce *any* of its laws" (Bedau 1969:22). AIDS activists are not likely, of course, to be in the forefront of advocating tax resistance to protest institutional indifference or denial of access to experimental drugs, since one primary motivation for activism is to direct more taxpayer money to the research efforts against AIDS. My point here instead is that acts of civil disobedience can assume coercive features to the extent that disruption rather than education is emphasized by activists.

In practice, there is likely to be a complex mix of education, provocation, and coercion, and indeed, as I suggested previously, AIDS activists may rely on more provocative or coercive measures as an instrument to achieve the possibilities for persuasion. There is, for example, an intriguing parallel between King and AIDS activists on the relation between illegal and legal tactics: "Nonviolent direct action seeks to create such a crisis and establish such creative tension that a community that has constantly refused to negotiate is forced to confront the issue" (King 1969:75). In King's view, then, as well as for some AIDS activists, the communal "crisis" and "tension" evoked by civil disobedience can facilitate mutual dialogue and even participation of the disenfranchised within the majority system.

Direct and Indirect Disobedience

A further distinction can be illustrated by contrasting Thoreau's refusal with a classical source for reflection on civil disobedience, Sophocles' play *Antigone*. In giving her brother a proper burial, Antigone *directly* violated the specific edict of the king, one she considered contrary to a principle of justice.

> Creon: "Now tell me, in as few words as you can, did you know the order forbidding such an act?"
> Antigone: "I knew it, naturally. It was plain enough."
> Creon: "And yet you dared to contravene it?"
> Antigone: "Yes. That order did not come from God. Justice, that dwells with the gods below, knows no such law. I did not think your edicts strong enough to overrule the unwritten unalterable laws of God and heaven, you being only a man" (Sophocles 1947:138).

Thoreau's action, by contrast, bore only an *indirect* relation to the objects of his protest. He was concerned, not with the validity of the poll tax law, but with the injustice of various social practices. Similarly, as Herbert Spiers acknowledges, the laws regarding trespassing and respect for property are not in themselves the focus of AIDS protests but are violated by activists to focus attention on more systematic injustices: "The laws that have been broken are, in the main, unrelated to the epidemic. . . . Such actions bring AIDS political issues to the fore . . ." (Spiers 1989:34). That is, unlike Antigone, King, and Gandhi, but like Thoreau, AIDS activists violate just laws to protest other unjust or inequitable social policies and practices, such as an inadequate provision of health care.

The indirect character of AIDS civil disobedience helps explain the highly symbolic and theatrical nature of such protests, for as James Childress has noted, "the communication of indirect resistance depends on a symbolic connection between the act and the cause" (Childress 1971:33). Die-ins or red tape do not so much rely in the suasion of reasoned moral discourse as on analogies and metaphors that strike the imagination and consciousness. The risk that theatrical, indirect disobedience runs is, however, suggested by Robert Brustein's criticism of similar tactics by some protesters during the Vietnam War: "[W]hat may have been originally stimulated by a desire to dramatize a cause for the sake of curing an injustice now often seems like theatre for its own sake, destructive in its aim, negative in its effect, performed with no particular aim in mind" (Brustein 1971:22).

Legal and Translegal Warrants

The traditions of civil disobedience in our culture have typically distinguished the warrants for acts of illegal public protest according to whether appeals for authorization are made to positive law, such as the U.S. Constitution, or to translegal sources, such as religion or morality. A prominent warrant for civil disobedience in many of its classical exponents, including Antigone, Thoreau, and King, is a translegal appeal, the notion that the validity of positive laws must be assessed by a higher moral standard and that laws that do not conform to this standard may be considered "unjust" and not binding on action. It is perhaps best exemplified by King, who was in effect drawing on classical political and religious distinctions: "One may well ask, 'How can you advocate breaking some laws and obeying others?' The answer is found in the fact that there are two types of laws: There are *just* and there are *unjust* laws. I would agree with Saint Augustine that 'An unjust law is no law at all.' . . . A just law is a man-made law that squares with the moral law or the law of God. An unjust law is a code that is out of harmony with the moral law" (King 1969:77).

This particular translegal appeal occasionally surfaces in the rhetoric of AIDS activists, but although some activists may have once been tutored in the practice of civil disobedience by an associate of King, their public discourse does not make any explicit attempt to locate the civil disobedience of AIDS within the moral parameters outlined by King. This is in part because the indirect nature of AIDS civil disobedience limits the utility of this kind of appeal. The particular laws typically violated by AIDS activists are not deemed unjust, and so the language of "unjust law" tends to be restricted more to antisodomy statutes rather than associated with AIDS-related legislation or policy. Passage of compulsory screening or quarantine measures might, of course, make this appeal more prominent in activist discourse.

This does not mean that other appeals, whether to warrants in positive law or to an immoral "state of affairs," are not available for AIDS activists. What is unclear, however, is whether activists have given sufficient attention to these alternatives. Spiers, a founding member of ACT UP, has observed that "there is not an articulated policy or justification" for civil disobedience among AIDS activists but nevertheless maintains that its use "falls well within established traditions" of political, legal, and moral reasoning (Spiers 1989:34). This latter claim remains to be examined, but in speaking with activists and reading their literature, one is often left with an impression that advocacy of civil disobedience is not combined with an acknowledgment that such acts cross a moral boundary, the obligation to obey the law, and require special justification. Civil disobedience is instead often portrayed as one of many alternatives in a spectrum of tactics that activists may employ to press their demands on the political and medical establishments, its use more conditioned by pragmatic circumstances than by recognition of its moral dimensions.

Despite his appeal to "established traditions," Spiers affirms that the civil disobedience of AIDS has a "unique" justification, the historical experience of neglect (Spiers 1989:34). It is not clear why this constitutes a unique moral orientation, since King of course advocated the cause of a historically oppressed people precisely in this fashion. The historical precedent frequently invoked by activists is not, however, the civil rights movement but rather the persecution of the Jews under Nazi Germany. That story of an oppressed people who did not prevail in resisting evil and injustice has for some activists furnished a hermeneutical frame by which to portray what is morally and existentially at stake in the AIDS epidemic and in civil disobedience as one practical response, namely, community survival. This point will become evident as we examine and reconstruct the patterns of justification by AIDS activists along moral criteria—just cause, last resort, reasonable expectation of success, proportionality, and limitation—embedded in the traditions of civil disobedience.

The Hermeneutics of Genocide

Just Cause

The fundamental, though not sufficient, criterion for the justification of civil disobedience is to justify the cause, "which usually consists of showing that a law or policy is unjust or that certain conditions in the society need to be rectified" (Childress 1971:169). The ends do have to justify the means, but this does not entail that the ends themselves are immune from moral scrutiny. Nevertheless, the overarching objectives of AIDS activists to "end the AIDS epidemic," to cite the language of

ACT UP, or the proximate end of equitable access to drugs and eventually therapies for AIDS should not be a matter of great controversy for our society.

The moral question raised by the standard of just cause is why activists believe achieving these objectives at least in part requires civil disobedience rather than conventional political methods. The obligation to obey the law may be limited, for example, by appealing to a "higher good: the amelioration of suffering and the saving of lives" (Spiers 1989:34). Yet, it is unclear why the practical conduct entailed by these imperatives is necessarily civil disobedience, since we engage in many activities to relieve suffering and save lives, such as the practice of medicine, that do not require illegal acts. I here want to reconstruct some claims of activists in a manner congruent with the idea of just cause in the traditions of civil disobedience.

A cause might first be considered "just" if it involves actions taken to *vindicate rights* that have been wrongfully denied. Thus, in the context of AIDS, it could be argued that, given the experience of historical neglect, the rights of PWAs to health care generally and to AIDS drugs specifically have been routinely denied. Civil disobedience may therefore be validated as a method to affirm these rights.

The difficulty with such an argument is that it seems to warrant a singular exception for PWAs, rather than bring their situation into conformity with the health care status and rights of other citizens. As illustrated by the scandal of 31.5 million medically indigent persons in this country, we have no guaranteed political-legal right to health care in our society. Without intending to condone, let alone endorse, this reality, my claim is that the justification of civil disobedience on the grounds that the positive rights of PWAs to health care have been violated assumes the validity of a right that our society has yet to acknowledge. Moreover, although there may be an accepted right to validated therapies, such as prescription drugs covered by insurance or Medicaid, it is far from clear that there is a right to *nonvalidated* therapies or experimental drugs. Hence, an argument that AIDS activists are justified in resorting to civil disobedience based on the denial of health care rights must first show both that the rights in question are recognized in social and political institutions and that PWAs have been singularly excluded from access to health care.[3]

A second interpretation of just cause that seems relevant to the civil disobedience of AIDS concerns the *protection of innocent persons from violent attack*. This reasoning would likewise focus on the historical failure of government and related public health agencies to "protect" adequately many of its citizens from the ravages of an epidemic.

On this account, civil disobedience would be grounded, not in the denial of a positive right to health care, but rather in the more fundamental negative right of self-defense. As Spiers has put it, "If only by its inaction and inattentiveness to the plight of afflicted people, the government betrays its fundamental disregard of some citizens' health and lives, then prima facie they are justified in taking extreme actions in their own defense" (Spiers 1989:34).

It is important to see that, on this account, the right of self-defense is claimed, not against HIV, but against *the government*. The contested issue here is how this institutional inaction might be construed as a form of "violence." How does the failure to prevent harm from a virus itself become a form of harm? That such a connection is in fact made by some activists, even if inchoately, is conveyed in their more evocative rhetoric. For example, reacting to then-President Reagan's first public address on AIDS, Kramer has written: "There's only one word to describe his monumental disdain for the dead and the dying: genocide" (Kramer 1989:158). Similarly, Spiers has maintained, "Passive genocide, by means of neglect, is believed by many activists to be *the correct characterization* of governmental policy on AIDS" (Spiers 1989:34; my emphasis). The use by some activists of the language of "murderer" to describe certain political officials or agency administrators, as well as "holocaust" or "apartheid" to characterize the cultural response to AIDS, likewise expresses a sense that the social context of AIDS is permeated by violence.

This hermeneutics of genocide raises three difficult substantive issues. The first involves the kinds of assumptions necessary to allow us to make conceptual sense of a phrase like "passive genocide." The moral point is actually the AIDS version of the common debate in philosophical ethics over whether there is a morally relevant difference between omissions and commissions, or between "letting die" and "killing." We may well grant that there are situations in which it is permissible to allow a person to die from the natural disease process of a terminal illness. Nevertheless, if death could have been prevented, and those in special and influential positions of authority (whether a physician, a researcher, or a politician) took no or insufficient action to prevent the death, then we might understand the death as "premature" and consider those who could have acted but did not as morally culpable and even causally responsible for the death. Since the outcome is death, the failure to act in such circumstances can be construed as the moral equivalant of directly killing a person.[4]

This scenario presents in microcosm what some activists believe to be true more generally about our culture's response, politically and scientifically, to AIDS. It assumes that much of the harm, misery, and suffering from AIDS could have been prevented by responsible leadership and responsive research. Yet, our common discourse about what constitutes an act of "killing" or "violence" not only focuses on the *outcome* of an act, such as death, but also on the *intention* behind the act. AIDS activists need to establish, then, that the indifference of various leaders and institutions toward PWAs and AIDS generally is motivated by an *intention to kill*. It is not at all clear, however, that such a position has been successfully established.

Some activists, to be sure, have seemed to make precisely this claim that indifference masks a lethal intentionality. For example, Kramer contends: "I have come to believe that genocide is occurring: that we are witnessing . . . the systematic, *planned* annihilation of some others with *the avowed purpose* of eradicating an undesirable portion of the population" (Kramer 1989:263; my emphasis). Yet, the tenuous nature of this claim is revealed by how Kramer subsequently contradicts himself: "Ronald Reagan, Dr. Bowen [former Secretary of Health and Human Services], Dr. Wyngaarden [ex-NIH director], doctors at the NIH and FDA, are equal to Hitler and his Nazi doctors performing their murderous experiments in the camps, *not because of similar intentions,* but because of similar outcomes" (Kramer 1989:270; my emphasis). However, if the claim about intentionality is abandoned, then the analogy itself seems seriously flawed.

In the hermeneutics of genocide, moreover, a second issue is why action taken in self-defense should be *limited* to civil disobedience; surely, if activists and the communities they represent are convinced that their experience of AIDS is analogous to the immeasurable evil of genocide or holocaust, then nonviolent disobedience seems a rather tame response. Two questions then emerge, namely, whether practices of nonviolent activism are fully coherent with the evocative rhetoric of activists and whether the rhetoric itself implicitly contains a warrant for crossing the boundary from nonviolence to violence. Kramer's call for riots, while not endorsed by activist groups, is at least coherent with this hermeneutical frame, for implicit in the language of genocide is a moral logic that requires more forceful action than civil disobedience.

A final consideration, related to the preceding point, is whether the hermeneutics of genocide is an *appropriate* interpretation of the cultural response to AIDS. There is a strong sense in which political and moral discourse about the disease is simply impoverished when the principal interpretative frames are appropriated from contexts such as Nazi Germany, in which several million people died involuntarily as a direct consequence of formalized policies of mass murder. This is not at all to recommend insensitivity toward those who have died and have suffered in various ways from the epidemic, both in this country and worldwide. However, compassion, that is, suffering with others, does not require a discourse about the disease that disservices our moral language and memory.

Last Resort

The functional and symbolic purposes of law in our society entail that its violation by acts of civil disobedience should be a last resort. That is, all other reasonable alternatives to redress wrongs and grievances, including appeals to political representatives, recourse through the courts, and legally permitted assemblies, protests, and demonstrations, should be exhausted before resort to civil disobedience is advocated. The historical narrative outlined above and the reasons given by activists for their actions suggest that for the most part AIDS activism has followed such a moral chronology, more confrontational tactics being adopted only after six years of silence from the nation's leading political official, accompanied by what appeared to be an interminable drug trial and review process. If at times perhaps not the only resort for activists, it is at least quite clear that civil disobedience was not the first alternative.

I indicated above that the public protest model, exemplified by civil disobedience, is designed in part to effect change through bringing about negotiation and dialogue, in which activists themselves assume consultative or advisory roles in the policymaking process. The difficult question activists now confront is whether, given the substantial expenditures for current research on AIDS, as contrasted with even five years ago, and given that policymakers and researchers have manifested a greater openness to community concerns, there now exist alternatives within the political and medical establishments that render the use of civil disobedience unnecessary. For example, now that PWAs and their advocates participate on the NIAID's Advisory Council, the AIDS Research Advisory Committee, and the AIDS Clinical Drug Development Committee (NIAID 1990:3), it seems reasonable to ask whether such channels would prove more efficacious in realizing the objectives of activists.

To be sure, from the standpoint of AIDS activists, whatever successes have been achieved, whether institutional enfranchisement or expanded drug distribution, are insignificant relative to the ultimate goal of eradicating AIDS. Moreover, to the extent that civil disobedience is seen as expediting political and regulatory changes, such successes will feed demand for similar actions. Nevertheless, one goal of a morally motivated movement of civil disobedience is to seek its own abolition over time due to changes in laws and policies.

Reasonable Expectation of Success

As I noted initially, public judgments about AIDS civil disobedience, both pro and con, invoke (almost exclusively) a criterion of effectiveness. Yet, such judgments are typically made retrospectively, while the standard of "reasonable expectation" requires prospective assessments. Evaluating the effectiveness of civil disobedience in advance necessarily involves two questions: *what* this tactic is designed to achieve and *whose* assessments count. This latter question is significant, since the prospect of success in civil disobedience will often hinge on a variety of moral and prudential factors beyond the control of activists, including the willingness of opponents to tolerate confrontational action. It is important then to consider several perspectives on success in the context of AIDS activism.

It would be unreasonable to expect the civil disobedience of AIDS to achieve the overriding objective of eradicating the epidemic, in a manner analogous to the effect like protests had in bringing America's involvement in Vietnam to closure. A lethal virus is not going to negotiate a peace treaty. There are, however, several more proximate goals that civil disobedience might accomplish, which could provide the conditions by which a successful war on HIV is waged. For example, the success of AIDS civil disobedience could be assessed with respect to its pedagogical purposes. The role of the public media is crucial in this respect, and so it is not surprising to find activists asserting that they have "concentrated on protests and civil disobedience that garner considerable media attention" or that "civil disobedience often succeeds in focusing major media attention" on such issues as access to treatments, health care, or health education (Novick 1989:36, Spiers; 1989:34). It may not make a difference to activists whether the ensuing attention is favorable or not (often it is not) so long as such issues are raised in a public forum.

A second reasonable expectation of AIDS activists might be the extent to which civil disobedience impresses the necessity for dialogue and coordination among several parties—policymakers, researchers, activist groups—that have previously worked at cross-purposes. At times, civil disobedience might be the direct instrument of bringing about a process of negotiation and consultation in which the activists themselves are invited to participate in the dialogue. In other instances, civil disobedience may be indirectly effective in that it makes noncon-frontational organizations that rely on conventional political channels more palatable as negotiating partners. As Alvin Novick has expressed it, "those who participate in civil disobedience may be understood as the 'bad guy' of a 'good guy-bad guy' team, for irritation and annoyance drive society to listen more sincerely to calmer advocates" (Novick 1989:36; Span 1989:D4). That is, even if more militant activists and protesters are excluded, civil disobedience may nevertheless work to instigate the consultative process necessary for a coordinated AIDS effort that achieves the goals desired by activists.

Is it reasonable to expect that civil disobedience will effect change, not only on initiating the negotiating process, but also on its outcomes, such as expanded programs of research, expedited review policies, and innovative drug distribution projects? It should be recalled here how ACT UP has retrospectively attributed changes in FDA policy directly to civil disobedience. As Carl Cohen has remarked, however, "deeply committed protesters are tempted to overestimate the effectiveness of what they do, crediting to their disobedience every change in the desired direction" (Cohen 1989:24). Indeed, AIDS policy changes are typically the fruit of the negotiating process, and acts of civil disobedi-ence may have only an indirect influence. That at least appears to be the view of prominent researchers, upon whom the success of AIDS activism is partially contingent. For example, Dr. Anthony Fauci, who as director of the NIAID is responsible for oversight of the ACTGs, has observed: "When they [members of ACT UP] were *just* protesting, they would often make medically or scientifically unreasonable de-mands. But over the past year, they've adopted a stance of well-in-formed articulate activism. They give us a very good grass-roots per-spective of the needs of the community and how what's available can best be applied to the people affected by the epidemic" (Crossen 1989:A9; my emphasis).

I have identified ways in which civil disobedience is portrayed as an *instrument* to achieve particular ends of AIDS activists. Even if the prospective realization of these objectives might be unreasonable, how-ever, civil disobedience might still be considered an effective means to express or *symbolize* certain values, such as solidarity with others, a community legacy of fighting for survival rather than passivity, or an unwillingness to accept death as an inevitable outcome from the dis-ease. This distinction between instrumental and expressive or symbolic civil disobedience can be illustrated by considering an issue on which AIDS activists do not speak with one voice.

The standard of effectiveness requires as a corollary that the means be carefully modulated to the ends sought, and on one account, "AIDS activists have proven themselves to be extremely conscientious in the planning and execution of their activities" (Spiers 1989:35). Yet another activist, who participated in the civil disobedience and protests against Burroughs-Wellcome, has commented: "Nine-tenths of [ACT UP's] actions aren't very well targeted. But, so what? If we want to vent our anger, I say, let us. No one dies because of us" (Crossen 1989:A9). It goes without saying that the latter approach flouts the criterion of *reasonable* expectation of success, construed instrumentally. Even if ineffective in that sense, however, civil disobedience may be a symbol of outrage against a political and medical system perceived to be unresponsive to the needs of PWAs.

A further caveat is that civil disobedience may make the prospect of success tilt toward the unreasonable. Although by its very dramatic nature, deliberate acts of lawbreaking will command media attention, in the eyes of those who are the object of the protest, whether politicians or health care administrators, civil disobedience may be viewed as an inappropriate form of intimidation in a democratic polity. A real risk run by civil disobedience is that it may alienate the very individuals whose participation is necessary to achieve objectives broader than the initiation of process and thus be counterproductive. As one AIDS researcher has commented, militant AIDS activism is "reaching a point of diminishing returns. The concern that many of us have had is that they [ACT UP] are so alienating, so disruptive, that people might leave the field" (Kolata 1990; Specter 1990).

Proportionality

At whatever level the prospects of success from civil disobedience are deemed reasonable, the anticipated gains must be weighed against the almost certain production of negative outcomes, including erosion of respect for the authority and bindingness of law, or what Cohen describes as "injury" to the social fabric that affirms the values of democratic process (Cohen 1989:25). In one respect, of course, for those who believe the only outcome of silence is death, any achievement of civil disobedience, or even mere participation in symbolic action, will constitute an overall benefit or gain. Nevertheless, the benefits of drawing media attention to AIDS issues may, for example, be offset if activists are portrayed as making "unreasonable demands" or acting in such a manner as to contribute to their further isolation. In addition, using civil disobedience as a method to effect changes in drug research and regulatory policy might be outweighed by the additional risks assumed by PWAs from nonvalidated drugs, including the risk of even earlier death.

Moreover, the standard of proportionality requires an inclusive accounting and should address how prospective goods and harms will be distributed among various persons and communities. The scope of moral concern must therefore be broader than activists and their communities. If, for example, activists are correct in directly attributing drug policy changes or access to more nearly adequate health care services to civil disobedience, these benefits need to be evaluated against the burdens imposed on others, especially third parties, by the disruption of legislative debates over, for example, benefits to volunteer firefighters, or the diversion of scarce health care resources from other needy patients, or the additional costs borne by taxpayers to fund expanded programs of research and health services.

Limitation

A final standard for moral assessment of civil disobedience is constituted by several different senses of limitation. One issue anticipated above concerns *discrimination* regarding the objects of acts of civil disobedience. If, for example, politicians and researchers are deemed primarily responsible for the plight of PWAs, it is morally unfair to engage in actions, such as disrupting commercial traffic, whose effects fall directly on third parties. Such methods use other persons merely as means or instruments to achieve the ends of activists.

A second sense of limitation is concerned with whether crossing the moral boundary from legal to illegal actions risks crossing a next line from nonviolence to *violence*. I have claimed that this possibility is implicit in the hermeneutics of genocide, and many activists have explicitly not ruled out the eventual possibility of violence, including "extensive damage to property, or . . . injury to people," depending on the subsequent course of the epidemic and the responsiveness of government and the research community (Spiers 1989:35). Other activists have raised the prospect of "armed resistance," and in a provocative passage whose implications for AIDS activism he does not elaborate, Kramer favorably contrasts the terror tactics of the Israeli organization Irgun with the passivity of gay men: "It was an underground guerilla army, and its members were extremely disciplined and daring. They started fires. They threw bombs. They kidnapped. They assassinated. They executed their enemies. They won" (Kramer 1989:191). The moral question confronting AIDS activists is where the line will be drawn beyond which they will not go to achieve objectives of public education and access to health care services; what kinds of tactics are truly methods of "last resort"? Needless to say, resistance that takes the form of violence requires a stricter burden of justification than nonviolent actions do.

It is also necessary to examine the *proportion* between particular acts of civil disobedience and the general objectives of AIDS activism. The sense of proportion is observed in nonviolent protests that target those institutions that can most effectively alleviate the health care dimensions of the epidemic, such as the FDA or NIH. It was clearly violated in the most infamous AIDS-related civil disobedience action, the "Stop the Church" protest jointly organized by ACT UP and WHAM! (Women's Health Action and Mobilization) at St. Patrick's Cathedral on December 10, 1989, to protest Roman Catholic teaching regarding condoms, safe sex education, and abortions. The demonstration, which drew some forty-five hundred persons, included die-ins staged during the homily of John Cardinal O'Connor, followed by screams of "Stop the Murder" and the crumbling of the communion wafer by one ACT UP member.

Although ACT UP's "Capsule History" does not mention the incident, other than to note that "111 people [were] arrested, 43 inside the cathedral for a dramatic 'die-in' at the Cardinal's feet," it reflects a heightened sense of the moral limits of civil disobedience that this disruption of a worship service was criticized even by prominent members of the coalition (ACT UP 1990:3; Handelman 1990:90,116). A morally vigorous civil disobedience campaign involves acknowledging that protests cannot be an end in themselves but must convey a constructive point to an audience who may not know or share the overarching objectives of activists.

Prospects for Public Discourse

As Cohen has argued, "the justification of deliberate law-breaking is never easy, and in a reasonably healthy democracy it is exceedingly difficult" (Cohen 1989:25). It is finally not clear that the civil disobedience of AIDS sufficiently meets the burden of justification constituted by the criteria of just cause, last resort, reasonable expectation of success, proportionality, and limitation. This assessment reflects assumptions about both the nature of civil disobedience and the nature of moral and political justification. Because civil disobedience is a public act with social consequences, the *audience* of justification cannot be confined to the communities activists represent but must necessarily be broadened to encompass the larger society. In this wider public discourse, it is highly unlikely that the polemical rhetoric of "genocide," or associated language of "holocaust," "murderer," or "apartheid," will resonate with any significance. Indeed, it is much more probable that the polemic will be dismissed *together* with the legitimate claims that lie behind it. The challenge for activists is to construct a public discourse about the disease that conveys both the experience of injustice and an invitation to discussion rather than polarization.

The hermeneutics of genocide raises as well suspicions about the sincerity and complicity of activists. It is not, I have argued, a fully coherent position to meet alleged institutionalized genocide with non-violent protests. Beyond this point, however, it is disingenuous to accuse the NIH of genocide, as in the May 1990 protest, for example, when prominent activists themselves have served as consultants and members of NIAID AIDS research committees. The discourse of polemic seems to erode the validity of the very proposals and policies activists have been instrumental in formulating, for they are then portrayed either as negotiating with the moral equivalent of a Mengele or as having been coopted by the institution.

The available opportunities to construct a health care system that is more responsive to the special needs of PWAs present a second challenge for activists, namely, determining whether their objectives will stand a greater chance of being achieved by working within the system or dissociating themselves from it. It is more than likely that the AIDS epidemic will not be eradicated in the immediate future; now that their voice has been and is being heard in policymaking, activists may serve a more constructive function through consultation rather than confrontation. This is not to say that a healthy society does not need protesting voices, but the reality of the matter is that when such voices are shrill, unrelenting, and uncharitable, they risk further isolation.

The moral and political task of activists is then to engage in genuine public discourse about AIDS with an audience broader than their own particular communities. But the prospects of public discourse first presuppose that activists and their communities are accepted by society, particularly as embodied in its political and institutional leaders, as constituting part of the "public" that can rightfully demand claims to social goods, including access to health care, and demand accountability when such claims are neglected or ignored. There is, then, a correlative civil responsibility to treat PWAs respectfully as citizens rather than as pariahs. It is perhaps not surprising that AIDS activists have felt compelled to be so shrill given their outsider status relative to the dominant cultural ethos. Indeed, it is the nature not only of HIV but also of values embedded in this ethos and in our institutions that has made AIDS so intractable.

Political officials have a public moral responsibility to exercise courageous leadership and statesmanship in addressing the societal challenges of AIDS. With the exception of former Surgeon General C. Everett Koop, a lone voice in a moral wilderness, few at the federal level have shown a capacity for anything other than trying to make AIDS an invisible disease. Symbolic actions can be important in shaping a social vision on AIDS; it is certainly commendable for public figures to visit pediatric AIDS care units, but an even more significant step would be visible meetings with representatives of the communities most afflicted by AIDS. Such actions not only would display political courage but also would convey to society that even its most disparaged citizens are not to be excluded from the community of moral concern. In this respect, it is distressing that many prominent federal officials, including President Bush, chose not to attend or address the Sixth International Conference on AIDS in San Francisco. Activists will surely see their absence as a sign that less than complete political commitment persists and that even after a decade of death and dollars, the medical and moral challenges of AIDS are not being seriously addressed. It is precisely such political distancing from AIDS that informs the adoption of civil disobedience and other disruptive tactics by activists.

In addition to symbolic actions, political leaders need to implement programs to ensure that PWAs receive an adequate level of basic medical care. This is admittedly a difficult task in an era of many demands for scarce resources. It is, however, a revealing sign of the moral integrity of a culture that, rather than abandon the ill to fend for themselves, it binds itself to the ill through practices of caring. For their part, pharmaceutical companies should not see in desperate patients an opportunity to increase profit margins but should make treatments available at reasonable cost and, perhaps with government support, provide subsidies to indigent patients.

We may view PWAs as victims of a lethal disease, but they are also often *moral victims,* for our cultural response to AIDS has often concentrated on solutions appropriate for an ideal world. In this imperfect world, however, the reality of addressing unassumed sexual responsibility, addictive drugs, prejudice, and even disease is unavoidable, and it is such a world that must be understood as constituting the legitimate concerns of activists. An openness to a genuine dialogue in the face of death will truly be revealing of the moral character of our culture.

NOTES

1. NIAID director Anthony Fauci issued a substantial document in advance of the demonstration refuting in some detail the "inaccurate statements, allegations, and demands" in ACT UP literature about the ACTG's accomplishments (NIAID: 1990).

2. At times, the language of civil disobedience is used rather indiscriminately, as in the following example: "Gay men and lesbians were accustomed to 'private civil disobedience' and had learned long ago to be defiant of law. . . . Oppression teaches people to dare to defy unjust laws" (Novick 1989:36). The conceptual reasoning here is that for those persons who have historically acted outside the law, civil disobedience regarding AIDS raises no new or distinctive set of moral considerations. Such an argument is misleading, however, to the extent that civil disobedience entails public rather than private acts and thereby has *social* ramifications and consequences, including the need for public justification, and also because it involves a willingness to assume, rather than evade, sanctions or punishment for legal wrongdoing.

3. This is not to deny that homosexuals have not been allowed to claim certain other civil rights, but issues of discrimination in the area of housing, employment, family life, etc., pertain more to "gay" activism than "AIDS" activism, a distinction AIDS activists have themselves insisted upon. The right to freedom from discrimination based on sexual orientation is, of course, based fundamentally in the negative right of privacy, whereas, as I have emphasized, the claim of a right to health care involves the assertion of a positive right.

4. In trying to account for the activist language of "genocide," "murderer," and "holocaust," I am attributing to activists an understanding of "violence" as an institutionalized condition of affairs and not simply a discrete act of directly killing a person. For an exposition of this general account of violence, see Harris 1974.

REFERENCES

ACT UP (AIDS Coalition To Unleash Power) 1990. *A Capsule History of ACT UP*, pp. 1–4.

Annas, George J. 1990. Faith (Healing), Hope, and Charity at the FDA: The Politics of AIDS Drug Trials. In Lawrence O. Gostin, ed., *AIDS and the Health Care System*, pp. 183–194. New Haven: Yale University Press.

Bayer, Ronald. 1983. Gays and the Stigma of Bad Blood. *Hastings Center Report* (April) 13(2):5–7.

Bayer, Ronald. 1989. *Private Acts, Social Consequences: AIDS and the Politics of Public Health*. New York: Free Press.

Bedau, Hugo Adam, ed. 1969. *Civil Disobedience: Theory and Practice*. Indianapolis: Bobbs-Merrill.

Brustein, Robert. 1971. *Revolution as Theatre*. New York: Liveright.

Chase, Marilyn. 1990. AIDS Activists in San Francisco Shout Down Secretary of Health and Human Services Secretary's Speech. *Wall Street Journal* (June 25), p. B4.

Childress, James F. 1971. *Civil Disobedience and Political Obligation: A Study in Christian Social Ethics*. New Haven: Yale University Press.

Childress, James F. 1986. Civil Disobedience. In James F. Childress and John

Macquarrie, eds., *The Westminster Dictionary of Christian Ethics*, pp. 94–95. Philadelphia: The Westminster Press.

Cohen, Carl. 1989. Militant Morality: Civil Disobedience and Bioethics. *Hastings Center Report* (November/December), 19(6):23–25.

Crimp, Douglas. 1989. AIDS: Cultural Analysis/Cultural Activism. In Douglas Crimp, ed., *AIDS: Cultural Analysis, Cultural Activism*, pp. 3–16. Cambridge, Mass.: The MIT Press.

Crossen, Cynthia. 1989. AIDS Activist Group Harasses and Provokes to Make Its Point. *Wall Street Journal* (December 7), pp. A1,7.

Eigo, Jim. 1989. Treatment and Data Update. ACT UP Memorandum, October 23.

Gross, Jane. 1990. Protest, Not Poignancy, Marks AIDS Gathering. *New York Times* (June 21), p. B5.

Handelman, David. 1990. ACT UP in Anger. *Rolling Stone Magazine* (March 8), pp. 80–90,116.

Harrington, Mark. 1990. Anatomy of a Disaster. *The Village Voice* (March 13), pp. 4,5.

Harris, John. 1974. The Marxist Conception of Violence. *Philosophy & Public Affairs* (Winter) 3(2):192–220.

Hilts, Philip J. 1990. 82 Held in Protest on Pace of AIDS Research. *New York Times* (May 22), p. C2.

Hughes, Kyle. 1990. AIDS Activists Protest at State Capitol. *Reporter-Dispatch* (March 29), p. A13.

King, Jr., Martin Luther. 1969. Letter from Birmingham City Jail. In Hugo Adam Bedau, ed., *Civil Disobedience: Theory and Practice*, pp. 72–89.

Kolata, Gina. 1990. Advocates' Tactics on AIDS Issues Provoking Warnings of a Backlash. *New York Times* (March 11) p. IV:5.

Kramer, Larry. 1989. *Reports from the Holocaust: The Making of an AIDS Activist*. New York: St. Martin's Press.

Kramer, Larry. 1990. A Call to Riot. *OutWeek* (March 14), pp. 36–38.

NIAID (National Institute of Allergy and Infectious Diseases). 1990. NIAID Responds to ACT UP Allegations and Demands. Office of Communications, NIAID, National Institutes of Health (May 16), pp. 1–6.

Novick, Alvin. 1989. Civil Disobedience in Time of AIDS. *Hastings Center Report* (November/December), 19(6):35–36.

Palca, Joseph. 1989. AIDS Drug Trials Enter New Age. *Science* (October 6), 246:19–21.

Shilts, Randy. 1987. *And the Band Played On: Politics, People, and the AIDS Epidemic*. New York: St. Martin's Press.

Specter, Michael. 1990. More Theatrics Than Science. *Washington Post Health* (June 26), p. 7.

Specter, Michael and Malcolm Gladwell. 1990. Activists Block Streets to Disrupt AIDS Conference. *The Washington Post* (June 20), p. A4.

Sophocles, 1947. Antigone. E. F. Watling, trans. *The Theban Plays*, pp. 126–162. Baltimore: Penguin Books.

Span, Paula. 1989. Getting Militant about AIDS. *The Washington Post* (March 28), pp. D1,4.

Spiers, Herbert R. 1989. AIDS and Civil Disobedience. *Hastings Center Report* (November/December), 19(6):34–35.

The Latest Word. 1990. *Hastings Center Report* (January/February), 20(1):56.

Thoreau, Henry David. 1962. Civil Disobedience. In Joseph Wood Krutch, ed., *Walden and Other Writings*, pp. 85–104. New York: Bantam Books.

Verhovek, Sam Howe. 1990. 80 Are Seized in AIDS Protest to Seek Funds. *New York Times* (March 29), p.B6.

8. AIDS and the Physician-Patient Relationship

ROBERT J. LEVINE

Do PHYSICIANS HAVE a duty to treat patients with AIDS? What an astonishing question! Not since the great plagues of earlier centuries has it been asked whether physicians must treat patients with any specific disease (D. Fox 1988; Rosenberg 1989). Physicians of the modern era had good reason to believe that this question was safely relegated to the archives of history. Astonishing or not, this is a question that has in recent years been asked very frequently. There has been a vast outpouring of commentaries, analyses, and policy recommendations in response to this question.

This chapter is not an attempt to respond directly to the question of whether physicians have a duty to treat patients with AIDS. Rather, it is an exploration of the social and professional settings in which the question is asked in order to facilitate understanding of why it is asked. This exploration is conducted in the form of a tour through the formation of the physician-patient relationship from the initial encounter to the maturation of the fully developed relationship. We shall notice that in every moment of this process the attitudes and behaviors of both physicians and patients are altered profoundly by such factors as fear, prejudice, and resentment of, e.g., unfamiliar and burdensome procedures. These alterations are displayed by comparing and contrasting the physician-patient relationship during the AIDS epidemic with the traditional relationship as it existed before the advent of AIDS.

Because our question is about the duty to treat, I pay particular attention to the attitudes and behaviors of the physicians.[1] I highlight those factors that cause many physicians to be hesitant and some even hostile about assuming this responsibility. If it were not for these factors, there would be no reason to ask about a duty to treat.

But this is not exclusively a story of the reluctant and unwilling physicians whom I believe are a minority group within the medical profession. And this is not only a story of patients who are either infected or at risk of infection with human immunodeficiency virus (HIV). No patient or physician can escape noticing that AIDS as a disease entity and the AIDS epidemic as a social phenomenon have had profound and far-reaching effects on the physician-patient relationship.

Before proceeding I acknowledge some of my relevant biases. The texture of the discussion in this chapter reflects my commitment to the position that good physicians experience a sense of responsibility with regard to serving patients—all patients, including those who have or who are at risk of contracting HIV infection. Their sense of responsibility typically derives from a recognition of what it means to be a physician and from a deep concern for the well-being of their fellow human beings—a concern that motivated them to become physicians in the first place. These are not the physicians who have asked or who have caused others to ask about whether there is a duty to treat patients with HIV infection.[2] Such physicians do not find the wellsprings of their sense of responsibility in the legalistic notions of rights and duties. Rather, they are more inclined to be responsive to such statements of ideals as: "Worthy to serve the suffering."[3]

Having said this, I must add that I am not without sympathy for some physicians who do not behave as I think a good physician should. It is hard to be a good physician when paralyzed by fear of infection or wearied to the point of burnout. This discussion will reflect my sympathy with such physicians just as it will reflect my antipathy with regard to the bigots.

The Physician-Patient Relationship

Mark Siegler, a physician-ethicist, has developed a model of the physician-patient relationship (1979), one that I find substantially valid and conducive to the purposes of this chapter. In this model there are four "moments": (1) the prepatient phase, (2) data gathering and data reduction, (3) physician-patient accommodation, and (4) the physician-patient relationship. For the sake of convenience they are presented as if they occurred sequentially. In the real world, however, real people may not follow this sequence; they may, from time to time, move from one moment to another and back.

The Prepatient Phase

In the prepatient phase, a person who is going about the everyday activities of life notices that not all is going well. Somehow life is not measuring up to expectations.

We all experience transient aches and pains, tiredness, weakness, apathy, upset stomachs, and the like. When we experience such perturbations, we may assign to them whatever meaning we choose. My stomach is upset because I overindulged in alcohol or pizza, because of anxiety, motion sickness, or "a bug."

How we deal with such disturbances is also up to us. We have the power to choose whether to take a nap or a vacation, to purchase an over-the-counter remedy or a copper bracelet, or to consult a friend, pastor, naturopath, social worker, physician, or philosopher. Such choices are influenced by diverse social, cultural, economic, and other factors (Siegler 1979).

Occasionally, the power to choose is wrested from one's hands. For example, if one suddenly collapses with a heart attack or a stroke, one will most likely be picked up by an ambulance and rushed to the nearest emergency room.

In our social system the power to ascribe meaning to disturbances and to choose how to deal with them often becomes a matter for negotiation with some person or persons with whom one has a relationship—e.g., one's friend, spouse, colleague, or supervisor. For example, I may say to my colleague that I cannot do my share of the work today because I am very tired. I may go on to explain that I am tired because I stayed up too late last night or I am worried about an ailing relative; this explanation will probably satisfy my colleague. However, if my lassitude persists, my colleague is likely to become less and less accepting of my explanations. At some point she is likely to suggest that I consult a physician. This may be, at least in part, an expression of concern for my well-being. It is also likely to represent an exhortation to secure legitimation of the sick role as described by Talcott Parsons (1951, 1972). What she is saying is this: "You can't use tiredness as an excuse for not doing your share of the work any longer unless it is due to some illness and that can only (or best) be decided by a doctor."[4] Such not-so-subtle coercive pressures are often as effective as an ambulance in moving people out of prepatient phase and into the office of a physician.

Data Gathering and Data Reduction

A person's decision to consult a physician reflects a judgment that the problem is or could be a medical problem. When the person arrives in the physician's office for the first appointment, the physician begins by performing the various maneuvers and procedures characteristic of the moment of data gathering and data reduction; she takes a history, performs a physical examination, and then usually arranges for the conduct of various laboratory tests. The purpose of these activities is to attempt to make a diagnosis. If these activities result in the diagnosis of a disease that accounts for the disturbance experienced by the person, the physician will consider this a "problem of clinical medicine" (Siegler 1979).

Let us recall that one of the reasons to consult a physician is to get legitimation of the sick role. To have one's problem diagnosed as being due to a disease is a crucial step in the legitimation process. Our tired person may return to the colleague who suggested consulting a doctor in the first place and say: "My doctor told me that my tiredness is due to iron deficiency anemia. All I have to do is take these pills and within a week or so I should feel better." This is a very happy outcome for all concerned. The person (now called patient) will be excused for a while from assuming a full share of the work load with full expectations of recovery.

Suppose instead that this person returns from a consultation with the physician to report: "My doctor says 'there is nothing wrong' with me. The problem is that I am not getting enough sleep. I am staying up too late moonlighting on another job." The colleague's response to this is likely to be much different. This person, lacking the physician's legitimation of his entitlements to the sick role, is likely to be seen as irresponsible—not living up to his social obligations. Consequently, he might consider not providing a full account of the physician's evaluation to his colleague. Whether or not he does, his desired collegial relationship is probably in jeopardy.

Let us now consider a third scenario. Suppose the diagnosis is HIV infection. What will he tell his colleague? This is particularly problematic if, as is so often the case, his colleague does not know he is in an "at risk" group. There is a high risk of jeopardizing his collegial relationship no matter what he does or does not tell her. She may have a groundless fear of infection through casual incidental contact with him or with things he has touched. She may recoil from association with "undesirables" such as gay men or intravenous (IV) drug abusers. She may assume that he is such an "undesirable" even if he was infected through a blood transfusion administered in the course of treatment for a peptic ulcer "earned" by worrying about his job. She may believe that the legitimacy of the sick role is tarnished if disease is "self-inflicted" through freely chosen behaviors. Thus, she might shun the HIV-infected gay man but not the "innocent victim" with hemophilia.

Such misconceptions about the nature of the infection and attitudes about the social worthiness of the infected or those at risk for infection, though unwarranted, are widely held. Persons in "at risk" groups, aware of these benighted attitudes and false beliefs, may thus choose against consulting physicians when they experience disturbances to their sense of well-being. Legitimation of the sick role, a motivating influence for most persons in our social system, is not among the benefits they may confidently anticipate. Unlike a diagnosis of iron deficiency anemia, which has the effect of preserving a desired relationship, a diagnosis of HIV infection may destroy it.

CONFIDENTIALITY

Let us now return to the initial encounter between physician and patient. Data gathering with the aim of diagnosing is pursued first through the taking of a history and the performance of a physical examination. In this moment the patient is expected to "bare all," both literally and figuratively. Patients routinely share with their physicians information of such a private nature they would not consider divulging it to most others, not even their closest friends and relatives. Such information may be withheld from the physician or disguised but only at the patient's peril; lack of candor may result in an erroneous diagnosis.

Confidentiality is, of course, crucial to the formation and proper functioning of the physician-patient relationship. This has been recognized since ancient times. The Hippocratic Oath includes this pledge: "What I may see or hear in the course of the treatment or even outside the treatment in regard to the life of men, which on no account one must spread abroad, I will keep to myself holding such things shameful to be spoken about."[5] In modern times the physician's general ethical obligation to maintain confidentiality is given the additional force of law. Given such assurances of confidentiality, the typical patient feels free to "bare all" with impunity. Whether he would feel so secure if fully informed about medical confidentiality, which Siegler (1982) has called a "decrepit concept," is beyond the scope of this discussion; the point is that he does.

By contrast, the person at risk for HIV infection has been put on notice by society that he must be very wary with regard to medical confidentiality.[6] Suppose he is diagnosed as having an HIV infection. In more than twenty states the doctor is required to report this to public health officials (Dickens 1990).[7] In many of these states such reports are followed up by contact tracing. Although public health officials are bound by confidentiality laws, the "contacts" are not. Thus it may become generally known not only that the patient is HIV infected but also that he is a member of some stigmatized group.[8] The consequences of such sharing of information can be very grave indeed (Novick 1984).

Even if he lives in a state in which HIV infection is not reportable, there is cause for concern; many states are considering changing their laws to require such reporting (Dickens 1990).

What if the physician decides that the patient's lover (or lovers) or needle-sharing contacts must be protected from contracting HIV infection through contact with the patient? What if the patient is unwilling to tell his intimate contacts of his infection or otherwise take steps to protect them from infection? The law is not at all clear on whether the physician is either required or permitted to warn or otherwise protect such endangered others or whether, on the other hand, the duty to maintain confidentiality should prevail (Gostin 1989a:48–50). This unsettled state of the law creates anxieties for both physicians and patients, anxieties that serve as disincentives to the formation of physician-patient relationships.

BLOOD TESTING

Once the history taking and physical examination have been completed, the time has come to draw blood for laboratory testing. Most physicians and most patients recall a time when this was a rather uncomplicated ceremony: "Just a little pin-prick," said the physician. Or, "This won't hurt a bit, dearie," said the laboratory technician. Now the situation is different.

Suppose first that the physician thinks there is no reason to "rule-out" HIV infection. Must she observe blood and body fluid precautions? Most hospitals and many medical societies have policies requiring that such precautions be taken universally with all patients whether or not HIV infection is suspected.

The physician may think, as so many do: "Isn't this foolish? One cannot be on 'red alert' all the time. If I could only pick and choose the occasions for observing these precautions, I would probably be much more rigorously attentive to the details of these procedures than I am now when I am virtually certain that there is no danger. Besides, am I not signaling to this patient that I may not trust him? After all, he did tell me that he has not engaged in any activity that would put him at risk for HIV infection.

"On the other hand, he probably knows of the medical society's requirement for universal precautions. There has been so much about this in the newspapers. If I do not observe them he may think that I am lax in my observance of other medical standards and lose confidence in me."

By now, gloves have been donned over recently rewashed hands and the bloodletting is in progress. As she changes tubes, a drop of blood splashes on her forearm. She stops to scrub it away with soap and water. "My goodness," thinks the patient, "she really is suspicious of me. I wonder if she is surreptitiously drawing blood for antibody testing. I know it's against the law, but. . . ." He watches the physician with increased anxiety as she inserts the used needle in a device designed to destroy it.

Suppose next that the physician thinks there is a reason to rule out HIV infection. She may think first, as too many do, "Is it worth the risk to me to draw his blood for HIV-antibody testing?" She knows that the risk to her is fairly small. Even if he is HIV seropositive, the risk of her becoming infected after a contaminated needle stick is in the range of 0.03 to 0.9 percent (Gostin 1989a:17). This is far less than the 12–17 percent risk after similar exposure to the blood of patients with hepatitis B infection even after passive immunization of the exposed person with immune serum globulin (Gostin 1989a:17).

But HIV infection is different not only from hepatitis but also from all other infections and diseases. There are certain attributes of HIV infection that strike fear in the hearts of physicians and other informed persons as no other condition does, not even the many diseases that are much more promptly and uniformly lethal.

HIV infection could cost this doctor her career (Gostin 1989a:13–14), her plans to have children, and probably her relationship with her spouse or lover. It would also quite likely have far-reaching implications in her ability to maintain social relationships, purchase life insurance, travel, and so on.

Having considered all this, this good physician decides to proceed with blood drawing for HIV antibody assay. Actually, she does not decide to proceed. This is what she would have decided with any other simple blood test. Although in principle, informed consent is required for any blood test, this requirement is rarely observed in medical practice.[9]

For HIV-antibody testing, by contrast, full-fledged informed consent is required by law in most jurisdictions (Gostin 1989b). Moreover, the policies of many institutions require that informed consent be supplemented by pretest counseling and that posttest counseling be provided when the results (either positive or negative) are delivered to the patient. Both physician and patient cannot fail to be aware of how different this is from all other superficially analogous experiences they have ever had. The patient who arrived in the physician's office expecting advice and assistance and, if necessary, to be "taken care of," is instead immediately alerted to his "right to be left alone,"[10] of the perils attendant upon accepting his physician's advice, and of the uncertainties inherent in diagnostic testing.[11] This is a stressful and unfamiliar way to begin a physician-patient relationship.

If the patient agrees to HIV-antibody testing, the physician may proceed. In these circumstances she may choose to escalate precautions by putting on a gown, mask, and goggles even though this is probably unnecessary and will certainly add to the patient's consternation. If the result is positive, the patient will be faced with a variety of problems, some of which have already been introduced and others of which will be discussed shortly.

If the result is negative, can both physician and patient relax? Not really. It is well known that seroconversion after infection is commonly delayed for several months and occasionally for over a year (Gostin 1989a:29). Depending on the circumstances, physician and patient may both find it necessary to adjust their behaviors to the possibility that there might be HIV infection even though the initial antibody test is negative. Some physicians have adjusted their behaviors irresponsibly. They have refused to treat patients with negative antibody tests based on their belief that mere agreement to allow antibody testing indicates that the patients are probably in some "at risk" group even though they have denied this.

What if the patient resists the physician's recommendation for antibody testing? The physician may attempt to persuade the patient to reconsider his negative decision, reminding him of the advantages of knowing his antibody status. Good physicians often engage in persuasion, coaxing patients, e.g., to lose weight, exercise more, stop smoking, or take all, not just some, of their medications, and so on. They do not stop at mere recitation of risks, benefits, and alternatives followed by a passive interlude of waiting for the patient's informed and unconstrained decision.

A recommendation to a patient to have an HIV-antibody test done may, however, be more complicated than advice to lose weight, to have a barium enema, or even to have open-heart surgery. The physician does not experience a refusal to have a barium enema as a potential threat to her personal well-being. She may proceed to persuade the patient to accept her recommendation with an untroubled conscience knowing that she has only the patient's interests in mind. By contrast, persuasion to accept an HIV-antibody test is complicated. She and the patient may each suspect that her motivation is partially or primarily a concern for her own well-being. Even if it is not, she may be concerned that the patient thinks it is. In a sense, then, these people are approaching each other warily with unspoken concerns about the other's willingness to relate openly and honestly.

She may, instead, recommend anonymous testing, that is, the patient may be referred to a laboratory where he will be assigned a unique number that cannot be linked to any personal identifier and thus learn his antibody status without anyone else knowing it (Bayer, Levine, and Wolf 1986; Field 1990:51–53). This solves some problems but creates some others. Simply knowing that one is HIV seropositive creates some problems for the patient, which are beyond the scope of this discussion (Novick 1984). The patient may choose either to keep his antibody test result secret from the physician or to inform her if she promises to keep it secret even to the extent of not entering it in his medical record. The problems associated with the first choice are obvious. Regarding the second choice, an agreement not to enter the result in the medical record is detrimental to the purposes of the medical record. Consultants and physicians covering during nights, weekends, and vacations may reach flawed judgments owing to incomplete or distorted information. This point notwithstanding, until recently, many hospitals and clinics had policies forbidding the physician to enter the results of HIV-antibody tests in medical records without the patient's consent.

Finally, in some circumstances, the physician may force the patient to submit to HIV-antibody testing even though he persists in his refusal.[12] This is, of course, a terrible way to build or continue a relationship.

Now that we have come to the close of the initial encounter between physician and patient, let us pause to consider what we have observed. Both have already found themselves in highly unfamiliar territory. It does not matter whether the patient has or is at risk for HIV infection, he is unable to escape noticing that this is unlike his previous initial encounters with physicians.

The physician and patient are approaching each other warily. Some physicians are beginning to wonder if it is worth it. Is it worth coping with the fear of infection? Is it worth investing all this time and energy in blood and body fluid precautions, in informed consent and pretest and posttest counseling (for a simple blood test), in dealing with conflicts of loyalties in the management of private information? Is this my duty?

The Physician-Patient Accommodation

In the first moment, the patient decided that his problem was or might be a medical problem; this is why he sought the initial encounter with the physician. In the second moment, the physician—by virtue of having made a diagnosis—concluded that the patient's problem was a problem in clinical medicine. This is, therefore, a problem that merits the professional attention of *a* physician. In the third moment the physician and patient engage in negotiations that might culminate in the formation of a physician-patient relationship. The goal of this moment is to determine whether *this* physician will be *this* patient's physician.

There are numerous and various reasons that may influence the choices of particular physicians and particular patients to form particular physician-patient relationships. The patient may decide not to continue with a particular physician because, for example, the physician has a poor bedside manner, seems incompetent, displays the wrong diplomas, lacks the proper hospital privileges, has too long a queue, or charges excessive fees (Siegler 1979).

The remainder of this discussion focuses on the factors that may influence the physician's decision. The physician must consider (Siegler 1979): (1) Am I technically competent to help this patient? (2) Is the quality of my interaction with this patient such that it might undermine my capacity to help him? (3) Can I agree with this patient about the goals of the therapeutic relationship and the means to pursue them? Let us consider how AIDS may influence the physician's responses to these questions.

TECHNICAL COMPETENCE

The centrality of technical competence in medical ethics is reflected in the fact that it is mentioned or suggested in three of the American Medical Association's seven Principles of Medical Ethics (1982). "A physician shall be dedicated to providing competent medical service (Principle I) . . . strive to expose those physicians deficient in . . . competence (Principle II) . . . obtain consultation, and use the talents of other health professionals when indicated" (Principle V). In some cases it is clear that the patient's medical problem requires the services of a particular type of medical specialist. For example, consider an internist's encounter with a patient who has abdominal pain. If the pain is due to appendicitis, the patient must be referred to a surgeon. If, on the other hand, the pain is due to a peptic ulcer, the internist is likely by virtue of her education and experience to be able (competent) to provide appropriate therapy.

In some cases the notion of competence requires more subtle interpretation. The abdominal pain might, for example, be due to irritable bowel syndrome. Although all internists are educated in how to manage this problem and most regularly see patients with this very common disorder, some are strikingly more successful than others in treating such patients (Siegler 1979). Similarly, some psychiatrists seem much more adept than others in treating patients with affective disorders.

According to the American Medical Association, technical incompetence is the only ethically valid reason to excuse a physician from the general obligation to provide medical services for HIV-infected patients (1988). In its 1988 statement on this subject the key sentence is: "A physician may not ethically refuse to treat a patient whose condition is within the physician's current realm of competence solely because the patient is seropositive."

There are, however, some physicians who wish to evade their responsibilities to "seropositive patients" on grounds of fear, prejudice (infra), or "emotional inability."[13] Some of these physicians apparently choose to remain technically incompetent—to omit HIV infection from their "current realm of competence"—in order to acquire a socially acceptable excuse for their avoidance of HIV-infected patients (Lewis, Freeman and Corey 1987).

QUALITY OF INTERACTION

Most physicians can affirm Siegler's (1979:31) observation:

Among my patients, there are some for whom I have a very deep affection, others whom I find agreeable, and those whom I frankly dislike. Although I strive to care for each of my patients to the best of my ability, there is little doubt that I am more effective as a person and as a physician with those patients I like. We resonate well together: they know how I am thinking and feeling, and I apprehend how they are doing more directly than in other cases. They know they have a friend as well as a doctor. These observations echo the eloquent passages of Dr. Lain Entralgo when he speaks of medical *philia*, a deep medical friendship, as being at the heart of the relationship between doctor and patient (Lain Entralgo 1969).

Among the several factors that may impair the quality of the personal interaction between physician and patient, two are especially relevant to the problems at hand: fear and prejudice.

FEAR

We have already considered the fear of infection that some physicians experience on the occasion of drawing one specimen of blood from a patient who might have HIV infection. These physicians may hesitate to accept patients with known HIV infection since, if they do, they will experience the same fear on each of the many occasions it will be necessary to perform some invasive procedure.

This fear of HIV infection is not limited to the fainthearted, to the inexperienced, or to the irrational or uncommitted. Listen, for example, to Gerald Friedland, a physician who is both highly experienced and deeply committed to the care of patients with AIDS (1989:68): "After seven years of working with AIDS patients, knowing well the statistical risks, I must admit that I remain frightened. When I notice a blemish on my skin, I can't help wondering if it could be Kaposi's sarcoma. I still interpret minor illness in myself as the beginning of the 'expected' HIV infection although rationally I know better."

Infection is not the only thing that physicians fear. Some are concerned that acceptance of patients with HIV infection would have detrimental effects on their practices. Patients might avoid such physicians for a variety of reasons: fear of contracting HIV infection in the physician's office from contaminated instruments or though casual contact with infected patients in the waiting room (Marshall, et al 1990); reluctance to sit side-by-side with such "undesirables" in the waiting room; fear that, if they go to an "AIDS doctor," they may be suspected of either having AIDS or being in an "at risk" group.

Some physicians are concerned that developing a reputation as an "AIDS doctor" will reduce their status in the medical profession (Arras 1988). They might be marginalized by their colleagues as were many of the "plague doctors" in Europe during the Black Death epidemics (D. Fox 1988).

PREJUDICE

Early in the course of the AIDS epidemic, several groups of people were identified as being "at risk" for the disease. By far, the two largest groups were and continue to be homosexual men and abusers of intravenously injected illicit drugs. In American society each of these groups is stigmatized. This term, as Jonsen reminds us, "designates a complex social and psychological process whereby certain persons are perceived as being without social value and even as threatening to the dominant society. They are marked (hence, the word *stigma,* which in derivation evokes the branding of a criminal) for exclusion from certain social benefits and interactions" (1990:158).

Several prominent persons have proclaimed publicly that AIDS is a punishment inflicted by the Supreme Being on such unregenerate sinners. They have asserted, and some continue to assert, that such sinners are getting what they deserve and thus merit no sympathy: "The wages of sin are death." Those who make this claim distinguish homosexual men and intravenous (IV) drug abusers from "innocent victims" such as children and hemophiliacs. Unfortunately, a substantial number of Americans seem to agree.

Even more unfortunately, a substantial number of physicians seem to embrace this attitude.[14] Kelly and his colleagues (1987) studied the reactions of physicians to two hypothetical male patients who were identical in all but two respects: Their diagnoses were either AIDS or leukemia and their "romantic partners" were named either Robert or Roberta. Physician respondents "considered the AIDS patient to be more responsible for his illness, more deserving of what has happened to him, to be experiencing more pain but less deserving of sympathy and understanding, more dangerous to others, and more deserving of quarantine." Further, they were "less willing to engage in conversation with an AIDS patient" than with one with leukemia, "less willing to attend a party where he was either present or had prepared food, . . . to work in the same office, . . . to renew his lease if he were a tenant, . . . to continue a past friendship and . . . to allow children to visit him" (p. 790).

In addition to sharing in the prejudicial attitudes held by an unfortunately large segment of the general public, many physicians have negative reactions and prejudicial responses to certain types of patients. The categories of patients that evoke these negative responses overlap only partially with those stigmatized by the general public.

"Admitted or not," says the psychiatrist, James E. Groves, "the fact remains that a few patients kindle aversion, fear, despair or even downright malice in their doctors" (1978:883). Such patients, whom Groves calls "hateful patients," are "those whom most physicians dread." Among the responses of physicians to such patients are "helplessness in the helper, . . . unconscious punishment of the patient, . . . self-punishment by the doctor, . . . inappropriate confrontation of the patient, and . . . desperate attempts to avoid or extrude the patient from the caregiving system."

Groves classifies hateful patients according to "four stereotypes":

"dependent clingers, entitled demanders, manipulative health-rejectors, and self-destructive deniers." Although patients with HIV infection may fit into any of these categories, just as patients with other diseases and problems do, there are two of these stereotypes that merit further consideration here: entitled demanders and self-destructive deniers.

The entitled demander uses "intimidation, devaluation and guilt-induction to place the doctor in the role of the inexhaustible supply depot" (Groves 1978:885). These angry people evoke in their physicians fear (e.g., of litigation) and counterattack. "The doctor's usual impulse . . . is a wish to point out suddenly and devastatingly that the patient has earned little, medically or in larger society, and deserves little" (p. 885).

There is a tendency among health professionals, particularly those who have no personal experience with relationships with individuals with HIV infection, to categorize such persons in general as entitled demanders. This image is reinforced by the oft-repeated display on television of "AIDS activists" disrupting scientific meetings, forming picket lines around buildings housing such federal agencies as the National Institutes of Health (NIH) and Food and Drug Administration (FDA), and demonstrating in the streets of cities on both coasts of the United States. Such demonstrations are characterized by the use of violent language—federal officials, for example, are greeted with loud chants of "Nazi" or "murderer."

This image is further developed in the frequent reports of litigation initiated by or on behalf of persons with HIV infection over breaches of confidentiality, entitlements to medical care or to payment for medical care, and entitlements to employment, immigration, public education, and so on.

Two additional factors that contribute to the image of the HIV-infected patient as an entitled demander will be discussed in subsequent sections: the controversies over the rights of such patients to receive investigational drugs and the nature of the debate about whether the physician has a duty to treat patients with HIV infection.

As we have already noticed, some physicians think that patients with AIDS deserve their unhappy plight. Implicit in this attitude is a perception of the patient as a "self-destructive denier." Before the advent of the AIDS epidemic, physicians had had ample frustrating experience with such self-destructive behaviors as alcoholism. "Yes, I will stay up all night controlling this patient's bleeding esophageal varices. But I know that as soon as he is discharged, he will resume his heavy consumption of alcohol. How can he be so self-destructive? How can he be so disrespectful of my efforts, *ruining my handiwork?*" With intravenous drug abusers, the physician has had similarly frustrating experiences with, e.g., bacterial endocarditis, hepatitis, and now HIV and opportunistic infections.

It is not clear whether continuing exposure through needle sharing or unsafe sexual practices presents any threat to the individual who has already contracted HIV infection. It is clear, however, that such behaviors present serious risks to others. We have already noticed how such continuing destructive behaviors create strains in the physician-patient relationship as the physician wonders whether the duty to maintain confidentiality is stronger than the duty to prevent harm to others.

Patients in "at risk" groups who appear not to have contracted HIV infection and who continue unsafe sexual practices or needle-sharing activities despite their physician's attempts to educate or admonish them to do otherwise will almost certainly be branded as self-destructive deniers. And how is the physician to react to teenage patients as they experiment with sex (usually unprotected) and drugs? Or to a heterosexual man who pays prostitutes double their usual fee for the privilege of not wearing a condom? Or to men and women who engage in extramarital sexual liasons? Such patients have always presented problems to physicians, but in the age of AIDS the stakes are getting higher.

Physicians are spending ever-increasing amounts of time exhorting ever-enlarging proportions of their patients to be monogamous or to use condoms or both. All too often the patients respond: "But insisting on a condom would be such a sign of distrust." Or, "having sex with a rubber is like taking a shower while wearing a raincoat."

"Self-destructive deniers," according to Groves, ". . . evoke all of these negative feelings [aversion, fear, counterattack, guilt and feelings of inadequacy] as well as malice and a secret wish that the patient will 'die and get it over with' " (1978:887).

Judith Lorber, a social scientist, uses kinder and gentler terms than Groves does to classify patients: "good patients and problem patients" (1975). Patients who are trusting, cooperative with doctors, nurses, and with hospital routines, and who complain only when it is medically warranted, are considered "good patients." Those who do not behave according to these "good patient norms" are labeled "problem patients."

> As other researchers have found, the better educated and younger patients tended to have more autonomous or deviant attitudes toward being a hospital patient. This study found that patients with deviant

attitudes tended to argue more with the residents, interns, and nurses, and to complain more about minor discomforts as a way of getting attention (p. 223).

Many patients with HIV infection are better educated and younger than most patients with other lethal diseases (Zuger 1987) and have more autonomous or deviant attitudes. Many are argumentative—e.g., over their rights to access to investigational drugs (infra)—or worse. Some have even attempted to infect their physicians and nurses by spitting at or biting them (Gostin 1989b:1047). Although such attacks on health professionals are unusual, stories about them are told repeatedly in hospitals, thus contributing to the image of patients with AIDS as problem patients. As Lorber has observed: "Possible consequences of being labeled a problem patient are premature discharge, neglect, and referral to a psychiatrist" (1975:213).

Early in the course of their acculturation into the medical profession, medical students and residents learn from their peers to categorize patients as either "interesting" or "uninteresting" and as either "ideal" or "despised" (Mizrahi 1986: 70–78).[15] Whether or not a patient is "interesting" is "almost solely determined by professional criteria relating to diagnosis; that is, the symptoms are the primary basis of valuation, and the outcome of the disease—whether it is curable—is the secondary basis" (p. 70).

Mizrahi quotes a prospective chief resident's outline of "patients whom the housestaff found frustrating":

> One, patients you take care of even though you can't make better; two, people you can make better but who won't follow your instructions; three, patients who resist your attempts at diagnosing; four, those who you can do the right thing for and the patient doesn't get better; and five, making a good diagnosis but not being able to do anything for the patient (pp. 71–72).

Until recently there was not much that physicians could do to "make better" the patient with AIDS. Even now, drug therapy can only postpone the inevitably lethal outcome. We have already noticed how and why some patients resist attempts at diagnosing HIV infection.

Further frustration was voiced by one of the interns interviewed by Mizrahi (p. 72): "There's very little [internal] medicine can do outside of infectious disease, and the things we can do something for are usually related to self-inflicted diseases. You tune them up and they go right back out and do it again."

Mizrahi's second system of classification—"ideal" or "despised"—is based upon the patient's social and behavioral attributes (1986:70). Ideal patients are described in such terms as *clean, articulate, cooperative,* and the like—most of which conform closely to "external systems of social status." Thus, persons of low social status are unlikely to be seen as "ideal patients"; as is well known, the poor and minorities are afflicted by HIV infection in disproportionately large numbers.

Mizrahi concludes:

> In summary, there were many categories of disparaged patients who were actively and visibly shunned by the house staff. First, there were the *self-abusers*: those with so-called self-induced disease, especially those brought on by alcohol, cigarettes, drug usage, and overeating. Second, there were the *system abusers*: those assessed as manipulators, malingerers, psychosomatic complainers ('crocks'), and demanders. Third, there were *housestaff abusers*: troublesome patients who are difficult, demanding, suspicious, disrespectful, hostile, or ungrateful and who are also often included in either or both of the first two categories (pp. 77–78).

To the extent that patients are categorized as either "uninteresting" or "despised" or both, they are increasingly likely to be "GROPed"; "GROP" is Mizrahi's acronym for Getting Rid of Patients.

Before we move on to the physician-patient relationship, it is worth reflecting on the power of this language: "hateful," "despised," "uninteresting," "self-destructive," "entitled demanders." Some of these are the terms physicians use in the literature of medicine. Others are terms social scientists use to describe the attitudes and behaviors of physicians. The language itself creates barriers to the accommodations that are a necessary prelude to the physician-patient relationship.[16]

The Physician-Patient Relationship

"The relationship is distinguished from the accommodation by its duration, depth and maturity. Although there are no formal signs to acknowledge its existence, physicians and patients usually recognize that their medical relationship has advanced and entered a new phase. . . . The essence of the doctor-patient relationship is the exchange of a deep bond of trust between patient and doctor" (Siegler 1979:35).

We have considered the importance of diagnosis to the patient in gaining legitimation of the entitlements of the sick role. Now it is time to examine another aspect of the institutionalized expectation system (Parsons 1951). There is an obligation upon the sick person "to seek *technically competent* help, mainly, in the most usual sense, that of a physician and to *cooperate* with him in the process of trying to get well. It is here, of course, that the role of the sick person as patient becomes articulated with that of the physician in a complementary role structure" (pp. 436–437; emphasis in the original). In the following paragraphs I consider in more detail the concepts of "technically competent help" and "trust."

TECHNICALLY COMPETENT HELP

The notion of "technically competent help," as envisioned by the medical profession, has many components, some of which were considered earlier. The one I discuss here is the scientific basis for recommendations of drugs for therapeutic purposes.

The technically competent physician generally limits her recommendations for therapeutic drugs to those approved for commercial distribution by the FDA. FDA, in turn, grants such approval only to drugs that have been demonstrated safe and effective through the conduct of randomized clinical trials (RCTs) (Kessler 1989). Physicians have become accustomed to thinking of the RCT as the "gold standard" for validating claims of therapeutic efficacy.

A problem with the federal drug approval process culminating in the RCT is that it takes a long time, typically seven to ten years after the initial discovery of the drug. Quite understandably, patients with AIDS have protested that this is too long in that it is much longer than their average life expectancy.

Early in the course of the AIDS epidemic, individuals with AIDS and those who speak on their behalf, including AIDS activists, began to take actions designed to bypass, alter, or exploit (in some cases) the drug approval process. With time their efforts have been increasingly successful.

A full account of these activities is beyond the scope of this discussion.[17] The following brief survey is designed to show how some of them have had an effect on the physician-patient relationship.

Before an RCT is begun, there are usually reports of preliminary uncontrolled studies indicating that the investigational new drug is effective. Often the drug appears to be far more effective than any standard or noninvestigational therapy (Levine 1986a:199–202). This was certainly the case in 1986 when the RCT comparing azidothymidine (AZT) with placebo was begun; at the time there was no drug known to be effective for the treatment of AIDS.

Patients who become aware of these preliminary reports often come

to regard these investigational new drugs as the "best available therapy" for them. Accordingly, many of them will go to great lengths in
their efforts to gain access to these drugs.

Until recently the only way to gain access to such an investigational
new drug was to enroll in an RCT. In 1986, patients with AIDS
recognized that enrollment in the placebo-controlled trial of AZT was
the only way to get a 50 percent chance of receiving what they believed
was the "best available therapy." Some of them—with the collabora-
tion of their physicians—falsified their medical histories so as to appear
to match the inclusion criteria for the RCT.

How does a physician react to a patient who requests falsification of
inclusion criteria? One hopes that a major component of the response
is compassion in the face of the patient's desperate situation. But if the
physician cooperates, she knows that she will be undermining the
validity of the RCT. Such an action strikes at the very heart of the
scientific basis of technically competent medicine.[18]

Such a request from a patient may create a necessity to return to
the negotiations characteristic of the physician-patient accommodation. Recall that one of the questions the physician had to address was
this: "Can I agree with this patient about the goals of the therapeutic
relationship and the *means* to pursue them?" The answer may be "No,
I cannot conspire to undermine the scientific basis of my profession."
If so, the relationship might come to an end.

Since 1986, largely in response to the effective political pressure
brought to bear by AIDS activists, patients have been able to gain
access to investigational new drugs through such mechanisms as
"treatment INDs" (Levine 1987b), "expanded access," and "the parallel track."[19] Since one of the criteria for eligibility for the parallel track
is "the patient does not meet the entry criteria for the controlled clinical
trials," physicians are now being called upon to falsify exclusion rather
than inclusion criteria.

Physicians have been able for many years to make investigational
new drugs available to some of their patients through the use of compassionate INDs (Nightingale 1981). In general, compassionate use of
investigational new drugs has not presented a major problem to physicians apart from a bothersome paperwork burden. Most commonly, the
compassionate-use mechanism is employed after the RCTs have been
completed while final action by the FDA to approve a drug for commercial distribution is being awaited.

By contrast, the new mechanisms for providing access may be employed very early in the drug development process before the RCT is
completed or, in some cases, before it is even begun. Moreover, whereas

compassionate use is usually recommended by a physician who under-
stands the drug well or entails referral to such a physician, the new
mechanisms are typically requested by patients who often know more
than the physician about the drugs and the rules for gaining access to
them. As they make their demands and appeal to the rules, they may
engage in behaviors characteristic of Groves' "entitled demanders" and
Lorber's "problem patients." We have already considered the consequences of being so perceived by physicians and other health professionals.

Many physicians experience anxiety over having to use drugs not
proved safe and effective. Some physicians have expressed concern
that early access will undermine efforts to conduct RCTs:

> If patients can get access to investigational new drugs outside RCTs
> why would any be willing to enroll in RCTs? We may never know
> whether the new drugs are safe and effective. These people are not
> merely uncooperative with my efforts to provide technically competent
> help for them, they are undermining my ability to provide technically
> competent help to anybody else.
>
> Even when they do enroll in RCTs they do things that threaten the
> validity of the RCTs. They share their drugs with each other so each is
> assured of getting at least some active drug (Levine 1990). They take
> additional drugs some of which they believe are therapeutic (although
> they are not even recognized as investigational by the FDA) and some
> of which are illicit drugs of abuse. How can anyone rely on the data
> developed in such RCTs?

TRUST

As Siegler put it, the "essence" of the physician-patient relationship
is "the exchange of a deep bond of trust between doctor and patient."
The patient is able to trust the physician because, among other reasons, the latter is bound ethically to a duty of loyalty (Ramsey 1970:2).
Legally, this is fiduciary relationship; a fiduciary is bound by law "to
the duty of constant and unqualified loyalty" (Holder 1983). But as we
have noticed, the physician who forms relationships with patients with
HIV infection or who are at risk for such infection is presented with a
variety of conflicts of loyalties. Is the physician to be more loyal to the
patient's confidentiality interests or to the duty to either prevent harm
to third parties or serve public health interest? Does loyalty to the
patient require the physician to cooperate in activities that will tend to
undermine the scientific bases of technically competent practice? How
is the patient to know how his physician will decide when confronted
with such conflicts? Can he really trust his physician?

If he is not certain that he can trust his physician, is it prudent to keep his part of the bargain—i.e., to cooperate? Should he "bare all" of his private behaviors? Should he let the physician know that he is not taking all his medications because he is sharing them with friends or that he is taking, in addition to the prescribed regimen, other drugs and remedies of untested merit? Can the physician trust this patient? When such a patient suddenly develops new symptoms and signs, should the physician suspect an interaction between the prescribed drugs and some other remedies taken surreptitiously, even if the patient denies taking other drugs?

BURDENS AND BURNOUT

Abigail Zuger writes from the perspective of a resident in internal medicine at Bellevue Hospital in New York City (1987). For her, the burdens of caring for patients with AIDS are more than abstract problems to be subjected to rational analysis, they are a lived reality She describes in vivid terms the helplessness and frustration experienced by residents who take care of patients with AIDS: "The patients are . . . the same age or younger than their physicians or nurses. They are very sick—they have raging fevers, enormous weight loss, severe shortness of breath. Medical science offers them no cure and few treatments that are more than feeble temporizing efforts" (p. 17). AIDS burnout "results from too many intense, emotion-filled relationships with young dying patients. . . . Residents become depressed, disillusioned with all medical intervention, quick to write 'Do Not Resuscitate' orders, slow to carry out other, less emergent, interventions. 'It doesn't matter; he's going to die anyway,' is their reductionist slogan" (p. 19). While the psychological phenomenon of "AIDS burnout" is common (Wachter 1986), Zuger states that the development of "unusual psychological strength" occurs at least as commonly.

Zuger identifies another feature of AIDS that tends to disrupt the physician-patient relationship. The opportunistic infections that afflict patients with AIDS are generally caused by "exotic pathogens," bacteria, fungi, and parasites with which their physicians have had little or no experience. Treatment usually consists of investigational drugs that are often quite toxic, difficult to obtain, and unfamiliar to most primary care physicians. Consequently, the management of patients during the frequent episodes of opportunistic infection must necessarily be directed by expert consultants. Thus, says Zuger, "AIDS patients are distanced sometimes to the point of estrangement from primary care givers inexperienced in their care" (p. 17).

The Duty to Treat

In light of the fears, anxieties, prejudices, conflicts, uncertainties, disruptions, and burdens we have considered so far, it is not surprising that many physicians hesitate to assume responsibility for the care of patients with HIV infection. Some of those physicians, wondering if they were ethically obligated to assume such responsibility, sought guidance by consulting the American Medical Association's Principles of Medical Ethics (1982): "A physician shall, in the provision of appropriate patient care, except in emergencies, be free to choose whom to serve, with whom to associate, and the environment in which to provide medical services" (Principle VI). Thus, it appeared that they were free to choose not to serve patients with HIV infection.

In the United States there is a very high value placed on the freedom to choose. A strong presumption in favor of this freedom to choose is reflected in law and in social practices. Liberty is identified in the Declaration of Independence as one of the "inalienable rights" with which we are endowed by the Creator. Thus, when some physicians assert a right to choose not to take care of patients with AIDS, it is not to be taken lightly.

The assertion of this right by physicians who were unwilling to serve patients with AIDS is what precipitated the great outpouring of commentary on the duty to treat to which I referred at the outset. No, these commentators argued, the physician has no such right. She or he has instead a duty to treat such persons. Because the articulation of this duty was developed in response to an assertion of a right to behave otherwise, the argument assumed an adversarial tone. This is typical of arguments grounded in considerations of rights and duties.[20]

In ethical discourse, the language of rights and duties yields powerful requirements to act in certain specified ways; such language is often used to force persons to perform actions they would not have chosen freely, to coerce unwilling behavior. If one has a duty to respond to a claim grounded in a right, one must respond, or else (Ladd 1979). The language of rights and duties is appropriate for an ethics of strangers—e.g., for transactions in the marketplace. It is not, however, a suitable vocabulary for the description of or prescription for the caring relationships we expect to develop between patients and primary care physicians. Indeed, an ethics of rights and duties not supplemented by some other considerations such as caring (Angoff 1990), relationality (Powell 1987), responsibility (Ladd 1979), virtues (Merrill 1990), or conscience (Jonsen 1990) has a tendency to impede the formation of satisfactory physician-patient relationships (Levine 1987a).

The AMA's promulgation in 1988 of a revised policy proscribing on ethical grounds a physician's refusal to treat patients solely because of HIV seropositivity was an important and praiseworthy action. It reaffirmed the medical profession's commitment to the service of patients —all patients—thus providing support and inspiration to those physicians who experience this sense of commitment. Moreover, it repudiated the position taken by some physicians that there are certain types of persons who are unworthy of medical attention.

But recall the reason that the duty to treat question was raised. It was because some physicians were unwilling to serve patients with HIV infection. What effect will the AMA's clear articulation of the physician's duty have on the behavior of these physicians? Perhaps it will result in the coercion of some frightened, prejudiced, reluctant, or burnt-out physicians to take care of patients with HIV infections. Now, if they do not, they can be cited and sanctioned for a breach of professional ethics. But what patient would want such a physician?

AIDS as a disease entity and the AIDS epidemic as a social phenomenon have had profound and far-reaching effects on the physician-patient relationship. As we have seen, the effects are felt by all physicians and all patients in every "moment" of their relationships. They are experienced by patients with and without HIV infection and by uninfected persons who either are or are not members of the so-called "at-risk" groups. At the very least, these patients notice that in their encounters with health professionals they are in increasingly unfamiliar territory where wariness in one party evokes wariness in the other.

We have looked in greater detail at the attitudes, anxieties, experiences, and behaviors of the physicians. Even those who willingly assume responsibility for treating patients with HIV infection experience, to recall some examples, fear of infection or of ostracism by colleagues or patients and resentment of "not completely rational" requirements for universal blood and body fluid precautions; they are threatened, e.g., by the need to use drugs that have not been validated scientifically and wearied by having to cope with so many "problem patients." Such experiences and others we have considered are very different from what these physicians anticipated when they chose to enter the medical profession.

And what about the other physicians? There are some who are for various reasons hesitant or reluctant to assume responsibility for taking care of patients with HIV infection. There are even some who either openly reject or surreptitiously evade this responsibility. It is because of these physicians that the question is so often raised about whether there is a duty to treat patients with HIV infection.

Although I have not attempted to respond to this question, I have suggested that an affirmative response does not help mitigate many of the problems that caused the question to be asked in the first place. While one can assert a duty to treat, one cannot argue coherently that there is a duty to be unafraid. Similarly, one cannot coerce empathy (or even sympathy) or any of the other feelings or attitudes that are essential to the development of caring relationships between physicians and patients.

AIDS has not only had extensive and troubling effects on what the physician-patient relationship is. It has also highlighted some of the shortcomings in our capacity to develop a stable social consensus about what it ought to be.[21]

NOTES

1. The central focus of this chapter is on the relationships of patients to primary care physicians such as family and general practitioners, many general pediatricians and internists, and some specialists in obstetrics and gynecology. Much of the discussion is, therefore, not applicable to physicians such as diagnostic radiologists, anesthesiologists, many surgeons, and others who typically have transient encounters rather than enduring relationships with patients.

2. Actually, some physicians who have willingly assumed responsibility for the care of patients with HIV infection have asked if there is a duty to treat. In asking this question they are not seeking guidance for their own behavior. They are instead expressing a concern about the attitudes and behaviors of their reluctant colleagues.

3. This is the motto of Alpha Omega Alpha, the leading medical honorary society.

4. The validity of the Parsonian vision of the "sick role" has been subjected to serious challenges (e.g., Brody 1987: 68–73). The validity of these challenges is beyond the scope of this chapter. Renée Fox provides a critique of some of these challenges, as well as an argument for the continuing substantial validity of the "sick role" (1989:35ff).

5. Reprinted in the *Encyclopedia of Bioethics*, p. 1731.

6. This consideration of medical confidentiality as it relates to patients who have or who are at risk for HIV infection is necessarily superficial. For more extended discussions see Gostin (1989a), Dickens (1990), and Edgar and Sandomine (1990).

7. Fully developed AIDS is reportable in all states and in the District of Columbia.

8. Although public health officials do not tell "contacts" the name of the infected

person, they often guess correctly. Incorrect guesses precipitate a different but equally vexatious set of problems.

9. In medical practice, consent to simple procedures such as venipuncture is usually presumed. It is rarely fully informed (Levine 1983).

10. Legally and ethically, the requirement for informed consent is grounded in the rights of persons to be left alone or to be self-determining (Levine 1986b:96–97).

11. Acknowledgments of uncertainty provoke strong feelings of anxiety in physicians and patients alike (Katz 1975:165–206).

12. In some jurisdictions the physician may insist on involuntary testing for HIV antibodies after accidental exposure to blood or body fluids (Closen et al. 1989: 610; Connecticut Public Act 89–246).

13. The AMA's initial "Statement on AIDS" recognized the doctor's "emotional inability" as an excuse from the general duty to treat patients with AIDS (Angoff 1990:39):

> Physicians and other health professionals have a long tradition of tending to patients afflicted with infectious disease with compassion and courage. However, not everyone is emotionally able to care for patients with AIDS. If the health professional is unable to care for a patient with AIDS, that individual should ask to be removed from the case. Alternative arrangements for the care of the patient must be made.

This exception was deleted from the 1988 revision of the policy statement.

14. For a survey of physicians' public expressions of prejudice against patients with AIDS and persons in the so-called at risk groups, see Angoff (1990: 5–15). For additional discussion of physicians' and other health care workers' attitudes toward AIDS patients, see Abigail Zuger's essay in this volume.

15. For extensive surveys of these and other reactions by residents to patients, see Mizrahi (1986) and R. Fox (1989: 108–130).

16. This language is actually rather mild compared with that used by residents to describe such patients (Mizrahi 1986:41).

17. For further discussion, see Levine (1990).

18. For a consideration of the ethical obligation of primary care physicians to cooperate with RCTs, see Levine (1986b).

19. A proposed policy statement, "Expanded Availability of Investigational New Drugs Through a Parallel Track Mechanism for People with AIDS and HIV-Related Disease" was published by the U.S. Public Health Service in the *Federal Register*, May 21, 1990.

20. The concept of rights is most characteristically employed in an adversarial context; as John Ladd has argued, "To have a right is to have a right against someone" (1979:74). The notion of duties is not necessarily adversarial. It becomes adversarial when linked with the concept of rights as it so often is in the literature of bioethics. My reference to a language or an ethics of rights and duties encompasses the concept of duties only when linked thusly to that of rights, e.g., a duty to respond to a claim grounded in a right. It does not include a duty arising from such other considerations as conscience or responsibility.

Not all commentary on the physician's duty to care for patients with AIDS has been grounded in considerations of rights and duties. Other considerations are emphasized by Zuger (1987), Arras (1988), Angoff (1990), and Jonsen (1990), for examples.

21. I thank Bruce Baker, Alan Mermann, Kathleen Nolan, and Frederic Reamer for their helpful suggestions based on reading an early draft of this chapter.

REFERENCES

AMA (American Medical Association). 1982. Principles of Medical Ethics. In *Current Opinions of the Judicial Council of the American Medical Association,* p. ix. Chicago: AMA.

AMA Council on Ethical and Judicial Affairs, 1987. Ethical Issues Involved in the Growing AIDS Crisis (revised, September 1988).

Angoff, N. R. 1990. Do Physicians Have an Ethical Obligation to Care for Patients with AIDS? M.D. thesis. New Haven: Yale University School of Medicine.

Arras, J. D. 1988. The Fragile Web of Responsibility: AIDS and the Duty to Treat. *Hastings Center Report* (April/May), 18 (2, Suppl.):10–20.

Bayer, R., C. Levine, and S. M. Wolf. 1986. HIV Antibody Screening: An Ethical Framework for Evaluating Proposed Programs. *JAMA* 256:1768–1774.

Brody, H. 1987. *Stories of Sickness.* New Haven: Yale University Press.

Closen, M. L., D. H. J. Hermann, P. J. Horne et al. 1989. *AIDS: Cases and Materials.* Houston: John Marshall.

Dickens, B. M. 1990. Confidentiality and the Duty to Warn. In L. O. Gostin, ed., *AIDS and the Health Care System,* pp. 98–112. New Haven: Yale University Press.

Edgar, H. and H. Sandomine. 1990. Medical Privacy Issues in the Age of AIDS: Legislative Options. *American Journal of Law and Medicine* 16 (1 and 2):155–222.

Encyclopedia of Bioethics, W. T. Reich, ed. 1979. New York: Free Press.

Field, M. A. 1990. Testing for AIDS: Uses and Abuses. *American Journal of Law and Medicine* 16 (1 and 2):33–106.

Fox, D. M. 1988. The Politics of Physicians' Responsibility in Epidemics: A Note on History. *Hastings Center Report* (April/May), 18 (2, Suppl.):5–10.

Fox, R. C. 1989. *The Sociology of Medicine: A Participant Observer's View.* Englewood Cliffs, N.J.: Prentice-Hall.

Friedland, G. H. 1989. Clinical Care in the AIDS Epidemic. *Daedalus* (Spring), 188 (2):59–83.

Gostin, L. O. 1989a. Hospitals, Health Care Professionals, and AIDS: The "Right to Know" the Health Status of Professionals and Patients. *Maryland Law Review* 48 (1):12–54.

Gostin, L. O. 1989b. The Politics of AIDS: Compulsory State Powers, Public Health, and Civil Liberties. *Ohio State Law Journal* 49 (4):1017–1058.

Groves, J. E. 1978. Taking Care of the Hateful Patient. *New England Journal of Medicine* 298:883–887.

Holder, A. R. 1983. Do Researchers and Subjects Have a Fiduciary Relationship? *IRB: A Review of Human Subjects Research* (January), 4 (1):6–7.

Jonsen, A. R. 1990. The Duty to Treat Patients with AIDS and HIV Infection. In L. O. Gostin, ed., *AIDS and the Health Care System,* pp. 155–168. New Haven: Yale University Press.

Katz, J. 1975. *The Silent World of Doctor and Patient.* New York: Free Press.

Kelly, J. A. et al. 1987. Stigmatization of AIDS Patients by Physicians. *American Journal of Public Health* (July), 77 (7):789–791.

Kessler, D. A. 1989. The Regulation of Investigational Drugs. *New England Journal of Medicine* 320:281–288.

Ladd, J. 1979. Legalism and Medical Ethics. *Journal of Medicine and Philosophy* 4:70–80.

Lain Entralgo, P. 1969. *Doctor and Patient,* F. Partridge, trans. New York: McGraw-Hill.

Levine, R. J. 1983. Informed Consent in Research and Practice: Similarities and Differences. *Archives of Internal Medicine* 143:1229–1231.

Levine, R. J. 1986a. *Ethics and Regulation of Clinical Research.* 2d.ed. Baltimore: Urban & Schwarzenberg.

Levine, R. J. 1986b. Referral of Patients with Cancer for Participation in Randomized Clinical Trials. *CA—A Cancer Journal for Clinicians* 36:95–99.

Levine, R. J. 1987a. Medical Ethics and Personal Doctors: Conflicts Between What We Teach and What We Want. *American Journal of Law and Medicine* 13 (1 and 2):351–364.

Levine, R. J. 1987b. Treatment Use and Sale of Investigational New Drugs. *IRB: A Review of Human Subjects Research* (July/August), 9 (4):1–4.

Levine, R. J. 1990. Human Experimentation: New Developments (1986–1989). In R. D. Gaare, ed., *BioLaw,* pp. R.213–R.235. Bethesda, Md.: University Publications of America.

Lewis, C. E., H. E. Freeman, and C. R. Corey. 1987. AIDS-related Competence of California's Primary Care Physicians. *American Journal of Public Health* (July), 77 (7):795–799.

Lorber, J. 1975. Good Patients and Problem Patients: Conformity and Deviance in a General Hospital. *Journal of Health and Social Behavior* 16:213–225.

Marshall, P. A., J. P. O'Keefe, S. G. Fisher, and A. J. Caruso. 1990. Patients' Fear of Contracting the Acquired Immunodeficiency Syndrome from Physicians. *Archives of Internal Medicine* 150:1501–1506.

Merrill, J. O. 1990. Telling Good Stories, Living Good Lives: Physician Virtues and the Doctor-Patient Relationship. M.D. thesis. New Haven: Yale University School of Medicine.

Mizrahi, T. 1986. *Getting Rid of Patients.* New Brunswick, N.J.: Rutgers University Press.

Nightingale, S. L. 1981. Drug Regulation and Policy Formulation. *Milbank Memorial Fund Quarterly* 59:412–444.

Novick, A. 1984. At Risk for AIDS: Confidentiality in Research and Surveillance. *IRB: A Review of Human Subjects Research* (November/December), 6(6):10–11.

Parsons, T. 1951. *The Social System.* New York: Free Press.

Parsons, T. 1972. Definitions of Health and Illness in the Light of American Values and Social Structure. In E. G. Jaco, ed., *Patients, Physicians and Illness: A Sourcebook in Behavioral Science and Health,* pp. 107–127. New York: Free Press.

Powell, P. M. 1987. Deciding for Others: Rights and Responsibilities in Medical Ethics. M.D. thesis. New Haven: Yale University School of Medicine.

Ramsey, P. 1970. *The Patient as Person.* New Haven: Yale University Press.

Rosenberg, C. E. 1989. What Is an Epidemic? AIDS in Historical Perspective. *Daedalus* (Spring), 118 (2):1–17.

Siegler, M. 1979. The Nature and Limits of Clinical Medicine. In E. J. Cassell and M. Siegler, eds., *Changing Values in Medicine,* pp. 19–41. Bethesda, Md.: University Publications of America.

Siegler, M. 1982. Confidentiality in Medicine: A Decrepit Concept. *New England Journal of Medicine* 307:1518–1521.

Wachter, R. 1986. The Impact of the Acquired Immunodeficiency Syndrome on Medical Residency Training. *New England Journal of Medicine* 314:177–180.

Zuger, A. 1987. AIDS on the Wards: A Residency in Medical Ethics. *Hastings Center Report* (June), 17 (3):16–20.

9. AIDS and the Obligations of Health Care Professionals

CARING FOR THE sick is a difficult and sometimes dangerous job. A fact of life for most of recorded history, this truth has been rediscovered by health care providers and patients of our own generation in the particular context of AIDS. Over the last ten years the disease has provoked an escalating debate over the obligations of physicians and other health care professionals to their contagious patients. Research has now established that human immunodeficiency virus (HIV) infection can be transmitted under some circumstances from patient to practitioner; data have also confirmed that many practitioners are reluctant to care for patients with AIDS, with some adamant in their refusal to do so.

Given the nature of the HIV infection and AIDS, are health care professionals who avoid these patients exercising a professional right or committing a moral outrage? Ongoing commentary on this question by practitioners, their patients, and medical ethicists has evolved into a substantial body of literature, which often, inevitably, transcends the specific context of HIV infection to explore the basic philosophic groundings of the health care professions. This discussion summarizes a variety of approaches to this issue proposed over the last several years, including historical and ethical models considered and practical concerns voiced as the AIDS epidemic continues to grow around the world.

Refusals to Treat

The young man had had diarrhea for months before he was admitted to the hospital with a bad case of dehydration. His physician was certain he had inflammatory bowel disease. However, during a hospitalization that stretched out for several months, the patient proved to be HIV positive with a virulent, untreatable intestinal parasite. By the time he was ready for discharge, he had a diagnosis of AIDS and required daily nutritional supplements administered through an intravenous catheter. He had lost the lease to his apartment, and his parents refused to have him at home. His medical insurance had lapsed.

The patient's doctor called the hospital's AIDS clinic. "I won't be seeing him anymore," he said. "When he's discharged I'm going to send him to you." Asked for a reason, he had many.

"I'm just not equipped to deal with those people," he said. "You know . . . my nurse . . . my other patients . . . the blood drawing . . . I have no social worker. . . . He needs transportation here. . . . I wouldn't know how to arrange it. . . . The AZT. . . . I'm not sure what those lymphocyte studies mean. . . . The office isn't set up for it. . . . It just wouldn't work out. I'm referring him to you."

The reluctance of physicians and other health care professionals to care for patients with HIV infection or AIDS has been documented in a variety of arenas. Early in the epidemic, avoidance and stigmatization of infected patients was commonplace on hospital wards, although formal documentation of these incidents is largely lacking (Zuger 1987). Subsequently, individual reports of medical care denied to patients with proven or presumed HIV infection began to appear in the lay press: a British physician summoned for a house call, for instance, refused to enter the sickroom of a patient with AIDS, and a number of cardiovascular surgeons in the United States declared their intent to test all patients preoperatively and cancel the surgery of any found to be HIV positive (Law 1987, *New York Times* 1987a).

Surveys of health care professionals conducted over the last several years have provided a more detailed picture of these attitudes and practices.:

• A survey of fifteen hundred American physicians in 1986 documented a disinclination to treat HIV-positive patients for a variety of reasons: "I would not knowingly treat a homosexual patient with AIDS, but I would treat patients who got the disease by blood transfusion and I would treat children with AIDS," commented one anonymous respondent (Ghitelman 1987).

• A survey of one hundred thirteen British dentists in 1986 disclosed that 42 percent of those polled would choose not to treat HIV-positive patients in their own offices. Between 20 and 30 percent of physicians and nurses polled in the same survey felt patients who were candidates for invasive procedures should be HIV tested and referred to "units specialising in HIV-positive patients" if HIV positive (Searle 1987).

• Fewer than 50 percent of 325 American orthopedic surgeons surveyed in 1986 agreed that an orthopedic surgeon was ethically obliged to operate on HIV-infected patients in all situations in which surgery was medically indicated; 11 percent felt the surgeon was not ethically obliged to operate even in emergency situations. In contrast, only 4 percent of the respondents had at some time in the past themselves declined to operate on HIV-infected patients (Arnow et al. 1989).

• In a 1986 survey of 258 house officers at two large New York City residency programs, roughly 50 percent of respondents were mildly, moderately, or extremely resentful at having to take care of AIDS patients; 25 percent stated they would stop taking care of AIDS patients if given a choice, and 24 percent felt that refusing to care for AIDS patients was not unethical (Link et al. 1988).

• Of approximately 4000 dentists polled in Chicago in 1987, only three were willing to accept new AIDS referrals (*New York Times* 1987b).

• Of 174 second-year medical students working in a large public New York City hospital in 1987, 7 percent felt they should have the prerogative of declining to take a history from a patient with AIDS, fourteen percent felt they should have the prerogative of declining to examine the patient, 32 percent felt they should be able to decline to draw blood from the patient, 10 percent felt that physicians should be allowed to decline care outright to patients with AIDS, and 48 percent felt that physicians should have the prerogative of declining care if the patient was assured care elsewhere (Imperato et al. 1988).

• In a poll of 2000 randomly selected U.S. households in 1988, 25 percent of respondents stated that if they discovered their own physician were treating someone with AIDS or with the AIDS virus, they would switch physicians (Gerbert et al. 1989).

These reports together delineate a prevalent reluctance among some health professionals to care for HIV-infected persons, although actual incidents of care withheld appear to be less common. Multiple factors are evidently responsible for this reluctance. Foremost among them is the risk HIV-infected patients may constitute to the health of the practitioner and the practitioner's family, but a host of secondary reasons are present as well. First, HIV patients are seen as a risk to the practitioner's livelihood, potentially jeopardizing relationships with noninfected patients. Second, HIV-infected patients are seen as difficult patients medically: their care may tax the immediate competence of primary health caretakers, requiring subspecialty consultation, specialized treatments, and unfamiliar medications that may be difficult to obtain, and may entail numerous unfamiliar side effects.

Third, although AIDS patients may survive for years after diagnosis, their course is often seen as inexorably downhill, rendering the considerable energy and effort expended on their behalf by health care providers "futile" according to some perspectives. Caring for the dying patient has always been an acquired skill and something of an acquired taste among health care professionals. And finally, HIV-infected patients are often considered undesirable simply by virtue of their risk groups: consciously or subconsciously, their caretakers may sort them into the subcategories of the "innocent victims"—pediatric patients, heterosexual contacts, those who acquired their infection from transfusion of blood or blood products—and the others, the male homosexuals or intravenous (IV) drug users who by implication are the culpable victims. Within inner city populations of HIV-positive persons, poverty, lack of medical insurance, and chaotic social circumstances may render them undesirable patients in some eyes as well.

A Historical Perspective: the Practitioners

The disease was so contagious that one caught it not just by attending the sick but also by looking at them. Men died without servants and were enshrouded without priests; fathers did not visit sons, nor did sons visit fathers; charity was dead, and all hope cast down. . . .

For the doctors there was neither profit nor honor in this disease. They dared not visit the sick, for fear of becoming infected. And when they did visit, they did little and earned nothing, for the sick all died. . . .

To survive there was nothing better than to flee the region before becoming infected. . . .But I myself, to avoid disgrace, did not dare absent myself, but with continuous fear preserved myself as best I could. Even so, near the end of the plague I developed a fever and a bubo: I was ill for a period of six weeks, so dangerously ill that all my friends thought I would die, but the swelling resolved and, treated according to my own principles, I escaped by the will of God.

—Guy de Chauliac,
Fourteenth century surgeon

Unique as the phenomenon of AIDS may be in the modern era, health care professionals have faced patients with new, frightening, and dangerous contagious diseases before. The record of these confrontations forms a background against which most ethical analyses of the developing encounter between the health care professions and AIDS have been set (Loewy 1986; Zuger and Miles 1987; Arras 1988, Kim and Perfect 1988). No single epidemic infectious disease of the past can be set as a precise analogy to HIV infection. Still, the stories of tuberculosis, smallpox, leprosy, plague, and other infectious scourges sometimes unexpectedly echo the story of HIV infection, down to the fact that these diseases often predominantly infect a most undesirable set of patients—the poor.

The history of the health professions' past encounters with dangerous contagious diseases has been explored on several levels. The reactions of individual practitioners faced with dangerous patients form a first level of analysis. The deontological context in which these reactions occurred forms a second: were individual reactions consistent with or at odds with the obligations created by the professional standards and public expectations of the time? Finally, a third level of analysis has consisted of the accommodations, both legislated and informal, reached between the health care professions and the public authorities to cope with the pragmatic details of epidemic disease.

The reactions of individual practitioners to contagious patients form an anecdotal record that begins in the ancient world. Thucidydes' account of the great plague of Athens in 430 B.C. confirms that occupational infection was part of the practice of medicine of that time: "For neither were physicians able to cope with the disease, since they at first had to treat it without knowing its nature, the mortality among them being the greatest because they were more exposed to it . . ." (Smith 1980:343). That occupational infection was not an inevitable part of the profession is illustrated by the story of Galen, physician to the Roman Emperor Marcus Aurelius in the second century A.D. When the plague struck Rome, Galen wrote in his memoirs, "I hastily set out from the city, going eagerly to my native country" (Walsh 1931:203). Only when the plague had resolved did he venture back to Rome.

When the bubonic plague swept through Europe in the fourteenth century, individual physicians continued to react in disparate ways. Some actually fled from their plague-ridden cities. Others remained behind but took a variety of precautions to avoid victims of the disease, from locking themselves in their homes, to standing outside plague houses shouting orders to the clergy caring for the patients within (D'Irsay 1927; Jonsen 1989). Still other physicians appear to have kept at their jobs: the roster of deaths as the plague proceeded through Europe included the chief physicians at the courts of the German emperor, the king of France, and the duke of Burgundy; five of the Pope's twelve physicians; and members of the medical faculties at the universities of Montpelier, Padua, and Paris (Gottfried 1983:117).

During the "Great Plague of London," the outbreak of bubonic plague in London in the winter of 1664–65, the behavior of individual physicians was similarly inconsistent. Nine physicians volunteered for plague duty and several others were appointed to this role by the government. These medical personnel who remained in the city were frequently the less prestigious practitioners who served the poorer classes, among whom the worst of the epidemic raged. In addition, a population of unschooled nurses grew up during that year, who administered much of the hands-on care of the plague victims, were widely distrusted, and were said often to abscond with valuables after the patient's death. Most of the remainder of London's physicians, apothecaries, and surgeons appear to have left the city until the end of the plague (Bell 1924:62,86–88). Among them was Thomas Sydenham, who was to become one of the most eminent physicians of the seventeenth century (Payne 1900:109).

The reaction of physicians confronting epidemic yellow fever in Philadelphia in 1793 was similar. Some well-respected practitioners fled the city—one only after he had caught the disease and was convalescent. Of those who remained behind, many, including the eminent Benjamin Rush, became ill with the fever themselves (Powell 1949). The same inconsistent behavior recurred during the intermittent outbreaks of epidemic disease in the United States in the nineteenth and early twentieth centuries. In some cases physicians fled from cities crippled by cholera, for instance, and in others they remained among the sick, with considerable mortality among them (Rosenberg 1962:68–69). In the 1918 influenza epidemic, the death rate among physicians was substantial, although possibly no greater than that of the general population (Friedlander 1990). Epidemic outbreaks of polio were diagnosed among the personnel of hospitals as recently as 1934; occupational acquisition of tuberculosis continues through the present (Gillam 1938; Geisler et al. 1986). No instances of individual physicians fleeing this or the other infectious epidemics of the twentieth century have been identified.

A Historical Perspective: The Profession

Much praise is also due to those worthy physicians who have remained at their posts at the peril of their lives, and adminis-

tered comfort and relief as far as in their power. Physicians are
justly considered as public property, and like military men, it
pertains to their profession to be occasionally in the way of
danger; hence they are bound by the ties of honor to be found
in their places in an hour when an exertion of their skill might
save the lives of thousands.

—Editorial in the *Federal Gazette*
(Philadelphia, 1793)

The record of individual practitioners throughout history has clearly
been contradictory with regard to the care given patients with contagious diseases. The context in which this ambivalence occurred forms
the next level of analysis: did the standards of medical practice accepted in the past enshrine the care of dangerous patients as a necessary professional activity, or were physicians considered within their
rights when they refused to undertake this duty? Ethicists and historians who seek to place the behavior of individual practitioners in some
normative context have concluded that, like the individual, the professions themselves were generally ambivalent toward this duty.

Again, this conclusion has ancient historical roots. The Hippocratic
corpus emphasized the physician's need to exercise discretion in undertaking the care of incurable patients—a class of patient into which
most of those striken by epidemics would fall (Edelstein 1967:96–97).
The physician's specified duty during an epidemic was only "to declare
the past, diagnose the present, foretell the future" (Jones 1923:1:165).
There is no specific injunction to remain among the ill. Similarly, the
Hippocratic Oath and the Prayer of Maimonides, the two major classical codes of medical practice that endure to this day, do not mention
this particular obligation.

During the Black Death, nothing written by medieval physicians
specifically addresses the issue of professional obligations. Physicians
writing about the disease instead urged their colleagues to take adequate precautions against infection: using gloves to hold a urinal, for
instance, and avoiding poorly ventilated rooms. Several repeatedly
mentioned that physicians *"debent curare infirmos"*—must care for
the sick. This phrase has been interpreted as a refutation of the powerful ancient tradition against accepting hopelessly sick cases and, by
some historians, as evidence of the moral obligation the profession felt
to care for victims of the plague (Amundsen 1977:414). However, no
more elaborate commentary on this obligation exists.

During the London plague of the seventeenth century, the public
appears to have expected physicians to assume some occupational risk

by remaining among the contagious; little evidence exists that this obligation was recognized within the medical profession. The "ethical code" issued by the Royal College of Physicians in 1543 had made no mention of a duty to remain among contagious patients. The only evidence that practitioners felt some professional rather than entirely personal or religious obligation to care for contagious patients is contained in a statement by an apothecary, William Boghurst, who cared for hundreds of patients during the plague:

> Every man that undertakes to bee of a profession or takes upon him any office must take all parts of it, the good and the evill, the pleasure and the pain, the profit and the inconvenience altogether, and not pick and chuse; for ministers must preach, Captains must fight, Physitians attend upon the Sick, etc (Payne 1894:59–60).

In nineteenth-century America a professional duty to treat contagious patients like that outlined by Boghurst became for the first time an established cornerstone of the medical profession. In 1793 Benjamin Rush had characterized his determination to stay with his patients as a religious personal obligation, while laymen such as the editor of the *Federal Gazette* had likened physicians to army men, "bound by ties of honor" occasionally to endanger themselves. Fifty years later, the founders of the American Medical Association codified these metaphors into a specific professional medical duty. "And when pestilence prevails," reads the Code of Ethics published by the AMA in 1847, "it is their [physicians'] duty to face the danger, and to continue their labors for the alleviation of the suffering, even at the jeopardy of their own lives" (AMA 1871:32).

This duty remained a part of the AMA's Code of Ethics until 1957, when, during the first jubilant years of the antibiotic era, it was deleted. In its place, Section VI of the AMA's revised code remained to indicate that: "A physician shall, in the provision of appropriate patient care, except in emergencies, be free to choose whom to serve . . ." (AMA 1986:ix). Until the emergence of AIDS, the issue was not further considered by professional medical or nursing organizations. In the long history of medicine, the specific injunction to care for dangerous patients had a lifespan of slightly over a hundred years.

A Historical Perspective: the Public Health

> The said master Giovanni shall not be bound nor held under obligation except only in attending the plague patients. . . .

namely, the doctor must treat all patients and visit infected
places as it shall be found to be necessary.
— Contract between Giovanni de Ventura and
the city of Pavia, May 6, 1479

Until the era of AIDS, then, the professional duty to treat contagious
patients was a relative innovation in the structure of the health care
professions. Although the lay public frequently decried the cowardice,
unreliability, the unscrupulousness of health practitioners in times of
epidemic disease, the professions did not respond directly to their
displeasure. Instead, careful accommodations were orchestrated between the professions and the public authorities based on a voluntaristic rather than deontologic approach.

In an insightful essay on this topic, Daniel Fox points out that the
history of modern health policy begins with the response of the leaders
of Italian city states to the intermittent epidemics of plague that per-
sisted in Europe from the fourteenth to the eighteenth centuries (Fox
1988). In some cases laws were passed forbidding physicians to leave
the city during plagues. More commonly, however, punitive measures
against members of the profession were avoided. Instead, alternate
personnel were deployed to perform the tasks necessary for the continued functioning of the community. Surgeons, considerably less prestigious than physicians at that time and frequently forbidden to practice
the arts of diagnosis and treatment, were occasionally dispatched to
plague hospitals to diagnose and treat the infected. At other times,
contracts were created between city officials and physicians — often
young physicians from the countryside — stipulating that, in return for
a home, a generous salary, and the promise of future citizenship, the
physician would care for plague patients, relieving more prestigious
colleagues of that responsibility.

For these plague doctors, heavily costumed, perfumed, and masked
according to the sanitary recommendations of the time, the disease
constituted an opportunity that could not be ignored. In return for
assuming the risks of the job, they were offered lavish financial recompense, as well as a chance to penetrate the otherwise quite restricted confines of the profession. Between visitations of plague, notes
one historian, medicine was a relatively prestigious calling in Renaissance Italy. During visitations of plague, it became considerably less
attractive. In place of well-to-do young gentlemen entering the profession, individuals whom the local physicians dismissed as "incompetent
foreign doctors," "idiots and mechanicals" rushed to apply for admission to the physicians' guild (Park 1985:36).

Negotiation between the civic authorities and the medical profession continued to underlie the care of citizens stricken with epidemic contagious disease up to and even after the mid-nineteenth century, when the internal codes of the profession took over. Plague doctors volunteered or were designated to serve; they availed themselves of all means of prevention available, from the robes and perfumes of the Renaissance to the more reasoned hygienic practices of the nineteenth century. Balancing the risks of succumbing to the illness against the ample material recompense they would receive if they survived, the plague doctors constituted a negotiated practical solution to a complicated ethical problem.

Ethical Models: The Professions

> A physician may not ethically refuse to treat a patient whose condition is within the physician's current realm of competence solely because the patient is seropositive.
>
> —American Medical Association
> Council on Ethical and Judicial Affairs, 1988

On all levels of analysis, then, the recorded performance of medical personnel at times of epidemic disease has been uneven. In the absence of any clear historic tradition, ethicists have necessarily approached the issue of the obligations of health care professionals to contagious patients from a variety of theoretical planes. At its most basic, the question of the obligations to "dangerous" patients is simply a facet of many broader analyses of the precise implications of the term "health care profession." Are professionals distinguished from the average worker in the nature of their obligations by the title of "professional"? Are doctors distinguished in obligations from the average human by that of "doctor"? In either of these roles, does the physician or health care professional necessarily assume an obligation to risk that exceeds that of his nonprofessional, nonmedical peers?

In exploring the elements of "calling," or vocation, that persist in the modern versions of the "learned professions," Gustafson has argued that "professional education and activity enable persons to competently exercise their callings, their moral motives" (1982:511). Professions, thus, are by implication moral enterprises, and professionals educated individuals whose vision of a larger good mandates that self-interest be transcended to some extent. This vision implies that the care of the HIV infected is to some extent part of obligations of all professionals. In an analogous discussion, Churchill has discussed the need for a "distinctive" professional ethic for physicians in addition to the legal, political, and personal values that govern the behavior of ordinary citizens. "A profession without its own distinctive moral convictions," he concludes, "has nothing to profess" (Churchill 1989:30). Again, a need is seen for an exclusive, specific moral code for health care professionals, with the implication that an additional layer of moral commitment presupposes a selflessness that would in turn mandate some commitment to the care of the HIV infected.

Despite these and other arguments, however, the modern professional codes that translate these theoretical expectations into concrete terms have not to date unequivocally confirmed the professional's duty to the HIV infected. Historical codes of practice had little to say about the obligations of physicians to contagious patients (vide supra); present-day codes are still being written and rewritten to the issue. Freedman has examined these addenda to American nursing and medical codes of practice regarding the care of AIDS patients, with occasional startling results. Whereas in the past, professional codes encompassed statements of the ideal and exemplary in practice, in the new AIDS-related addenda "the ethical stance of the average practitioner of limited altrusim" (1989:25) has instead been given voice. The American Nursing Association, for instance, states that in situations of "minimal risk," it is generally "morally obligatory" for a nurse to care for patients with AIDS. The definition of "minimal risk" and the obligations of the nurse in other situations are, however, specifically left to the individual nurse's judgment. The American Medical Association's statements on AIDS are similarly tepid. An initial 1986 statement by the AMA's Council on Ethical and Judicial Affairs noted that "not everyone is emotionally able to care for patients with AIDS" and sanctioned the referral of these patients elsewhere by health professionals "unable" to care for them. A subsequent statement issued in 1987 emphasized that HIV infection itself was not a legitimate reason for refusal of treatment but nonetheless continued to refer to physicians "not able" to care for the HIV infected for unspecified reasons. Contrasting these carefully worded phrases with the AMA's ringing exhortations of 1847: "And when pestilence prevails, it is their duty to face the danger." (AMA 1871:32), Freedman deplores the evolution of codes that simply mirror acceptable practice habits rather than seek to reform them into exemplary traditions. The sensibility of the broader good in Gustafson and Churchill's vision of the health-care professional are, as yet, not to be found in the professional codes under which these professionals operate in the United States.

Other ethical analysts have approached these issues from a different perspective on the obligation entailed by membership in the health care professions. The majority of these analyses have dealt with the specific situation of physicians, whose professional activities are generally self-designated, rarely defined or clarified by contractual agreement with an employer. Both of the two most familiar models of health care presently used to structure the physician's role in modern American medicine support the medical profession's obligations to HIV-infected patients in some limited respects. Neither of them, however, has strongly supported the individual physician's role in this effort (Zuger and Miles 1987).

The vision of the relationship between patient and physician as a contract, in which medical care becomes a commodity provided by physician to patient under a consensual voluntary agreement, allows either party to freely refuse to establish a relationship with the other. Once the relationship is established, however, the contract model of medical care imposes certain constraints on the physician. The care provided to the patient must be of acceptable quality according to the standards of current medical practice. The patient may sever the contract at any time; the contract cannot be severed by the physician, however, unless the patient is given adequate notice to contract with another acceptable physician. In the context of HIV infection, the contract model of care translates into an obligation for physicians to continue to care for HIV-infected patients with whom relationships have already been established. Referrals to other physicians acceptable to the patient and refusals to enter into care relationships with new HIV-infected patients are acceptable under this model.

A second model of health care increasingly advocated for modern medical practice, particularly in the United States, is based on the premise that all individuals are endowed with the right to basic health care. A correlative duty is thus imposed on the medical profession to provide that care. Individual physicians are, however, subject only to indirect obligations by this model in regard to details of their practice. Those employed in public hospitals and emergency facilities are mandated by the conditions of their employment to accept all individuals seeking their services. Other physicians, free to choose their work settings and their patients, may practice as they like. As long as other colleagues and facilities are available to fulfill the profession's obligation to society, an individual physician's participation in this goal is unnecessary. In the context of HIV infection, this model imposes no restriction on the freedom of the individual physician, in the absence of a medical emergency or a set of job stipulations, to care for the individual HIV-infected patient, provided alternative routes to health care exist for that patient.

Ethical Models: The Practitioners

> Does pestilence, like a sweeping flood, desolate the city, and hurry thousands into the dark confines of the narrow house? Lo! foremost in the front and fury of the storm, periling his life to save his friends, stands the good physician, the thoroughly furnished, the well-balanced physician.
>
> —Thomas Mitchell,
> professor of medicine, Transylvania University, 1842

The harsh, somewhat entrepreneurial conception of medicine that underlies the models of medicine outlined above, and their laissez-faire implications for the health care of the HIV infected, has deeply disturbed ethicists probing this issue. Uniformly, they have pointed out that certain intangibles historically inextricable from the roots of the medical profession are omitted from these modern models and yet still continue to imbue the modern profession. For many participants, both patients and physicians, the profession still retains some of its original mystical investitures, a vocation rather than a business, a primarily moral rather than primarily commercial enterprise (Osmond 1980). When this spiritual and moral overlay is applied to the structure of modern medicine, the individual physician's duty to treat HIV-infected patients has been strongly upheld in a number of analyses.

Zuger and Miles (1987) urged that the dimensions of modern medicine be extended through a return to a virtue-based medical ethic, a conception first enunciated in the classical world. This model casts the physican as a moral agent possessed of certain virtues necessary for membership in the medical profession. The virtues of courage, integrity, and commitment necessarily belonging to all true physicians would mandate that all physicians care for all HIV-infected patients as they would any other, irrespective of more specific details of contract and context. An individual obligation would exist for all members of the profession, voluntaristic in the sense that all true physicians would care for these patients voluntarily, and those declining would thereby be declining further membership in the healing profession.

Pellegrino (1987), citing the variable definitions of virtue and frequent scarcity of that commodity in general, has advocated a narrower expectation of the virtues inherent in the profession: he suggests that altruism, or effacement of self-interest, be acknowledged an obligatory part of medical practice. This necessity, in his formulation, results from several realities of medical practice. First, in his view the ill are vulnerable and powerless entities, rather than the actively independent contractors envisioned by the champions of the contract model of medical care. Second, medical knowledge is not a commodity privately owned by the physician and dispensed at will: it is a trust, conferred by society on some citizens through innumerable sanctioned invasions of the privacy of others, to be used exclusively for society's benefit. The oath taken at graduation from medical school publicly acknowledges this trust, establishing the physician as a public servant with a necessary degree of self-effacement in that role. As a fire requires suitable professional activity by a firefighter, in Pellegrino's view, so an HIV-infected person needing care requires suitable professional activity by a physician: a necessary mitigation of self-interest is generated by the parameters of the job.

Arras has urged a consideration of the physician's duty to contagious patients as part of a historical tradition that lives and endures despite the petty contradictory details of physicians' actions and reactions in times of plague. He argues that a continuum of traditional moral goals has always been implicit in the profession, including a duty to treat contagious patients, despite the inconsistent performance record in evidence historically. According to this conception, "physicians, if queried about their commitment to accept risk in the line of duty, would simply respond, 'this is who we are; this is what we do. Those who fail to treat are cowards and not true physicians' " (1988:13).

Specifically considering the question of whether physicians are obliged to treat patients with AIDS, Emanuel (1988) similarly focuses on the distinction between physicians and ordinary citizens. While ordinary citizens have no active obligation to any unrelated individuals, including those with AIDS, physicians are engaged in an enterprise distinguished from that of others by its primary professional goal of healing the sick rather than pursuit of wealth or other, more commonplace aims. By enrolling in the profession the physician has acquired the obligation to tend the sick: "The obligation is neither chosen nor transferable, it is constitutive of the professional activity." The care of persons with AIDS is simply a particular application of this general rule.

In contrast to this variety of arguments affirming the physician's duty to treat the HIV infected, arguments supporting the right of physicians to refuse to treat these patients have been infrequently advanced. Largely, the advocates of the physician's right to refuse have relied on a strong arbitrary defense of the physician's right to autonomy, generally supported by more concrete concerns. "To coerce a reluctant surgeon into operating on a specific patient may not only distort his judgment but also cause him to perform technically inferior surgery," point out two proponents of the physician's right to choose whom to treat (Pottenger and Siegler 1987). Others have cited primarily statistics of risk that they deem excessive (Day 1989); "acceptable" levels of risk approximated by more theoretical reasoning have not been worked out in these arguments.

AIDS and Magnitude of Risk

> Pious statements from higher-ups . . . about the treatment of patients with AIDS do not cut it. It is one thing to treat a patient who has AIDS, and quite another to come into direct contact with that patient's blood.
>
> —American physician, 1988

The moral mission of health care is thus generally agreed to uphold the duty of health care professionals, physicians in particular, to treat contagious patients needing their care. The situation of AIDS requires, however, a more detailed and pragmatic analysis than philosophy can supply. As outlined above, reluctance to care for patients with AIDS is a multifactorial phenomenon. While the roles prejudice and laziness play in this reluctance need little further commentary, the role of fear must be more objectively addressed. Although a general duty toward contagious patients clearly exists, no ethicist would uphold this theoretical principle to the extent that reckless or suicidal risks are mandated to be a part of every physician's calling. As quantitative estimates of risk are increasingly becoming a part of clinical decision making, so their utility in ethical discussions is essential to tether the principle to the practice. Only with these considerations can the abstractions used in the ethical analyses offered above be defined.

The magnitude of risk involved in caring for patients with HIV infection or AIDS is still being delineated as experience with the infection mounts. Several facts have been firmly established. The virus cannot be transmitted by "casual contact" with infected patients: handshakes, coughs, sneezes, and utensils such as forks, hairbrushes, and stethoscopes will not transmit it from one person to another. However, situations in which the blood or body fluids of an infected person are inoculated through the skin or onto the mucous membranes of another do have the potential for transmission (Friedland and Klein 1987). For health care professionals, then, the risk of acquiring HIV infection can thus be dichotomized initially into "zero" and "not zero" categories. For some, occupationally acquired infection simply will not occur despite their membership in the health care professions: psychiatrists and other physicians who perform no invasive procedures belong in this category, as do nurses who perform no bedside nursing functions, dietitians, social workers, and most therapists.

For other health care professionals, occasionally or regularly exposed to the blood or secretions of HIV-positive patients, the occupational acquisition of HIV infection remains a small but finite possibility. These at-risk individuals are members of a variety of disciplines: house officers, internists, nurses, and laboratory technicians may draw or process blood from patients; paramedical personnel are exposed to the blood and secretions of trauma victims; dentists, surgeons, and pathologists regularly explore blood-filled environments in their work. For none of these professionals is parenteral exposure to HIV inevitable: gloves, goggles, gowns, and "careful" needle-using behavior theoretically shield them from contact with the virus. For all of them, however, the risk of inoculation remains inherent in the fallibility of all protective measures presently in use: gloves tear, test tubes break, needles are hastily placed or misplaced.

Quantitation of the risk of occupational HIV infection thus depends on the prevalence of HIV infection in the treated population, the frequency of accidents that may lead to exposure, and the efficiency of transmission inherent in each exposure. Investigations into each of these variables have led to only very preliminary results. HIV prevalence varies widely from area to area: some hospitals may see cases only infrequently, while elsewhere a sizable minority of all emergency room or hospitalized patients may be infected with HIV. Needlesticks are frequent accidents on hospital wards, particularly among inexperienced personnel. Gloves are punctured regularly during surgery, with cited frequencies ranging from 2 percent to 30 percent of surgical procedures (Sims and Dudley 1988; Gerberding et al. 1990). Of those parenteral exposures to HIV that have been studied, approximately 1 in 250 (0.4 percent) has transmitted the infection; the rate at which exposure of mucous membranes to infected blood results in the transmission of infection appears to be considerably lower (Marcus et al. 1988; Becker, Cone, and Gerberding 1989).

Is the risk delineated by these numbers a small risk or a large one? It has been described as both. One study has estimated that, depending on locality, it places physicians between police officers and firefighters in magnitude of yearly risk of occupational-related fatality (Rosenberg, Becker, and Cone 1989). In comparison with the spectrum of other health-care-related occupational hazards this risk is similarly difficult to interpret. Compared with the risk of acquiring hepatitis B from a single exposure to highly infectious blood (approximately 15 percent), the risk of acquiring HIV from a needlestick is tiny, although the consequences of infection are more severe. When other infrequent occupation-associated risks are considered—that of being throttled by a violent patient, for instance—the risk of HIV acquisition becomes in comparison more substantial (Patterson et al. 1985; Hagen, Meyer, and Pauker 1988).

Do these numbers cause the duty to treat HIV-infected patients to cross the threshold from duty to supererogation? These first efforts to quantitate the risk of treating HIV-infected patients are as yet too cursory to have been included in many ethical analyses of the subject. Emanuel (1988) has attempted to factor magnitude of risk carefully into his schema by considering the situation of an orthopedic trauma surgeon practicing in San Francisco (estimated forty needlesticks per year, of which 33 percent carry HIV infection, and a maximum of 1 percent may transmit the infection) whose estimated yearly risk of acquiring HIV infection is thus 12 percent, or virtually 100 percent in ten years of this variety of medical practice. Clearly this risk is excessive; it contrasts dramatically with a soldier's less than 3 percent risk of dying in combat during a year of active duty in the Vietnam War. No ethical analysis would uphold a professional's obligation to perform under these odds.

On the other hand, several practical points must be added to this variety of quantitative ethics. First, Emanuel's numerical estimates of health care professionals' risk have yet to be validated by the actual incidence of observed occupational infections. These incidents continue to occur as sporadic, tragic accidents; a secondary occupational epidemic of AIDS among at-risk health professionals now ten years into the original epidemic has not been seen, nor, according to more careful studies into the nature and preventability of intraoperative blood exposure accidents, is it likely to occur (Gerberding et al. 1990, Henderson 1990). Also to be remembered is the fact that situations of excessive risk do not abrogate all obligations to HIV infected: "treat" is, again, a word with a spectrum of definitions. The professional in a situation of excessively high risk has no obligation to remain in that situation; an obligation to treat HIV-infected individuals endures, however, with the risk reduced to acceptable proportions. Sharing the infected patient load with other professionals, eliminating unnecessary exposures, and using the most effective precautions possible may all contribute to this goal.

The HIV-infected Physician

> Health workers must not deny care to the victims of this com-
> plex human nightmare. But if we are to be in the front lines,
> then we must make sure that we are better protected in all
> respects. I am living proof that it can happen to any of us. And
> no other health worker should have to go through what I have
> endured.
>
> Physician with occupationally acquired AIDS, 1989

In the short history of the AIDS epidemic, the figure of the HIV-infected health professional has raised a complex tangle of reactions on the part of both the professions and the public. Reports of occupationally acquired infection have accumulated in parallel with reports of physicians who sustain devastating social and professional losses on divulging their HIV infection to patients, colleagues, or employers (Applebome 1987; *New York Times* 1988). Irrespective of route of acquisition of infection this phenomenon merits careful ethical analysis; in the context of occupationally acquired HIV infection it becomes integral to any discussion of health care professionals' duty to treat HIV-positive patients.

The ideal Hippocratic physician was a godlike entity ("He should look healthy, and as plump as nature intended him to be; for the common crowd consider those who are not of this excellent bodily condition to be unable to take care of others") (Jones 1923:2:311). Symbolically, the HIV-infected practitioner violates this ideal. The deep human need to believe that caretakers are impervious to the infirmities they treat is no less true in our time than in Hippocrates': much of the hostility HIV-positive practitioners have evoked may be traced to their de facto betrayal of this need. In addition, the certainties that shield the civil rights of other HIV-infected individuals—in particular, that they constitute no risk to the health of client or colleague in the workplace—may not uniformly apply to infected health care workers. Whereas antidiscrimination legislation is increasingly invoked to protect the employment of HIV-infected persons, the situations of infected health care workers must be examined more carefully.

As in the analysis of risks HIV-infected patients constitute to practitioners, the risks infected practitioners constitute to their patients dichotomize immediately into "zero" and "not zero" categories. Those providers having no contact with the blood or body fluids of patients, and thus no risk of acquiring infection from patients, have similarly no risk of transmitting their own infection to patients. For them, the details of their employment are irrelevant as long as they remain able to perform their jobs. Other practitioners, however, who are in intermittent contact with patients' blood or mucous membranes, do create the theoretical risk that a conglomeration of accidental circumstances may result in transfer of blood from practitioner to patient. Again, the risk forms a spectrum, from the virtually impossible chance that a series of superficial needlesticks might transfer practitioner's blood to patient, to the more realistic possibility that a scalpel wound during surgery might inoculate a quantity of infected practitioner's blood into a patient's wound.

This spectrum of risk has as yet little magnitude: only isolated cases of patients who may have been infected by an infected health care practitioner have been reported. Magnitude of risk arguments are thus yet to be created for this scenario; by the same token, however, they are less important in this context than the simple acknowledgment that a risk may conceivably exist. Whereas assumption of some degree of risk is inherent in the calling of physician, it has no formal correlate in the calling of patient. Physicians and, by analogy, other practitioners operate under a time-honored enjoinder to do their patients no harm. In reality, of course, the harms a practitioner may constitute to a patient's health are legion, engendered by deficiencies ranging from carelessness to incompetence to substance abuse, in addition to influenza, hepatitis B, and other, less notorious, more easily transmitted infections than HIV. The ethical principle remains, however, that practitioners who knowingly place patients at any risk, however vanishingly small, are violating a basic code of their practice.

The legal and practical sequelae of this ethical principle are still evolving. In a recent analysis, Gostin (1989) argues that the inherent risk of HIV transmission to a patient is sufficient to be "taken seriously" even before the first incident of this transmission occurs. He rejects, however, both mass screening of practitioners and voluntary disclosure of HIV serostatus as possible means to this end. Expecting patients to make an "informed decision" regarding continuing under an HIV-positive practitioner's care is tantamount, in the midst of an ongoing public hysteria over AIDS, to demanding professional suicide. Systematic screening of physicians, operating room nurses, and other high-risk personnel by hospitals or regulatory boards is rendered impractical and ethically dubious by the same standards that have thus far precluded the mass screening of other populations. Only case-by-case deliberation by medical rather than judicial experts—if necessary, delimiting the infected professional's involvement in surgery or other invasive procedures while insuring privacy, confidentiality, and continued professional functioning—forms a viable solution to the problem.

Despite this reasoned analysis, the crippling irony of the facts has not been lost on high-risk professionals: those practitioners at greatest risk of occupational acquisition of HIV infection are those at greatest risk of its serious impact on their livelihood. Many of these professionals have become increasingly frustrated by what they forecast is the inevitable outcome of present trends—that surgeons, prohibited by prevailing ethical norms from screening their patients for HIV, will soon be subject by frightened patients to compulsory HIV screening themselves. They point out that in an abbreviated ethical algebra of "quid pro quo," they are victimized by ethical principles that oblige them to treat HIV-infected persons, yet confer no corresponding obligation on society to compensate for the injury they risk. Their instincts are, hence, to protect themselves by refusing to acknowledge a duty to treat, until compensatory protections are offered (Dudley and Sims 1988).

Various specific compensations have been proposed in answer to these points. They range from general calls for research into and development of better protective materials for gloves and sheaths for needles to more specific recommendations for measures within the professions' present grasp. Many voices, including the particularly poignant ones of physicians who have become HIV infected through occupational exposure, have called for improved disability insurance and worker's compensation benefits for all potential victims of accidents such as theirs (Cooke and Sande 1989; Cadman 1990). A formal acknowledgment by hospitals, medical schools, and leaders of the profession that the risk is a real one would offer considerable psychological support to those assuming that risk. A change in the prevailing work ethic of hospital wards, in which inexperienced students and residents are often dispatched to perform procedures they have never carefully learned how to do, would offer both psychological and practical benefits. Most authorities agree that the implementation of these measures will allow health care workers at risk to approach that risk with more reasoned, less emotional reactions.

The Developing Accommodations of AIDS

The same passions which made these regulations necessary
rendered them ineffectual.

—Edward Gibbon

As in the historical models cited above, the developing encounter between the health care professions and AIDS has involved individual actions, professional expectations, and pragmatic accommodations. Perhaps not surprisingly, these interactions have to date been remarkably consistent with the ambiguous precedents set during past epidemic diseases. Individual practitioners have reacted to the disease in inconsistent ways: overt refusals to provide care to the HIV infected have been relatively infrequent; covert refusals couched in referrals, delays, and failures to adhere to accepted standards of medical care have been more common. Major professional associations have issued emphatic but not always unqualified statements supporting the duty of the professional to care for HIV-infected patients. Patient advocate groups and the lay press have emphasized a duty to treat more strongly.

To date, however, these exhortations have not been reinforced by either professional or civil liabilities attached to the individual's refusal to comply. Rather, as in the past, an incentive rather than punitive system is evolving to reconcile the brewing conflict between public expectations and professional performance. A new generation of "plague" practitioners has evolved within the professions, who, like their medieval predecessors, have found a variety of compensations for the danger and difficulty of caring for these unpopular patients. For some, the pleasures of serving a particularly needy and appreciative population stand as rewards in themselves. For others, attractive salaries, prestige in a competitive research community, and a kind of folk-hero status in the popular press have constituted some of the more tangible rewards for plague duty in our time.

Unfortunately, this time-honored voluntaristic accommodation between society and medicine represented by a cadre of plague doctors and nurses may not achieve its intended goals today. The competence to treat and cure disease, considerably more potent in the medicine of our time than ever before, cannot be ignored in any formulation of a duty to treat HIV-infected persons. For possibly the first time in history, standard, rigorous medical care will make a substantial difference in the length of life and the quality of life experienced by victims of an epidemic disease. Thus, the evolution of a dichotomized community of medical professionals, only a fraction of whom are experienced, comfortable, and competent in the highly technical and rapidly evolving clinical care of the HIV infected, is unlikely to serve society's goals as the epidemic expands over the next decade (Bennett et al. 1989; Kobylak 1989).

This consideration constitutes a powerful argument against allowing the informal voluntarism of prior epidemics to develop in this epidemic as well. Optimally, however, an unprecedented policing of the professions will not arise as a necessary alternative. Rather, it is to be hoped that as medical treatment of the disease becomes more effective, and means of protecting health care professionals from occupational injury more potent, members of the professions will rediscover the individual commitments to healing that originally impelled them to their roles.

REFERENCES

AMA (American Medical Association). 1871. *Code of Ethics Adopted May 1847.* Philadelphia: Turner Hamilton.

AMA. 1986. *Current Opinions of the Judicial Council of the American Medical Association, 1986.* Chicago: AMA.

AMA. Council on Ethical and Judicial Affairs. 1988. Ethical Issues Involved in the Growing AIDS Crisis. *JAMA* 259:1360–1361.

Amundsen, Darrel W. 1977. Medical Deontology and Pestilential Disease in the Late Middle Ages. *Journal of the History of Medicine* 32:403–421.

Aoun, Hacib. 1989. When a House Officer Gets AIDS. *New England Journal of Medicine* 321(10):693–696.

Applebome, Peter. 1987. Doctor in Texas with AIDS Virus Closes His Practice Amid a Furor. *New York Times* (October 1), p. B8.

Arnow, Paul M., Lawrence A. Pottenger, Carol B. Stocking, Mark Siegler, and Henry W. DeLeeuw. 1989. Orthopedic Surgeons' Attitudes and Practices Concerning Treatment of Patients with HIV Infection. *Public Health Reports* 104(2):121–129.

Arras, John D. 1988. The Fragile Web of Responsibility: AIDS and the Duty to Treat. *Hastings Center Report* 18(2):10–20.

Becker, Charles E., James E. Cone, and Julie Gerberding. 1989. Occupational Infection with Human Immunodeficiency Virus. *Annals of Internal Medicine* 110(8):653–656.

Bell, W. G. 1924. *The Great Plague in London in 1665.* New York: Dodd Mead.

Bennett, Charles L., Jeffrey B. Garfinkle, Sheldon Greenfield, David Draper, William Rogers, W. Christopher Matthews, and David E. Kanouse. 1989. The Relation Between Hospital Experience and In-Hospital Mortality for Patients with AIDS-related PCP. *JAMA* 261(20):2975–2979.

Cadman, Edwin C. 1990. Physicians in Training and HIV (letter). *New England Journal of Medicine* 322(19):1392.

Churchill, Larry R. 1989. Reviving a Distinctive Medical Ethic. *Hastings Center Report* 19(3)28–34.
Cipolla, Carlo M. 1977. A Plague Doctor. In Harry A. Miskimin, D. Herlihy, A. L. Udovitch, eds. *The Medieval City*. New Haven: Yale University Press.
Cooke, Molly and Merle A. Sande. 1989. The HIV Epidemic and Training in Internal Medicine: Challenges and Recommendations. *New England Journal of Medicine* 321(19):1334–1338.
Day, Lorraine. 1989. The AIDS Epidemic from a Surgeon's Viewpoint. *Orthopaedic Review* 18 (suppl.):35–38.
D'Irsay, Stephen. 1927. Defense Reactions During the Black Death, 1348–1349. *Annals of Medical History* 9:169–179.
Dudley, H. A. F. and A. Sims. 1988. AIDS: A Bill of Rights for the Surgical Team? *British Medical Journal* 296:1449–1450.
Edelstein, Ludwig. 1967. The Hippocratic Physician. In Owsei Temkin and C. Lillian Temkin, eds., *Ancient Medicine: Selected Papers of Ludwig Edelstein*, pp. 96–97. Baltimore: The Johns Hopkins Press.
Emanuel, Ezekiel J. 1988. Do Physicians Have an Obligation to Treat Patients with AIDS? *New England Journal of Medicine* 318(25):1686–1690.
Federal Gazette. 1793. Editorial. Philadelphia, Pa. (October 5), p. 3.
Fox, Daniel M. 1988. The Politics of Physicians' Responsibility in Epidemics: A Note on History. *Hastings Center Report* 18(2):5–10.
Freedman, Benjamin. 1989. Health Professions, Codes, and the Right to Refuse to Treat HIV-infectious Patients. *Hastings Center Report* 18(2):20–25.
Friedland, Gerald H. and Robert S. Klein. 1987. Transmission of the Human Immunodeficiency Virus. *New England Journal of Medicine* 317(18):1125–1135.
Friedlander, Walter J. 1990. On the Obligation of Physicians to Treat AIDS: Is There a Historical Basis? *Reviews of Infectious Diseases* 12(2):191–203.
Geisler, P. Jan, Kenrad E. Nelson, Ray G. Crispen, and Vijai K. Moses. 1986. Tuberculosis in Physicians: A Continuing Problem. *American Reviews of Respiratory Disease* 133:773–778.
Gerberding, Julie Louise, Cary Littell, Ada Tarkington, Andrew Brown, and William P. Schecter. 1990. Risk of Exposure of Surgical Personnel to Patients' Blood During Surgery at San Francisco General Hospital. *New England Journal of Medicine* 322:1788–1793.
Gerbert, Barbara, Bryan T. Maguire, Stephen B. Hulley, and Thomas J. Coates. 1989. Physicians and Acquired Immunodeficiency Syndrome: What Patients Think About Human Immunodeficiency Virus in Medical Practice. *JAMA* 262(14):1969–1972.
Ghitelman, David. 1987. AIDS. *MD* (January), pp. 91–100.
Gibbon, Edward. 1932. *The Decline and Fall of the Roman Empire,* vol 1. New York: Modern Library.
Gillam A. G. 1938. *Epidemiological Study of an Epidemic Diagnosed as Poliomyelitis, Occurring Among the Personnel of the Los Angeles County General Hospital During the Summer of 1934*. Washington D.C.: U.S. Government Printing Office (Public Health Bulletin no. 240).
Gostin, Lawrence. 1989. HIV-infected Physicians and the Practice of Seriously Invasive Procedures. *Hastings Center Report* 19(1):32–39.
Gottfried, Robert S. 1983. *The Black Death: Natural and Human Disaster in Medieval Europe*. New York: Free Press.
Gustafson, James M. 1982. Professions as "Callings." *Social Service Review* 56:501–515.
Hagen, Michael D., Klemens B. Meyer, and Stephen G. Pauker. 1988. Routine

Preoperative Screening for HIV: Does the Risk to the Surgeon Outweigh the Risk to the Patient? *JAMA* 259(9):1357–1359.

Henderson, David K. 1990. HIV-1 in the Health-Care Setting. In Gerald F. Mandell, R. Gordon Douglas, Jr., and John E. Bennett, eds., *Principles and Practice of Infectious Diseases*, 3d ed., pp. 2221–2236. New York: John Wiley.

Imperato, Pascal James, Joseph G. Feldman, Kamran Nayeri, and Jack A. DeHovitz. 1988. Medical Students' Attitudes Towards Caring for Patients with AIDS in a High Incidence Area. *New York State Journal of Medicine* 88(5):223–228.

Jones, W. H. S., trans. 1923. *Hippocrates: Collected Works*. The Loeb Classical Library. Cambridge, Mass.: Harvard University Press.

Jonsen, Albert R. 1989. The Duty to Treat Patients with AIDS and HIV Infection. In Lawrence O. Gostin, ed., *AIDS and the Health Care System*, pp. 155–168. New Haven: Yale University Press.

Kalivas, James. 1988. Do Physicians Have an Obligation to Treat Patients with AIDS? (letter). *New England Journal of Medicine* 320(2):121.

Kim, Jerome H. and John R. Perfect. 1988. To Help the Sick: An Historical and Ethical Essay Concerning the Refusal to Care for Patients with AIDS. *American Journal of Medicine* 84(1):135–138.

Kobylak, Lester J. 1989. Do Physicians Have an Obligation to Treat Patients with AIDS? (letter). *New England Journal of Medicine* 320(2):121.

Law, Carl Edgar. 1987. Are British MDs Shirking Duty with AIDS Patients? *Medical Tribune* (June 17), 28(23):1.

Link, R. Nathan, Anat R. Feingold, Mitchell H. Charap, Katherine Freeman, and Steven P. Shelov. 1988. Concerns of Medical and Pediatric Officers About Acquiring AIDS from Their Patients. *American Journal of Public Health* 78(4):455–459.

Loewy, Erich H. 1986. AIDS and the Physician's Fear of Contagion. *Chest* 89(3):325–326.

Marcus, Ruthanne and the CDC Cooperative Needlestick Surveillance Group. 1988. Surveillance of Health Care Workers Exposed to Blood from Patients Infected with the Human Immunodeficiency Virus. *New England Journal of Medicine* 319(17):1118–1122.

Mitchell, Thomas D. 1842. *The Good Physician*. Lexington, Ky. The Observer and Reporter Office.

New York Times. 1987a. Heart Surgeon Won't Operate on Victims of AIDS (March 13), p. A11.

New York Times. 1987b.AIDS Clinic Being Weighed by Chicago Dental Society (July 21), p. B4.

New York Times. 1988. Right to Bar Treatment by Any with AIDS Virus Weighed (September 16), p. B7.

Nicaise, F. ed. 1980. *Guy de Chauliac: La Grande Chirurgie*. Paris: F. Nicaise.

Osmond, Humphrey. 1980. God and the Doctor. *New England Journal of Medicine* 302(10):555–558.

Park, Katherine. 1985. *Doctors and Medicine in Early Renaissance Florence*. Princeton, N.J.: Princeton University Press.

Patterson, William B., Donald E. Craven, David A. Schwartz, Edward A. Nardell, Jean Kasmer, and John Noble. 1985. Occupational Hazards to Hospital Personnel. *Annals of Internal Medicine* 102(5):658–680.

Payne, J. F., ed. 1894. Boghurst, William. *Loimographia*. Published in *Transactions of the Epidemiological Society of London*, vol. 13. London: Shaw.

Payne, J. F. 1900. *Thomas Sydenham*. New York: Longmans Green.

Pellegrino, Edmund D. 1987. Altruism, Self-Interest, and Medical Ethics. *JAMA* 258(14):1939–1940.

Pottenger, Lawrence A. and Mark Siegler. 1987. Surgeons' Obligations to Treat HIV-infected Patients. *Proceedings of the Institute of Medicine of Chicago* 40:81–82.

Powell, J. H. 1949. *Bring Out Your Dead*. Philadelphia: University of Pennsylvania Press.

Rosenberg, Charles D. 1962. *The Cholera Years: The United States in 1832, 1849, 1866*. Chicago: University of Chicago Press.

Rosenberg J., Charles E. Becker, and James E. Cone. 1989. How an Occupational Medicine Physician Views Current Blood-borne Disease Risks in Health-Care Workers. *State of the Art Review of Occupational Medicine* 4(Suppl.):3–6.

Searle, E. Stephen. 1987. Knowledge, Attitudes, and Behaviour of Health Professionals in Relation to AIDS. *Lancet* 1:26–28.

Sims, A. J. W. and A. J. F. Dudley. 1988. Surgeons and HIV. *British Medical Journal* 296:80.

Smith, C. F. trans. 1980. *Thucydides: History of the Peloponnesian War*. Cambridge, Mass.: Harvard University Press.

Walsh, Joseph. 1931. Refutation of the Charges of Cowardice Made Against Galen. *Annals of Medical History* 13:195–207.

Zuger, Abigail. 1987. AIDS on the Wards: A Residency in Medical Ethics. *Hastings Center Report* 17(3):16–20.

Zuger, Abigail and Steven H. Miles. 1987. Physicians, AIDS, and Occupational Risk: Historic Traditions and Ethical Obligations. *JAMA* 258(14):1924–1928.

10. AIDS and Privacy

FERDINAND SCHOEMAN

ISSUES OF PRIVACY surface in nearly every dimension of AIDS, from diagnosis, to treatment, to epidemiology, to prevention. A sampling of issues includes topics like reporting human immunodeficiency virus (HIV) infection to public health agencies, confidentiality of the therapist-patient relationship, and the duty, on the part of the individual or public health authorities, to disclose one's condition to a sexual partner, surgeon, employer, or insurance provider. No group in society is more vulnerable to both biological and social repercussions of a disease than those infected with HIV. Tragically, some aspects of protecting the privacy of those who are HIV infected have frightening potential for others who understandably wish to avoid contagion, as well as for those who recognize the social costs of the increasing numbers and changing profile of AIDS victims. AIDS, as we will see, is destined to have as much impact on the contours of our notion of privacy as computerization of records and the legalization of abortion did.

Conflict and the inevitability of unmet and haunting needs is nowhere more manifest than in the case of AIDS. AIDS is a lethal disease that is communicable in controllable ways. To think of it as a fatal disease invokes one pattern of normative responses: sympathetic and protecting attitudes. To think of it as a condition that is communicable in a controllable way invokes another set of normative responses: those attributing accountability for harming others. Being sick diminishes one's accountability for some things—things over which one has impaired capacity. The negligence or recklessness involved in infecting another with HIV is *not*, however typically the result of impaired capacity (*United States v. Sergeant Nathaniel Johnson, Jr.*).[1] A person who deserves compassion for having a disease *may* also deserve admonition for acquiring or condemnation for transmitting it. Spouses or partners of those HIV infected may have cause for complaint on either ground.

People infected with HIV have much to fear besides the disease. Because of the association of AIDS with promiscuity, primarily homosexual but also heterosexual, or the self-abandonment connected with intravenous (IV) drug usage, any adult with AIDS is suspected of degeneracy. One in five Americans regard those with AIDS as deserving their suffering because of their immorality (Blendon and Donelan 1988). Homophobia is widespread in the United States, and the intrusion of AIDS as a public health problem has in many people's minds lent legitimacy to hostility toward gay individuals (Goleman 1990). The level of public ignorance about the disease, the deficiency of scientific understanding surrounding aspects of its transmission, and the general hysteria about AIDS mean that people diagnosed as HIV positive must face social, economic, and medical hurdles no one with such dire medical prospects should have to confront. These prejudices extend to those who care for AIDS victims and even to the dwellings of those with AIDS. A diagnosis of HIV infection, or even a suspicion of this, is sufficient in some cases to deprive people of housing, employment, life and health insurance, social tolerance, routine and even emergency medical treatment like mouth-to-mouth resuscitation, schooling, social contacts, friendships, the right to travel in and out of countries—a social identity.

Studies of public attitudes toward those with AIDS make crystal clear the social consequences AIDS sufferers will confront (Blendon and Donelan 1988). One in four questioned in a survey indicated that he or she would refuse to work with someone with AIDS; the same percentage believe that employers should be able to fire employees with AIDS; 39 percent of people surveyed agreed that public school employees should be dismissed if found to have AIDS. In 1988, 18 percent felt that children with AIDS should be barred from school. Nearly one-third indicated that out of concern for their own children's health they would keep their children from attending schools that admitted children with AIDS. In surveys conducted in 1987, a substantial minority (between 21 and 40 percent, depending on the wording) favored isolating people with AIDS from the general community, from public places, and from their own neighborhoods. Panic over the prospect of becoming contaminated is even widespread among health professionals (see Zuger's essay in this volume). Also widespread is skepticism about the accuracy of risk assessments promulgated in the best medical journals. Tragically, fear of discrimination is itself an important obstacle to both greater epidemiological understanding of HIV transmission and implementation of public health measures aimed at minimizing HIV infection.

Further complicating the terrifying social and medical dimensions of HIV infection is the awareness of having been infected by and/or potentially infecting those with whom one is most intimate. This is a moral burden few could find anything but crushing. And yet, discovering and revealing one's own HIV status threatens this source of meaning and support perhaps more than any other.

Conceptual Foundations of Privacy

Because of the way AIDS is transmitted and because of the social, financial, and medical consequences of being identified as HIV positive, it is no wonder that AIDS and privacy intersect at every dimension of the disease. Let us turn our attention to some of the foundational issues related to privacy, beginning with the meaning of privacy.[2] There are broader and narrower conceptions of privacy. On the narrower range of conceptions, privacy relates exclusively to information of a personal sort about an individual and describes the extent to which others have access to this information.[3] A broader conception extends beyond the informational domain and encompasses anonymity and restricted physical access. Thus far the characterizations allow a sharp contrast between privacy and autonomy. Embracing some aspects of autonomy within the definition of privacy, it has been defined as control over the intimacies of personal identity. At the broadest end of the spectrum, privacy is thought to be the measure of the extent an individual is afforded the social and legal space to develop the emotional, cognitive, spiritual, and moral powers of an autonomous agent. An advocate of one of the narrower conceptions can agree about the value of autonomous development but think that privacy as properly defined makes an important but limited contribution to its achievement.

Privacy is important as a means of respecting or even socially constructing moral personality, comprising qualities like independent judgment, creativity, self-knowledge, and self-respect. It is important because of the way control over one's thoughts and body enables one to develop trust for, or love and friendships with, one another and more generally modulate relationships with others (Fried 1960). It is important too for the political dimensions of a society that respects individual privacy, finding privacy instrumental in protecting rights of association, individual freedom, and limitations on governmental control over thoughts and actions (Benn 1971). Finally, it has been argued that privacy is important as a means of protecting people from overreaching social (as opposed to legal) pressures and sanctions and is thus critical if people are to enjoy a measure of social freedom. This is a dimension of privacy I return to below.

Respecting privacy does not commit us to elevating it above all other concerns. We respect privacy even when we abridge it provided we do so for good reason. What I shall be arguing as we proceed is that HIV status is to be regarded as private information about a person, deserving protection, unless there is "a need to know" on someone's part that in the circumstances makes withholding information unreasonable. In assessing the need to know, we have a responsibility to use the best available information about risk factors. What is protected in one informational context may be unprotected in another. Assessing whether a risk is reasonable is not just a function of the probability of harm. Relevant too are the consequences of abstaining from that behavior and the alternatives available for achieving similar objectives.

In assessing the need to know, many factors depend for their strength on social perceptions, ones that can vary over cultures and within a culture over time and circumstance. They can also vary over class and gender within a culture. By offering some examples of the variability of these standards, we can recognize that many acts we would regard as intrusive, others would not so regard. For instance, in some cultures that place a high premium on the virginity of brides and consummation of marriage as initiating the married state, the first act of intercourse between the man and woman is publicly monitored (Stone 1979). In colonial New England, people were required to live within a household, thinking it improper that a person not be supervised in his private affairs. There was a village officer, the tithingsman, whose role was to pry into the private lives of people to ensure compliance with local social standards (Flaherty 1972). In some communities within the contemporary United States, having a child out of wedlock would be something important to conceal. In other communities, it is the norm. We can and should be sensitive to the class, cultural, and even gender differences in attitudes toward the importance of treating something as private. Inevitably, policies in a pluralistic society will grate against some sensibilities. however judicious the policies are.

Privacy and Sexually Transmitted Diseases

As the discussion of AIDS and privacy proceeds, some additional theoretical categories will be introduced. AIDS is not the first disease to raise privacy issues. Most states require that a test for venereal diseases

be made prior to marriage (Krause 1986:43–44) and that a doctor
certify that the partners either are free of disease or have it in noncom-
municable stages. All states have public health laws that require reporting sexually transmitted diseases (STDs). Most states do not deal
with AIDS or the presence of the HIV antibody as falling under public
health regulations pertaining to STDs proper, though they usually have
equivalent regulations for AIDS.

> As of July 1989, a total of 28 states required health care providers to
> report cases of persons infected with HIV to their state public health
> departments. The clear trend is toward reporting of HIV infection, with
> many states having such proposals before their legislatures (Gostin
> 1990a:1962).

Although it is certain that one major route of infection is through
sexual contact, there is concern that if AIDS or HIV infection is treated
as an STD, requiring reporting, those who are infected with HIV will
face additional social, medical, and economic isolation in addition to
the ravages of the disease (Gostin 1990a). Ironically, treating AIDS as
an STD would automatically engage those confidentiality requirements
associated with the relevant public health laws.

Privacy and AIDS

The range of privacy issues that arise in the AIDS environment is
bewildering (Gostin 1990a). These include confidentiality in relationships with health professionals and disclosure of HIV status to insurers
and employers, to state health agencies, to family members or sexual
or other partners where transmission is a possibility, to schools, and to
residential settings of almost any kind, including correctional facilities.
Privacy arises as an issue in considering proposals for HIV screening
and in partner notification.

AIDS also has an impact on consideration of public norms that
govern private relationships. AIDS and privacy intersect not only for
the health care provider, the state, and the HIV-infected person but
also for people in their ordinary and informal contact with others. The
law both reflects and influences the moral and social rules governing
these ordinary and informal contacts. Because AIDS is typically transmitted under circumstances that lie somewhere between the intimate
and the private, we tend to think that enforceable public standards are
not quite the appropriate levers for directing conduct. This attitude
about public standards in private relationships is something I will
reconsider. Especially I will want to consider how privacy norms oper-

ate vis-à-vis moral norms in general. Clarifying this relationship will help us discern which norms are applicable and what they impose or permit.

The standards I employ are those associated with our responsibility not to harm people, the state's responsibility to maintain public health, and our responsibility as members of society for maintaining practices of social trust and caring. At times the consequences of being guided by one of these standards frustrate the influence of the others.

The specific issues I cover in this essay are: (1) responsibility of therapists (including physician, psychologist, social worker) to disclose confidentially obtained information to another person who may be in danger because of behavior of the HIV-infected patient; (2) how privacy and social norms interact to modulate levels of social control related to endangerment of people; (3) the responsibility of a person to warn others of his potential transmission of HIV; (4) the responsibility of people in social and professional settings to volunteer information about their own or their children's HIV status; (5) the responsibility of the state to trace contacts through which HIV may have been transmitted; and (6) the use of HIV status and risk factors to determine health insurance eligibility. These topics encompass both legal and purely social norms. They encompass the individual's relationship to the state, to professionals, and to other citizens.

There is no pretension on my part to regard this range of topics as exhaustive or my consideration of the issues I do discuss as offering the last word on them. I do intend the discussion to acquaint readers with a range of significant privacy issues related to the AIDS crisis, alert them to relevant ethical dimensions of the issues, and offer some arguments for how these issues should be resolved on the basis of the current informational context. Little in life seems to change as dramatically as the horizon of information on HIV.

Privacy and the Therapeutic Context

In discussing limitations on the confidentiality privileges thought appropriate in the therapist-patient relationship, various forms of disclosure could be at issue. There could be disclosure to governmental health agencies, local, state, or federal. There could be disclosure to those who might help the patient, like physician or parent. There could be disclosure to those who might be or might have been endangered by the patient, like a sexual partner. Finally, there could be disclosure to courts, various criminal justice agencies, or those who might threaten the patient's welfare in other respects, like a health insurance provider or people seeking civil damages in court. In the discussion that follows, I am primarily concerned with disclosures to those medically endangered by contact with a patient. Here a case can be made for abridging the patient's privacy on the basis of someone else's need to know of her own risks.

Therapists counseling patients at various stages of HIV infection are aware of dangers their patients at times have posed for others. While some would maintain that the confidentiality of the therapist-patient relationship insulates the therapist from responsibility for those endangered, others would argue that such a restriction would violate the therapist's social responsibility. In this section I discuss the responsibility of the therapist in the context of a relationship with an HIV-infected patient who poses a danger for others. This issue brings us right to the heart of the conflict discussed in the beginning of this paper between seeing a person as ill and seeing a person as a threat to others.

Apparently, a person who confesses to his priest that he has contracted a contagious disease that he might infect his fiancée with is not entitled to confidentiality vis-à-vis his priest's communications with his fiancée.

> Catholic teaching holds that a man forfeits any vow of professional secrecy about an incurable and contagious venereal disease through his intent to act in a way that might gravely injure his bride (Regan 1943).

Analogously, the *Tarasoff* cases (*Tarasoff v. Regents of the University of California* 1974, and *Tarasoff v. Regents of the University of California* 1976) and subsequent others that have raised similar issues establish a duty to warn and protect potential victims of patients undergoing therapy (Lewis 1986, Fulero 1988). Is this a reasonable basis for uprooting a profoundly significant confidential relationship? To address this question and apply it in the therapeutic relationship, we will consider some additional material on the foundations of respect for privacy. I will draw some distinctions whose relevance for the scope and limit of therapist-patient confidentiality will become clear.

There is no one answer to why privacy is important; in different settings, privacy is important for different reasons. Some of our activities, particularly those connected with bodily or biological functioning or malfunctioning, are associated with privacy norms: elimination, sexual reproduction, illness. Such norms, though widespread and diverse, are not universal. Still, for us they are associated with respect for people, perhaps connected with practices that obscure some of what we share with lower animals.

Privacy norms governing such activities or areas of life are not typically directed to providing those carrying out these functions discretion about how to manage. Instead, these functions, though carried out in private, are traditionally strictly governed by norms that were internalized when young and vigorously sustained on pain of shame. Let us call the privacy norms that are so regulated *discretionless privacy norms*. In the case of discretionless privacy norms one has a duty *not* to present certain faces of oneself in public. The point of this restriction is decidedly not liberation from social control.

Next comes an area of life that is highly regulated but one in which the discretion of how to carry out the objectives is left to the agents. Parent-child relationships characteristically fall into this category. The authoritative discretion parents are accorded in raising their children is rationalized on the grounds that it is to be exercised solely for the purpose of promoting the child's best interest. People will disagree about what does promote the child's interest, and it is in this area of interpretation that a parent is afforded her discretion. Let us call the privacy norms that permit discretion in the achievement of a given objective *narrow privacy*.

Finally, norms that restrict access of others to a person or to a sphere of life may be in place to enable wide discretion in behavior and interpretation of roles. This discretion encompasses discretion both in the ends to be achieved, something lacking in the narrow privacy domain, and in the means by which the ends are to be reached, something shared with the narrow privacy domain. Today we think of the privacy associated with intimate adult relationships as entitled to this full measure of discretion. It is not merely that gratuitous surveillance by others is regarded as out of bounds, as is the case in the discretionless and narrow discretion domains. It is that the couple is thought to be at liberty to develop the relationship as they see fit and to explore possibilities that suit the contours of their individual personalities. Let us call such privacy norms *wide privacy norms*.[4]

Now we can locate the therapist-patient relationship on this spectrum of privacy norms. I argue that therapeutic relationships fall into the middle region, the region of narrow privacy norms. The privacy and discretion afforded the therapist-patient relationship must be exercised to serve specific goals, and it is not up to the therapist and patient to develop other goals or interpret the goals already embraced in eccentric ways. Or at least, it is only within these confines that the relationship becomes socially and legally privileged. Lest one think this is too confining a restriction, recall that this is no narrower discretion than that regulating the parent-child relationship, one that offers considerable latitude in interpreting where the child's good lies and that allows the development of considerable personal and interpersonal meaning within its confines (Schoeman 1989).

In the therapist-patient relationship, anything that does not serve the patient's interest within the general bounds recognized as socially responsible is out of line, a misuse of the discretion, a violation of the relevant norms. Though privacy norms protect many violations from public exposure, this does not redeem their character as violations.

Another consideration that the parent-child relationship shares with therapist-patient relationship has to do with the notion of social responsibility. Parents are entrusted to use their discretion to promote their children's welfare. But parents are also responsible for raising their children to be decent and law-abiding citizens. Just as a person's own welfare can conflict with what is right for her to do, so a parent's regard of her child's welfare can conflict with her attitude about what it is right for the child to do or to become. It could be, for instance, in a child's long-term best interest to be coached on how to cheat in certain endeavors. Nevertheless, we think it wrong for parents to promote the child's interest through such advice. This illustrates that there is a complex goal or a complex set of side constraints that govern parents in the discharge of their responsibilities to promote their children's welfare.

A therapist operates also to promote the welfare of the patient in the context of standards of social decency. Central to our understanding what it is to help someone is a compatibility with a measure of social responsibility. The way the notion of helping works, we are helping only when we do so in a way that is socially responsible. We do not "help" a child molester by teaching him how to get away with abusing children, even if that is the advice he seeks. People for whom helping them is actually inconsistent with respect for others are people we are willing to change but not willing to serve. We tell them, and sincerely believe, that changing them will help them, but that claim is beside the point. For whether it helps them or not, changing them is the first priority.

This distinction between the patient's welfare and social welfare applies very directly to AIDS counseling. The therapist-patient relationship may take on a value in its own right, independent of the relationship serving the patient's narrowly therapeutic interests. But the privacy and confidentiality privileges associated with the relationship are not warranted because of this additional meaning. Confidentiality privileges are afforded because it is presumed that in this way the patient's welfare is promoted in a socially responsible manner.

In claiming that therapists are bound by principles of social responsibility, am I also saying that therapists are best thought of as agents of the state?[5] The question suggests a conflation between the political and the moral. Principles of social responsibility may require therapists to circumvent political requirements, as when a therapist illegally informs a patient about birth control or abortion. Nevertheless, ideally we would hope that the standards that the state expects therapists to adhere to are morally appropriate. If there is no discrepancy, then acting in a way that is socially responsible is coincidentally acting in a way that the state endorses or requires. Furthermore, the therapist is there to assist the patient. To discuss constraints on this does not undermine the point of the relationship, though the constraints do reveal something about it. What they reveal is that a therapeutic relationship requires a sense of distance from the patient. This distance is required for professional judgment and presupposed in our practices of according professional privileges.

So now we recognize some structure in the account of privacy that pertains to patient-therapist relationships. Unlike spousal intimacy, the patient-therapist relationship is not primarily an end in itself but a vehicle to enable the patient to respond to problems with professional help in the context of limitations on the costs to others that providing such help can exact.

One might object on the grounds that parent-child privacy is not just there for the purpose of promoting the child's interests but has an independent dignity founded on the intimacy of the parent-child bond (Schoeman 1980). So similarly, one might extrapolate, the therapist-patient relationship can also involve intimate sharing, and insofar as it does so, it deserves the respect with which norms of privacy can grace a relationship.

There is something to be said for this objection, but it goes only so far as there is consensus between therapist and patient, just as it extends in the parent-child relationship only so far as there is consensus between parent and child. For if there is discord between parental and child will, then the parent is accorded authority only insofar as the parent acts in (her interpretation of) the child's best interest. That is why in many contexts children can obviate the requirement of parental consent by establishing to another objective evaluator that the child's interest is served by not involving the parent.

So in the therapist-patient relationship, it is assumed that there is a convergence of interest *and* that this convergence has already passed whatever moral thresholds responsible social agents will recognize. Therapists are not entitled to help patients shirk fundamental social responsibilities.

Someone might object to this bald claim, suggesting that lawyers are entitled to benefit their clients and work with unconditional confidentiality rules that seem blind to standards of social responsibility. To the extent that lawyers are at liberty to act as "hired guns," their practice has been subjected to intense criticism (Luban 1988). But independent of that, the comparison is more complex than suggested.[6] The therapist, we are presuming, is required to breach confidentiality, to prevent a serious harm that threatens. Rule 1.6 of The American Bar Association Model Rules of Professional Conduct allows (though does not require) lawyers to breach confidentiality "to prevent the client from committing a criminal act the lawyer believes is likely to result in imminent death or substantial bodily harm." Rule 3.3 of this same code makes lawyers responsible for assuring that false evidence is not presented to a court. If the lawyer is not effective at persuading the client to withdraw false testimony, the lawyer is then duty bound to disclose the fraud to the court.

Still, unlike psychotherapists, it is *not* clear that attorneys are required to act to protect potential victims of their client's violent intentions. In *Hawkins v. King County* an attorney was held not liable for failure to notify officials at his client's bail hearing of his client's dangerousness and was held not liable for failure to notify his client's mother, a victim of his client's dangerousness. Nevertheless, *Hawkins* is different from *Tarasoff v. Regents* in three important respects. The defendant in *Hawkins* did not have specific indications of the direction of his client's dangerousness. He only knew that he was dangerous to himself and others. The defendant in *Hawkins* was not in a position to make a specific evaluation of his client's dangerousness; it is something he learned from others. Third, the victim of the client's aggression was as much aware of the client's dangerousness as the attorney was. If the fact situation had been different in *Hawkins*, the outcome might also have been different.

A difference between the lawyer-client relationship and the therapist-patient relationship is that the right to representation at a criminal trial is a constitutional right. No similar constitutional right is recognized for medical or psychological services. Furthermore, a lawyer's client faces criminal prosecution wherein the full power of the state is aimed at convicting and then punishing him. The therapist in reporting an endangering of others is not acting in response to a threat to her patient posed by the state. Though there may be consequences of the disclosure for her patient, the point of the disclosure is not to hurt the patient. Reporting statutes and judicial decisions require that health agencies and endangered persons be notified, not that the police or prosecutors be notified.

Above, we established that the privacy accorded a therapeutic relationship is aimed at an outcome: promoting the patient's welfare within the context of social responsibility. Realizing this aim helps us situate the confidentiality privileges associated with therapy. The confidentiality of the patient's condition does not preclude the therapist from taking steps to ensure notification of those endangered by the patient. Therapists should notify public health officials who in turn would notify those put at risk. Those endangered have a need to know of their vulnerability, and this need warrants breach of confidentiality.

Which behaviors constitute a risk that therapists must take responsibility for notifying others of their risks? Here we can use as a standard the following: if it is unreasonable for a patient to fail to inform others of a life-threatening risk, then the therapist owes it to these other persons to notify them of the risk. In a later section of this paper I discuss when it is unreasonable for people not to inform others of risks they pose to them.

Social Norms and Ethical Standards

In this section I discuss when privacy may be abridged in order to promote important social objectives not well managed otherwise. I begin with a discussion of when privacy barriers are appropriate to protect people from social pressure and when not. I then relate the sense of social urgency over controlling some domain of life to the therapist's duty to maintain confidentiality. I present this section keeping in mind the ambivalence toward people with AIDS or HIV infection who act in ways that endanger others, as discussed in the opening section of this paper.

Over the past few years we have witnessed a change in attitude over matters like rape—stranger, acquaintance, and even spousal varieties; spouse abuse; child abuse; and sexual molestation of children. Social and legal privacy barriers were thought to stand in the way of public recognition and response to these serious and widespread forms of victimization. I would like to consider the dynamics of such a change and ask whether analogous change is appropriate in areas related to the transmission of AIDS. Specifically, I am interested in whether social pressure might be used to advantage to change what people find acceptable in behavior and the ways privacy norms can be modified to modulate this social pressure.

Instead of thinking of some matter as either private or not private, we should think that privacy is relative to various people and to various relationships or roles. We have multiple relationships with people, and some topics that are appropriate in one context are not in others. One major reason for structuring the social world in terms of domains or spheres is to regulate the social pressures that can be applied to a person. Thus we think that certain issues are none of some people's business, even if there is a point to their prying.

Why do we have such barriers? First of all, many of the things we might narrate to others about aspects of our lives, personal or not, do not merely provide information but also structure involvement. When there is no prospect for involvement, the information is out of place. For instance, if I tell an acquaintance that I am having domestic problems, I am probably doing this to occasion understanding and support. At the very least I expect concern for my plight and perhaps sympathetic and constructive advice. If there is no prospect for these, I have misjudged. Nor would it be a better world if people were to think it appropriate to relate everything to everybody. Narrations that call for understanding or concern based on a sense of trust would be stripped of their human aspect if we were to disassociate the informational from the caring and interpersonal aspect (Schoeman 1984b).

Second, we have social freedom to the extent that there are diverse opportunities to find support and mutual aid from others. These opportunities depend on what one might call value entropy: the lack of a single, authoritative, hierarchical perspective from which all of one's life is assessed. Instead we live in a context of diverse value principalities. We may fare well in some, not so well in others. But to the extent that we can find support in some, we are liberated from the need to succumb to the demands of others for many of the benefits that are important to our life. Suppose that in one area of life I am not what others would most desire. In my private life I can be an alcoholic or an atheist, gay or someone who fails to support his children. People who relate to me at work as co-workers need not, should not, take into account for purposes of work, what I do evenings (on the assumption that I am always sober at work or when on call).[7] To the extent that a person can engage in life one dimension at a time and be evaluated in terms of the dimension-relevant norms, that person is less subject to the distaste others feel toward one in other dimensions. This restriction of judgment to domain-relevant criteria enables people to be freer socially to be other things in other contexts.

How transparent should some aspect of life be vis-à-vis another? So far I have been intimating that for the sake of social freedom, areas of life should be as opaque vis-à-vis one another as feasible. To the extent that we find some behavior very dangerous, social attitudes toward the behavior tolerant, and legal punishment rather ineffective, then we have a good candidate for increasing social pressure against the behavior.

Increasing social pressure involves two stages of potential action. First we might count on people in domain-related areas to impose social costs on the person for disregarding values or norms important to the association. For instance, those within a profession may enforce their local standards on an individual, realizing that violations to the profession harm them all or violate something socially important. Here we want people to recognize that others whom they associate with will treat them critically if they transgress this boundary. Those associated will think that what is at issue is in their domain of concern and will express this to violators.

Privacy protects people from others by specifying and defining when others have a right to involve themselves in persons' behavior or even withdraw their association from them because of their behavior. Such social pressure is necessary for groups themselves to be effective social agents. Groups require social pressure to maintain organization and direction that can often be achieved only by expecting sacrifices from their members. Generally it is important to the prospect of social freedom that whatever judgment and pressures take place within an associational frame, they take place *only* within the relevant field.

Sometimes, however, such field-restricted review is not effective in keeping enough people from behaving in harmful ways. Then it is possible to draw in extra artillery by seeking support from nonrelevant areas. This is a way of raising the costs for behavior that is particularly harmful but not yet socially identified as legitimizing field-independent response. This is a way of closing off escape routes, diminishing the social freedom to engage in this behavior. For instance, if someone is guilty of sexually molesting children, we might expect that many would not want to associate in any way with this person, even though molesting has no direct bearing on other domains of the offender's life.

Before taking this route of field-independent social pressure, other methods can be employed, education being chief among them. But as with the case of AIDS, teenage pregnancy, rape, and child molestation, epidemics of these phenomena survive intensive educational efforts. Whatever is lacking in people's understanding of AIDS, it is not the fact that some sexual practices represent statistically perilous acts. To the extent that we can show that education is ineffective, then we have a basis for introducing more intrusive measures involving social pressure.[8]

There is evidence that in the case of HIV transmission, education had and has appreciable but limited effect. Significant percentages of gays continued to frequent bath houses and sex clubs, where unsafe sex was practiced as a "release" from the pressures of life-threatening diseases, and continue to practice unsafe sex at least some of the time.

Of even more concern was new data on gay sexual behavior generated by the first professionally designed random survey of San Francisco homosexuals. The study, undertaken by Research & Decisions, a prestigious marketing firm, found that 12 percent of local gay men had gone to a private sex club at some point during the month of August [1984]. During the same period, 1 in 10 gay men had gone to a bathhouse. The fact that so many gay men continued attending the facilities, despite the unprecedented publicity about their dangers, argued against the notion that baths would close for lack of business if gays were educated about AIDS (Shilts 1987:481).

A study conducted in 1983 by two San Francisco psychologists found that 15 percent of gay respondents said that they had stopped passive anal intercourse; 20 percent said that they were engaging in oral-anal contact (rimming) less often, and 28 percent had discontinued it all together. This leaves 52 percent undeterred in this activity. The study showed that gay men knew what put them at risk for AIDS, and yet "62 percent engaged in high-risk sex at the same frequency—or more often—than before they found out about AIDS. Only 30 percent reduced their risk behaviors" (Shilts 1987:260).

According to a study conducted by the San Francisco AIDS Foundation, in late 1989, 30 percent of the gay and bisexual men surveyed reported engaging in unsafe sex practices within the month of the survey. Men between the ages of eighteen and twenty-nine were particularly prone to unprotected anal sex, with 36 percent of this group reporting such activity within the year. Identified as particularly vulnerable were newcomers to the city, men in primarily gay relationships, and young men (Recent Reports 1990:4). Also distressing is the fact that the harm HIV can and does cause is less appreciated by people at risk living in areas not *yet* as hard hit as New York and San Francisco by the AIDS epidemic.

There is also accumulating evidence coming from counselors of those with AIDS that at-risk groups that are eager to distinguish themselves from gays, like bisexual men or hemophiliacs, disassociate themselves from vulnerability to risk factors connected to HIV infection (Exoo 1990; see also Bell's paper in this volume).

Information is widespread if not universal, but motivational impetus is frequently missing. We have to recognize and respond to this failure in rationality, not pretend that we are different sorts of creatures than we find ourselves to be. I am suggesting that one way to address the motivational issue is through social pressure. If it can work effectively by being employed exclusively in behavior-relevant domains, then it should be restricted to that domain. If it is not effective in that domain, it should be broadened in source. This second move involves removing privacy barriers.

Now let me relate this sense of urgency to the therapist-patient relationship. Here I suggest two things. First of all, setting standards for professionals can have an impact on public consciousness of right and wrong and on motivation to do what is right. Breaching confidentiality norms or changing expectations to acknowledge the import of breaching confidentiality in itself can make a statement about what is tolerable behavior. Therapists legitimately worry that if it is known that they have a duty to report certain problems a patient might raise, then people will not feel free to relate these problems, and there will be *less* constructive attention afforded the problems.[9] Alternatively, it may have the impact of raising a sense of public urgency that there is a problem in the first place.

Second, the greater the sense of urgency in the public expression of concern over a problem, the greater the sense on the part of the therapeutic community that a problem must be faced from the perspective of social welfare, as well as from that of client welfare. This means that the professional standards adopted in the area of disclosure will be more weighted to the concerns of the society than would otherwise be the case. My point is that therapeutic standards of disclosure affect public attitudes, and public attitudes in turn affect therapeutic standards. The more it seems unthinkable for therapists not to take responsibility for informing people at risk because of HIV infection of their own patients, the greater the public sense will be that strict standards of care apply in the possible transmission of a life-threatening disease.

To the extent that therapists feel that the costs of warning and reporting are gratuitously harmful to their patients, they will err on the side of not reporting. Socially constructive responses to a problem are helpful not just for those suffering directly from the problem but also for those who are potentially its victims. Therapists would be more willing to report and notify partners if they were to have confidence that their patients would not face discrimination on being reported.

The Individual's Duty to Warn

In the last two sections, I addressed the question of what responsibilities therapists have to breach confidentiality and protect those endangered by patients with AIDS. I fit this analysis into a discussion of the

aspects of the therapist-patient relationship that warranted privacy
protections and a discussion of how privacy works to modulate social
control over a domain of behavior. In this section, I discuss what
responsibilities a person has to warn others whom he may be endangering because of his HIV infection. Since this often arises in the
context of a sexual relationship, I focus here on standards of care that
are enforceable despite arising in a private setting. Later in this essay I
consider social but nonlegal standards related to our notion of caring
for others.

Conditions of trust and intimacy that are worth respecting should
be transparent, in that if partners were to be more fully informed of the
other, the basis of the trust and intimacy would not be undermined
(Baier 1986). Should this ideal be imposed by those not party to the
relationship? Could not the information be misleading, or might not it
be aberrational, or does it presuppose too much rationality in the agents?
How does it affect matters when the behavior in question is life threatening?

What responsibilities does a person who knows he is or might be
HIV infected have toward those he might transmit the virus to? Let us
restrict our attention here to those who would not willingly be part of
an interchange in which HIV might be transmitted. As this relates to
privacy, we might ask more specifically whether the intimacy or privacy of the relationship might bar public or legal accountability on the
part of someone who transmits the virus.

A further refinement of the question is in order. What we are here
concerned with is what standard the state will impose if it is addressed
to resolve a dispute between parties disagreeing over the proper standard of care. This involves, not surveillance on the part of the state into
relationships where it is not invited, but a response to a complaint
brought by people who were sexually intimate, even within the context
of marriage.

Although not dispositive of the moral, the legal framework for assessing liability between sexual partners for transmission of disease is
relevant. The leading relevant case here is *Kathleen K. v. Robert B.*
(1984). The California Court of Appeals held that the constitutional
right of privacy does not "insulate one sexual partner who by intentionally tortious conduct causes physical injury to another."

Kathleen K. alleged that she contracted genital herpes, a contagious
and debilitating condition for which there is at present no cure, as a
result of sexual intercourse with Robert B. at a time when he knew or
should have known that he was a carrier. She also alleged that Robert B. misrepresented to her that he was free from venereal disease and

that she relied on his assertion. Robert B. alleged that his right to privacy precluded a court's intrusion into the case, its jurisdiction in this domain.

The court found that Robert B.'s right to privacy was not absolute and was subordinate to the state's fundamental right to enact laws that promote public health, welfare, and safety. The court cited penal statutes covering consensual sexual acts, registration of convicted sex offenders, laws relating to paternity, even to marital rape legislation, to illustrate its jurisdiction in the private domain.

Recent Minnesota and New Jersey cases, *R.A.P. v. B.J. P.*, and *G.L. v. M.L.*, respectively, would allow a person to claim damages against a former spouse for transmitting genital herpes *during the tenure of the marriage*. Recovery is permitted on the basis of a duty to refrain from acts that might transmit a disease or minimally warn the spouse of her contagious condition. The New Jersey court endorsed the position that courts were instrumental in defining the level of care spouses owe one another.

The Supreme Court of Ohio (*Mussivand v. David*) held that if person A has a venereal disease and is having an affair with a married person B but has not informed B of his condition, A owes *B's spouse* notification of his, B's spouse's, vulnerability to the disease. (The duty A owes *B* was not an issue in this case.) Anything less subjects B's spouse to an unreasonable risk of contracting the disease, making A liable for damages.

These cases illustrate that sexual intimacy brings with it an enforceable standard of care despite being located within the private precincts of life. Most of the cases mentioned involved a risk of contracting genital herpes. Because the risks associated with AIDS are so much more threatening than those associated with herpes, there is every reason to think that the standard of care expected of those who might transmit AIDS will be more vigorously applied than that expected of those who might transmit herpes (Gostin 1990a; Lambert 1990).[10]

The standard of care required by law is implicit in public attitudes toward what people in intimate relationships owe one another. In one study of people who presented themselves at an STD clinic, when offered confidential HIV testing, 79 percent accepted; 71 percent of those accepting the test offered as a reason concern for transmitting HIV to their sexual partner(s).[11]

The intimate or delicate nature of many aspects of AIDS transmission is a real barrier to frank discussion of risk factors. Not surprisingly many people about to embark on a sexual relationship would not regard it as fitting to discuss prospects for transmission of venereal disease in general or HIV in particular. The more such issues are discussed in public contexts, the more people will in fact feel comfortable in raising them in private contexts without feeling as if they are doing something offensive and unreasonable. Very clearly people need more incentives or fewer inhibitions in taking safety precautions related to sexual behavior and frank sexual conversations. Much about our social upbringing disposes us to feel skittish about broaching such topics even with people we know well. More open discussion of such issues in schools, homes, churches, and other settings of exemplary social norms will go some way toward facilitating open expressions of concern when it is important to do so in sexual settings. The less prevalent the ravages of AIDS are within a community, the less awareness there will be that such privacy barriers are dangerous.

Disclosure to Those in Professional and Social Relationships

In this section I address the question of when information about one's HIV-positive status is unreasonably withheld from those with whom one has a professional or social relationship.

Despite a climate of mistrust of official information, real gaps in knowledge, and paranoia over contracting AIDS from casual contact with the HIV infected, policies must be based on the best information available, realizing its prospects for being revised. Policies should not be grounded on beliefs or fears that contradict documented findings. Democratic governments will have difficulty in maintaining such standards when the public is seriously misinformed about communicable diseases.

Privacy is especially critical in highly irrational contexts, like that evoked by the fear of AIDS. If we think that people armed with some information will behave irrationally, we might think that their claim to the information is less pressing than it would be if they were to sensibly appreciate the relevance of the information available.[12]

Those employed in certain professions who are seropositive might endanger others. For example, say an anesthesiologist or a dental hygienist is seropositive. Does that person have the duty to inform the employer, other members of the surgical team, *and* the patients of his condition and let the employer, colleagues, or patient decide whether the risk is worth taking? On the basis of current understanding, the risks of transmission of HIV from health care worker to patient are extremely remote.[13] Furthermore, whether an act is characterized as risky depends not only on the chances of harm but also on associated costs of abstaining. It is not that we expect people to avoid behavior that puts others at risk but that we expect them to avoid behavior that puts others at unwarranted risk. Whether a risk is unwarranted depends upon the context and feasible alternatives. For the occasional patient who does get infected through this low-risk activity, there is no reasonable standard of care that was violated.

I would argue that employees in general and health professionals in particular do *not* have a duty to inform their colleagues, customers, patients, or their employers of HIV-infected status on the basis of the following considerations: (1) Professional standards for procedures used by these practitioners should not be based on the accident of whether people bother to have themselves tested for HIV infection. (2) There does not seem to be a general measure of additional endangerment in the case of HIV-infected health care providers, and if there were, procedures would have to be changed to address this endangerment in a way that does not apply only to those tested. (3) There is a great deal of public hysteria about AIDS, and in this climate details about actual risk factors play an appallingly marginal role in social response. As evidence of the hysterical character of the social response, people seem more frightened by the prospect of shaking hands or doing business with someone infected with HIV than they are by the prospect of HIV infection through unsafe sexual practices.[14] This concern extends to health care workers, as well as to others (Henry et al. 1990).

To whom do people owe information about seropositivity? Once again it depends on the environment. Suppose that I reasonably fear that informing my dentist and doctor of seropositivity would result in their terminating services to me and that I would be left without medical services up to the time I displayed full-blown symptoms of AIDS? One might first say that informing them of seropositivity is not optional because they need this information to serve my interests and to protect their own. But the hypothesis is that many practitioners would use this information, not to help me, but as a basis for denying me further services because of unfounded fears on their part. Provided this were a way of protecting others, then their response might be reasonable even if it did not help me. But, as I will show, since the prospect of protecting others by denying me service is negligible, it falls out as a factor.

Here I would permit withholding of information under certain circumstances, objectively determined: (1) The standards in the profession are such that they know that they should take precautions with patients, aware that some percentage of their patients are seropositive without knowing it. (2) The objective risks of transmitting the disease through regular interchange, when proper general precautions are taken, is so low that not informing the service provider is not treated as negligent or reckless behavior. I have tried to formulate this standard of nondisclosure to satisfy two objectives: no one, including the health care provider, is put at unreasonable risk when following standard procedures,[15] and the patient faces serious risks of loss of medical treatment for non-AIDS-related problems and general health maintenance if he were to disclose his seropositive condition.[16]

In the case of schools and residential settings, like correctional facilities and group homes, the standard for disclosure should be "the need to know" standard even if HIV testing is performed as a matter of course on all residents. This need to know must be based on a realistic prospect of significant benefit accruing to the infected on the one hand or a realistic prospect for protecting others from infection on the other. While there *may* be some point to the medical staff's being informed of HIV-positive status, there is usually no advantage to anyone if the HIV-positive status is revealed to anyone else. Rather, the danger is that this information will be used as another basis for victimizing those afflicted and must be calculated into a judgment of whether there is discretion on disclosure of HIV status. In this context it is to be noted that instances of discrimination against those with AIDS are *increasing* despite the public's becoming better informed about transmission of HIV (Hilts 1990). *It is reasonable to think that those caretakers who claim to have a need to know of a person's HIV-positive status will be situated to help those with AIDS, or those who might contract HIV infection from those with it, and accordingly should be specially trained to manage in this role.* Otherwise, the pretense that this is for the benefit of anyone at all is farfetched and pregnant with abuse.

Next, let us consider a social and nonprofessional relationship. Suppose my four-year-old child is seropositive. Do I owe it to his friends to inform their parents that my child, the child their children play with, is seropositive? Do I owe it only to those who would take it calmly and rationally to inform them? Unfortunately, they might respond by saying they personally have no problems with their child associating with my child but that once it becomes known that my child has AIDS, their children will be ostracized by the *other* children, and that this is not a fate they can subject their children to in good conscience. These parents, to show their good will, can offer to help organize school understanding groups that, if successful, would facilitate general acceptance or at least tolerance of my child in all contexts.

Here it is less clear that the irrationality of others should be discounted. It can seem problematic to *not* inform the other parents precisely because of the irrationality of other people's responses. It would violate a trust to not inform these parents of what *their own* children might face in terms of harassment and ostracism. One can only hope that their understanding of the isolation they fear will promote sympathy on their part to help ensure that my child is not ostracized.

But just as privacy is not always the paramount value, respecting a trust is not always the most important value to respect. What about a parent who judged that her child's plight made that, and not other people's autonomy or confidence in one's forthrightness, her priority? After all, it is not that they are at risk of contracting the virus. So long as they are not endangered in this respect, why must they be informed? Adding further to this perspective, the parent of the infected child could more indirectly protect the friends of her child by encouraging the introduction of informational presentations at the school her child attends so that parents and children's responses will be measured by understanding.

Like most policy issues related to AIDS, information is useful here. The underlying basis of parental fears has to do with fear of transmission of AIDS through casual contact. Studies show that sharing facilities like beds, toilets, bathing facilities, and items likely to be soiled by saliva or body fluids provide no clear instances of conversion from seronegativity to seropositivity. Also, activities like hugging, kissing on cheeks or lips, and biting similarly provide no evidence of seroconversion. Even health care professionals who work with AIDS patients show *no* greater proclivity to seropositivity than the general population does, despite contact with blood, feces, vomit, and other fluids from infected patients (Friedland and Klein 1987).

Because the fear is based on misinformation about AIDS transmission, and because there is no appreciable danger of infection to others, and because one can try to deal with the social dangers indirectly, and finally because of the real needs of her own child, it is legitimate for the parent *not* to inform her child's playmates' parents. Their interest in knowing is not as compelling as maintaining discretion with the parent of the infected child. Still, it might be unwise not to inform for two important reasons: (1) It will be hard for the child to keep secret something so important to his life prospects like seropositivity, or development of AIDS-related complex (ARC), or AIDS. (2) When the child will need the most support, once the AIDS symptoms occur, the child's friends or their parents may feel they have been betrayed by not being informed and reject further contact for the lack of respect and trust shown them through nondisclosure.

Some of the positions I have advocated thus far may seem surprising and even inconsistent. I have required those who are HIV infected to notify sexual partners, but not playmates or health care workers, of their risk factors. What is due here is an explanation of why sexual partners have a duty to warn partners of their condition, even if they restrict themselves to safe sexual practices, while people coming in for dental, medical, surgical, or educational services do not. After all, the risk of transmitting HIV through heterosexual, vaginal intercourse, particularly in the direction of female to male, though real, is not very high for a very wide variety of cases. The difference can be elaborated along a variety of dimensions.

The first differentiating factor is statistical. Even though the prospects of transmitting HIV in one heterosexual sexual encounter, particularly one involving "safe" sex precautions, is small (on the order of 0.0002) (Hearst and Hulley 1988),[17] as far as we know it is greater than the chances of transmitting HIV in professional contexts like routine dental care and much greater than the chance of transmitting it in daycare or school contexts. In the case of daycare or school, there is negligible chances of transmitting HIV.

How does sex compare with surgery, with respect to transmission rate of HIV? It is estimated that the risk of transmitting HIV through surgery at a hospital that serves a community at high risk for AIDS is one infection in eight years, during which time tens of thousands of operations occur. This extrapolates to a transmission of infection rate to less than one in eighty years at a hospital that serves a community with HIV infection at less than 3 percent, a rate characteristic of many hospitals in the United States, *provided recommended precautions are taken* (Gerberding et al. 1990:1791).[18]

The current best estimate of seroconversion on the part of health care workers who suffer exposure to body fluids of HIV-infected patients is 0.42 percent, or 42 out of 10,000 (Marcus 1988). This figure is for health care workers who suffered needlesticks and exposure to blood on open sores or to the mucous membranes. Furthermore, there are some figures available for the exposure rate, both parenteral and cutaneous, during surgical procedures: 1.7 percent parenteral exposure, 4.7 percent cutaneous exposure (Gerberding et al. 1990:1789). It is reasonable to assume that of the cutaneous exposures, less than one quarter were to open wounds or to mucous membranes. This gives us a combined rate of 2.9 percent who suffered needlesticks or exposure of patient's blood to worker's open wounds or mucous membranes. When this exposure rate is multiplied by the seroconversion rate just cited, the total risk of conversion comes to 0.0001. This is half the rate of HIV transmission involved in safe heterosexual sex. And one can assume that risk of transmission during surgery is higher than during other medical procedures.

Second, particularly in settings like the dentist chair or the surgical theater, where there is some even remote prospect of transmitting HIV, there are standards recommended for dealing with *all* patients, recognizing that people with HIV may not know or even suspect that they have been infected. These standards go along with specialized training. A recent study of exposure to risk of surgical personnel to patients' blood during surgery concludes about a hospital staff that deals with a high percentage of high-risk patients and that abides by strict precautions that "no evidence was found to suggest that preoperative testing for HIV infection would reduce the frequency of accidental exposure to blood" (Gerberding et al. 1990).[19]

Third, there is professional review of medical settings to ensure that standards of care are researched, debated, and publicized; clearly there is no similar monitoring of sexual encounters. We legitimately have higher expectations of professionals than we do of ordinary citizens.

Fourth, there are gradations of trust between people in different relationships or capacities.[20] Generally in a therapist-patient relationship, the responsibilities go from the therapist in the direction of the patient, the latter being the more vulnerable. Some may not feel that this is true if the patient is HIV positive. But even conceding this, the general understanding of what is owed is colored by the typical situation. In social and intimate relationships, the responsibility is symmetrical. As argued earlier, sexual intimacy is minimally associated with standards of not harming the partner.

Finally, we regard provision of medical services as more important than sex. Accordingly, greater risks can be justified in facilitating medical services than in facilitating sex.

These observations support the judgment that the risk for transmission of HIV to health care providers not informed about one's HIV status is not unreasonable.[21]

Two related issues may occasion changes in the judgments so far offered. There is the possibility of treatment for those exposed to the blood or fluids of HIV-infected people to lessen chances of seroconversion. Studies are under way that will test whether azidothymidine

(AZT) treatments reduce the risk of seroconversion on the part of those recently exposed. If these prove significant in reducing the 0.42 percent noted, that would be a point in favor of disclosure of HIV status, at least once it is noticed that an exposure occurred.

Second, a sense of intense distress on the part of health care workers exposed to HIV blood or fluids is being reported. Henry et al. (1990) report:

> When asked about their emotional response to their HIV exposure, 11 (55%) of 20 health care workers reported severe acute distress and 7 (35%) of 20 reported persistent moderate stress. Five (25%) of 20 reported significant impact on their sexual relations and 6 (30%) of 20 quit their jobs as a result of exposure.

This finding among health care workers, those who can be expected to be best informed about HIV, presents as clear a picture as one could desire of the danger to others those infected with HIV are perceived as posing. This realization should intensify our commitment to keeping confidential a person's HIV status. It should also intensify our commitment to doing something to help those who become exposed while providing care for the HIV infected. The sorts of accommodations that would be of material help are enhanced life and medical insurance policies, additional research on what poses risks for health care workers and on whether various postexposure treatments could be effective, implementation and enforcement of high standards of protection for health care workers so that fewer are exposed, and counseling for those exposed.

One additional issue should be sorted out here. Physicians and dentists legitimately believe that unless they are aware of a person's condition, they cannot effectively and responsibly perform their job. The prospects of proper diagnosis and treatment are seriously compromised by their being kept ignorant of significant health factors like HIV-positive status. Does recognizing this alter the balance in favor of a duty to disclose to health care providers?

Although medical personnel do have a significant personal and professional stake in performing their jobs successfully, it does not follow that they have a right to information that will help them in this objective. To take an analogous case, suppose a person with a serious bladder infection tells his physician he is not sexually active. He may be most unwise in doing this and hurting himself in the process, but we would not say he has violated the physician's rights or that he had a duty to inform his physician of his condition.[22] I emphasize that I am talking about the minimal enforceable standard we can expect from someone. One might nevertheless think it wrong or unfair not to notify one's physician of one's positive HIV status, for the physician's sake, for one's own sake, and for the sake of a relationship of trust between the patient and physician. For reasons indicated above, the failure to notify does not put the physician at unreasonable risk, even though it may put the physician at some small risk.[23]

Partner Notification

Gostin and Curran (1986) and Brandt (1990) have reviewed some proposals related to compulsory control of AIDS. Very sensibly, Gostin and Curran propose a five-tier test for assessing screening programs:

> 1) the selected population should have a significant reservoir of infection so that there are no disproportionate numbers of uninfected persons having to submit to intrusive testing procedures; (2) the environment within which the population operates must pose a significant risk of communication of the infection; (3) knowledge of the results of testing should enable the authorities to take precautions to reduce the spread of infection which would be effective and which would not otherwise be taken without that knowledge; (4) the critical consequences of the testing and precautions should not be disproportionate to the benefits; and (5) no less restrictive or intrusive means of achieving the public health objective of screening are available (1986:24).

These authors then recommend *against* statutory partner notification as a public health response to AIDS. The authors suggest that little advantage for public health could be the result of such tracing. The absence of a vaccine or cure, on the one hand, and the long incubation period on the other, they argue, distinguishes AIDS from syphilis. The extended incubation period in the case of AIDS could easily involve trying to recall sexual or IV drug partners from three or more years back. Furthermore, they argue compulsory tracing would work against public health objectives by undermining patient/physician confidentiality and thus inhibit those with health worries from seeking medical advice.

This last point would count against partner notification for any disease, syphilis included. And, as I pointed out, similar claims were made for requiring reporting of suspected cases of child abuse; the subsequent history of the requirement does not seem to bear out this a priori reasonable prediction. Partner notification for STDs includes confidentiality safeguards. Such safeguards are reported to be well respected, with prospects for exposure being extremely remote (Wykoff et al. 1988).

Despite fears of confidentiality violations, critics have not documented breaches as partners have been traced for other sexually transmitted diseases. Public health officials claim that they have maintained strict privacy for the 117,000 patients whose diagnosis of AIDS have been reported to state health agencies (Lambert 1990).

Furthermore, partner notification for STDs does not involve release of the name of the informant who might have infected another to those notified. Rather, public health reports of those with STDs are maintained in strict confidentiality.

But what might be the health benefits of tracing when there is no vaccine or cure and the incubation period is potentially very extended? The answer seems simple. Notify people who might not otherwise suspect that they could be infected so that they (1) can regulate their own sexual practices in light of the new information; (2) have themselves tested for HIV infection; (3) avoid donating blood or sperm or avoid becoming pregnant until assured of HIV-free status; and (4) keep themselves posted about factors that might inhibit onset of disease for those who are seropositive. The claim of conflict of partner notification with public health objectives does not seem borne out by a review of the factors. Just the opposite seems the case. Spending resources on people who have already had contact with an HIV-antibody-positive person provides opportunities for the most focused and efficient expenditure of counseling and information services. Finally, partner notification provides some of the most valuable insights into practices that promote the spread of the disease; these insights lead to recommendations that could be life saving on a large scale (Wykoff et al. 1988).

Gostin and Curran (1986) also concern themselves with the potential for self-incrimination involved in compulsory tracing.[24] In many states homosexuality, IV drug usage, and even extramarital sex are illegal. There are serious problems this concern raises, but they do not present insuperable difficulties to either public health or civil liberties. To achieve public health goals, we might offer limited criminal immunity to someone who infected another knowing that the contact endangered the partner. But then also, if it could be shown at some future time that this person, subsequent to being notified of seropositivity, engaged in practices that put others at serious risk for contracting AIDS, then some measures, as unobtrusive as necessary, should be taken to ensure that this person ceases posing life-threatening risks to others.

With respect to self-incrimination related to reporting sexual contacts or sharing of needles, there is a parallel to statutes requiring reporting child abuse. In the case of *People v. Younghanz,* Younghanz claimed that California's child-abuse-reporting act interfered with his right to seek a cure for his illness. Whether a cause or effect of his mental breakdown is disputed, but connected to this breakdown was a protracted sexual relationship with a deaf-mute, borderline mentally retarded daughter, beginning when she was eight years old. Younghanz also contended that the disclosure requirement is unconstitutional because it compels him to incriminate himself and turns his psychologist into an agent of the state.

The court held that the duty of the psychologist is to report suspected cases of abuse, not investigate the abuse. Because much that is revealed to the psychologist need not be revealed to authorities, the abuse-reporting statute does not inhibit the psychologist in providing therapy and it maintains treatment as the principal reason for soliciting information from the patient.

What conditions should initiate tracing? Any confirmed seropositive person should be asked to name people he or she might have infected and the names of blood banks or sperm banks, if any, to which he has sold or donated body fluids. Should the tracing be voluntary or compulsory? A problem in making it compulsory is that there is a great deal of difficulty in establishing that a person who says he has completely forgotten with whom he shared needles or with whom he had risky sex is willfully withholding information. Still, the fact that a law will rarely be used does not mean that it indirectly does not serve a purpose. It helps to set or reaffirm a standard of public morality (Zimring and Hawkins 1973).

Suppose that a person claims he has provided all the names of people he might have infected, but it is found out later, somehow, that a person with whom he was living at the time or until recently or for an extended period was not mentioned. Then evidence of willful withholding of potentially life-saving information could be used in a criminal prosecution for violating health laws, provided full disclosure was treated as mandatory and not voluntary. Might such a statute have adverse consequences for effective tracing? It is hard to see why people would be more compliant with a request when it is unenforceable than when it is.

I should register a concern I have about my argument here. Given that cooperation on partner notification applies only to those who have been tested positive for HIV and that testing is by and large voluntary, it exposes people who have themselves tested to a measure of liability not shared by those who are either less interested or more worried in what they might find out by being tested. I confess I do not have a satisfactory answer to this.

There are widespread public fears that disclosure of seropositivity to the health department will mean not just that people who might have been made vulnerable to AIDS will be notified but also that employers, insurers, and others will be notified of one's health status. Here again we should insist, not just that confidentiality statutes that pertain to health agencies will be enforced, but also that policies will be based on evidence and not on fears unsupported by evidence. If health agencies have upheld their confidentiality requirements, public perceptions to the contrary should not be a basis for weakening reporting and tracing requirements.

Still, concern about exposure of people who are HIV positive is serious because of the devastating social consequences those known to be infected with HIV face. The prospect of such consequences provides many physicians with reasons not to comply with reporting statutes, provides groups of people at high risk with reasons not to have themselves tested, and provides people who suspect HIV infection in themselves with reasons not to seek professional help. What this shows is that widespread confidence in the confidentiality of a reported diagnosis of AIDS, or even of HIV infection, would have major epidemiological, scientific, and personal benefits.

One must differentiate between discrimination that results from public disclosure of positive HIV status, whatever the source, on the one hand, and discrimination that results from public disclosure on the part of public health agencies that received confidential reports of a person's HIV status. So long as the discrimination is not the result of public health agency disclosures, it cannot be argued that the initial reporting and the subsequent partner notification are the cause of the discrimination. In other words, the fact that those with HIV are discriminated against is not a reason to resist reporting and partner notification if these are not the basis of the information that leads to the discrimination.[25]

As of 1987 only three states and the District of Columbia had enacted legislation controlling the use of HIV-antibody test results. In the area of partner notification, federal legislation placed limitations on the disclosure of information obtained under programs authorized by the Public Health Service for prevention and control of STDs, including AIDS (Matthews and Neslund 1987:346). As of the end of 1988, eleven states required tracing of sex partners of those with AIDS (Lambert 1990).

Some suggest that rather than rely on the hit-or-miss effect that tracing generates, everyone who is even mildly suspicious of having been infected should come in for confidential testing. The first problem with this is that there are many people who are at risk of being infected but who are not even vaguely aware that they are at risk. Second, with nearly a whole population at least remotely at risk for AIDS, having many non–high-risk people tested will mean first of all a large number of false positives. Third, it will mean that the poor and uneducated, now the most likely victims of HIV infection, will not be notified of their real risks because there will be no tracing.

Privacy and Health Insurance

Another important privacy issue related to HIV notification arises in the area of health insurance. Those who write health insurance policies argue that people who are HIV infected or at higher risk for HIV infection, just like those at higher risk for a variety of other health-related conditions, should be expected to bear the higher costs of their situation. Insurers argue that it is reasonable for them as private businesses to assess premiums on the basis of risks. They argue also that payment in accord with differential risk is only fair to millions in need of health insurance who are not at risk for AIDS and will be priced out of the market if they have to shoulder the burden for treating a disease as costly as AIDS (Clifford and Iuculano 1987).

On the other side of the issue of charging differing premiums for those whose characteristics or behavior puts them at risk for AIDS is the concern that the notion of pooling risks is the point of insurance. If insurance rates were tailored to exactly those conditions one will face, there would be no point in involving an insurance company. As more and more conditions become predictable, through identification of genetic and social markers, provided insurers can insist on being apprised and assess rates accordingly, the whole notion of risk would become vestigial from the world of insurance.[26]

One aspect of the practices insurers follow in assessing risks is the prying into personal details of people's lives in potentially offensive ways. What differentiates potentially offensive prying from actually offensive prying is the evaluation of the need for the prying. Unmarried men, people engaged in certain professions, people living in certain areas, maybe even people who read certain literature—these people will be excluded altogether from or priced out of health insurance.

In this context one can consider differing sorts of information that insurers might inquire about and the privacy issues raised by these: HIV status, sexual or drug practices and those of one's sex partner or partners, handicaps, psychological stability, city and neighborhood in which one resides, occupation, and marital status. Clearly some of these are more intimate and sensitive sorts of information than others. The Red Cross, in screening blood donors, asks about HIV status, sexual and drug practices, recent travel, and other intimate matters. What keeps this inquiry from being offensive despite being intrusive is the clear relevance of the information to ensuring a safe supply of blood.

Can the insurance industry claim the same need to know as the blood banks? In the case of blood banks, lives are at stake. In the case of insurers, profits and overall insurance rates are at stake. It may be inappropriate that in an area as critical as health insurance the drive for profits overshadows health needs of citizens. If urgent health needs are not being met by current practices, then the claim that the need to know requires disclosure of intimate information comes to seem less credible in the case of insurers than in the case of blood banks. Here I am not discrediting the claim of the insurer but noting that it is less pressing than some.

Is the prying different in the case of HIV than in the case of other matters insurers require as a basis for setting rates? We expect and largely accept that insurers make assessments for risks. If insurers can evaluate our risks by marital status, by occupation, by age, by level of education, by habits like exercise or smoking, by physicians' reports, and by blood and urine tests for other identifiable markers, why not for potential for HIV?

Even though AIDS is a terrible affliction, it is not the only horrifying affliction that befalls people. Since insurers are permitted to require testing for other terrible conditions, it is unclear why they should be precluded from testing for AIDS-related conditions, as well as from writing exceptions into their policies for preexisting conditions. Insurers react to HIV susceptibility the way they react to most conditions. Outside the AIDS context we accept these policies without complaint. What makes normal policy offensive when directed toward HIV?

Clearly something else is going on in the case of HIV. What this something else is can be identified as follows: a major flaw in the way private insurance works, a flaw that typically affects those without political influence, has affected a politically active and articulate segment of the population. The privacy abridgments that end up causing people to lose coverage are not peculiar to AIDS but are made manifest only through the activities of AIDS activists. As a population we see more clearly what these policies mean in human terms in the case of AIDS. The best policy response to the systematic failures in health coverage is to protect information that is characteristically used to deny coverage for those at risk for AIDS. Requests for this information to be used in this way may be unreasonable.

Finally, what if insurers, in the normal course of events, and without prying, come to know that a person they are covering is HIV infected? Either diagnoses submitted by physician or drugs prescribed may leave little doubt. Here without intrusive prying a person's positive HIV status becomes known to them. Can the insurer then terminate coverage or place the insured person in a risk pool that encompasses only those with expectations of catastrophic health care needs? If the issue were genuinely and exclusively one of privacy, the answer would be yes. But for reasons just elaborated, the restriction on privacy was not motivated primarily on nondisclosure but on making health care benefits available to those most at need. Accordingly such discoveries would not be a proper basis for changing insurance rates.

I mentioned at the outset that in cases of real moral conflict we are haunted by needs and concerns that cannot be addressed because of the pressing nature of the other values involved. Tragically, this is what we confront commonly when we consider the needs of those infected with HIV in cases where people legitimately raise privacy concerns.

The fact that people infected with HIV may be thought to be living under a death sentence, both physically and socially, argues in favor of respecting the privacy interests of these people to the extent possible. Being so fated, however, does not release these people from standards of decency and care they owe others. After all, if AIDS is horrible to endure, it is horrible to transmit. A person's right to privacy concerning his HIV-positive status is properly abridged when doing so represents the least invasive and most efficient means of protecting others from contracting or spreading the disease.

We cannot afford to be anything but compassionate in our policies toward those infected with HIV. But because of the physical and social ruin this infection occasions, we cannot afford to be ambivalent toward those who unreasonably risk infecting others or who will not share information that can literally save lives.

I have discussed many reasons for thinking that the objectives of public health (preventing diseases and saving lives) and personal responsibility (holding people to a standard of care for others) are compatible and mutually enforcing. Furthermore, I suspect that if we are faced with an apparent conflict and opt for the public health objective, we risk diluting people's general sense of decency and community concern, an effect that indirectly and in the long run may cost more lives than are saved by responding expediently. But here we are in the area of almost complete speculation, where little in the way of evidence or argument counteracts individual prejudice.

ACKNOWLEDGMENTS

I express appreciation to Robert Ball, Nora Bell, Nathan Crystal, Patricia Conway, Linda Kettinger, Susan Lake, Robert Post, Bosko Postic, Frederic Reamer, Laurence Thomas, and Deborah Valentine for valuable discussions and resource materials that helped me develop an understanding of issues related to AIDS. Frederic Reamer has been an ideal editor, offering wise comments and constructively prodding me on numerous issues that arose in the myriad versions of this paper. The paper owes much to his care and commitment to making it the most valuable contribution it can be. I also thank Sara Schechter-Schoeman, Miriam Schoeman, and Dmitri Schoeman for a very helpful discussion on issues of AIDS and health insurance.

NOTES

1. *United States v. Sergeant Nathaniel Johnson, Jr.* upholds Sergeant Johnson's conviction for aggravated assault for attempting to engage in anal sex while knowing his condition to be HIV positive—making his semen deadly.

2. For a collection of much of the best writing on privacy along with a philosophical overview of this literature, see Schoeman (1984a). For a review of the philosophical dimension of central privacy issues, see Schoeman (1984c).

3. There is an even narrower conception, one that limits the range of privacy to personal information that is "undocumented."

4. One criterion of the difference between the narrow and the wide privacy norms can be phrased in terms of the distinction between a role and a relationship. While a role is relatively limited in the range of responses thought appropriate and the ends to be achieved, a relationship is treated as more flexible on both counts. Our standing as a parent is role governed insofar as we owe our children certain attitudes almost independently of how they behave; our standing as a spouse is much more responsive to the actual behavior of the partner (Greenhouse 1986).

5. I am indebted to Robert Post for suggesting that I address this question.

6. I am indebted to Nathan Crystal and Robert Post for coaching me on the intricacies of the lawyer-client confidentiality privilege.

7. There are, of course, jobs (the pope and the president are examples) for which it is important to be a certain kind of person in addition to having certain skills available when at work.

8. Regarding education as ineffective in reducing risk of HIV transmission to a "tolerable" level is not a reason to abandon educational efforts. As Nora Bell argues in her paper in this volume, education about significant health risks is important in

a democracy independent of whether most people modify their behavior in light of the efforts.

9. Some researchers have pointed out that this has not been the impact of child-abuse-reporting requirements, though where states change public health regulation to require reporting of HIV infection, numbers of people presenting themselves to be tested decrease, at least temporarily.

10. Marc Christian, Rock Hudson's long-term companion, "won a multimillion-dollar award from Rock Hudson's estate in a suit alleging that the movie star lied about his illness and continued having unsafe sex" (Lambert 1990:15A). Because Mr. Christian was not HIV infected, the basis of the award must have been infliction of emotional distress and violation of a duty to inform *(Christian v. Sheft)*.

11. Personal communication, Dr. Jeffrey Jones, Disease Control Division, South Carolina Department of Health and Environmental Control.

12. It is often the case that we deny people information because providing it conflicts with public policy goals or serves no useful social purpose, despite serving an apparently personal purpose. Youthful offenders and first-time offenders diverted into rehabilitation programs are protected from the stigma of a criminal past by having their previous arrest records expunged. Jurors at the trial stage are denied information about the accused, like evidence of a previous criminal record, because it might dispose them to respond to something besides the evidence of the relevant case. And indeed, medical records are typically treated as confidential, and both professional ethics and tort law enforce maintenance of this standard.

13. For discussion of risk of exposure during surgery, see Gerberding, et al. 1990.

14. Numerous studies find little change in extramarital sexual patterns occasioned by fear of AIDS. Blendon and Donelan (1988) provide evidence of people fearing infection from casual contact. Kegeles, Adler, and Irwin (1988) and Mc-Cusker et al. (1988) provide evidence of the marginal impact of AIDS information on reforming sexual practices, particularly among those most at risk.

15. Evidence for this claim is discussed below.

16. Someone might here want to distinguish between elective and nonelective surgery vis-à-vis duty to disclose.

17. Hearst and Hulley (1988) estimate the rate of transmission of HIV infection (male to female) to be no higher than 0.002 assuming one act of unprotected vaginal intercourse and assuming no genital ulcers. This value drops to 0.0002 with the use of a condom and spermicide.

18. Gerberding et al. (1990) acknowledge that the exposure rate may well be influenced by the precautions taken by surgical teams working at a hospital known to work with high-risk populations.

19. Gerberding et al. (1990) report that the exposure rate to the blood of a patient undergoing surgery was nearly equal for those perceived to be at high risk for HIV infection and those perceived to be at low risk: forty-one exposures per one thousand hours of surgery compared with thirty-seven exposure per one thousand hours of surgery.

20. I am grateful to Sara Schechter-Schoeman for suggesting this point.

21. I am grateful to Susan Lake for an illuminating discussion and for supplying some key points for the analysis on this point.

22. In this range of cases we would be unsympathetic if a patient eventually sues a physician for malpractice if a mistake results from the concealment.

23. I am glad to avoid the issue of whether privacy legitimates a person's lying to a physician about one's HIV status if asked directly.

24. In South Carolina, there is an exception to the maintenance of confidential-

ity of health department records on HIV infection when the information is relevant to a criminal prosecution. But even here, the prosecution must prove a compelling need, and in considering the merits of this claim, "the court must weigh the need for disclosure against both the privacy interest of the test subject and the potential harm to the public interest if disclosure deters future Human Immunodeficiency Virus-related testing and counselling or blood-organ, and semen donation." The person whose diagnosis is being requested is then entitled to a hearing to rebut the prosecutor's claim of compelling interest, and this hearing itself is private, unless requested public by the subject, and the proceedings themselves will not be recorded by the subject's name (Section 44-29-136, Laws of South Carolina). Other exceptions to confidentiality include: release made for medical or epidemiological information for statistical purposes in a manner that conceals individual identities, release made to control and treat STDs, release made to protect health or life of any person, and release of HIV-positive status of minor to school superintendent of school district and school medical professionals. Release of medical and epidemiological information is permitted with consent of persons identified (Section 44-29-135, Laws of South Carolina).

25. I am indebted to Susan Lake for this point.

26. We would be an indecent society if someone did not pay for the health needs of those afflicted with AIDS, up to the point where spending more would deprive others similarly in need. To make this level of care possible, risks have to be spread out over the population. If private insurers will not cover for these sorts of risks, then the government will have to cover them, charging taxpayers for the costs. There is no avoiding the fact that individuals at low risk will have to cover those at high risk. It can happen in the context of private or public insurance, but it cannot be avoided without succumbing to indecency. In this rendition of the issue, the same pool of people ends up paying anyway for those with HIV-related medical needs. The costs for given individuals or classes within the pool may change depending on whether they come from taxes or from insurance premiums. The demographics of AIDS may suggest that an increasing percentage of AIDS victims will not be those who would have had private health insurance. This leaves the population at large responsible. This realization would suggest that the insurers should be free to collect the information they think relevant since the government should be there for those not covered by private insurers anyway.

REFERENCES

Baier, A. 1986. Trust and Antitrust. *Ethics* 96:231–260.

Benn, S. 1971. Privacy, Freedom, and Respect for Persons. In F. Schoeman, ed., *Philosophical Dimensions of Privacy: An Anthology*, pp. 223–244. New York: Cambridge University Press, 1984.

Blendon, R. and K. Donelan. 1988. Discrimination Against People with AIDS. *New England Journal of Medicine* 319:1022–1026.

Brandt, A. 1990. Sexually Transmitted Disease: Shadow on the Land, Revisited. *Annals of Internal Medicine* 112:481–483.

Christian v. Sheft. 1988. Super Ct. LA Cty: *AIDS Literature Reporter* (June 24).

Clifford, K. and R. Iuculano. 1987. AIDS and Insurance: The Rationale for AIDS-related Testing. *Harvard Law Review* 100:1086–1825.

Exoo, G. 1990. Ladson, SC, Rest Area Interviews: Summary (April 26). A study funded by the Unitarian Universalist Social Concerns Grants Panel.

Flaherty, D. 1972. *Privacy in Colonial New England.* Charlottesville: University Press of Virginia.

Fried, C. 1960. Privacy. In F. Schoeman, ed., *Philosophical Dimensions of Privacy,* pp. 203–222.

Friedland, G. and R. Klein. 1987. Transmission of the Human Immunodeficiency Virus. *New England Journal of Medicine* 317: 1125–1135.

Fulero, S. 1988. *Tarasoff:* 10 Years Later. *Professional Psychology: Research and Practice* 19: 184–190.

G.L. v. M. L. 1988. 550 A.2d 525 (N.J. Super. Ch.)

Gerberding, J., C. Littell, A. Tarkington, A. Brown, and W. Schechter. 1990. Risk of Exposure of Surgical Personnel to Patients' Blood During Surgery at San Francisco General Hospital. *New England Journal of Medicine* 322:1788–1793.

Goleman, D. 1990. Studies Discover Clues to the Roots of Homophobia. *New York Times* (July 10), p. B1.

Gostin, L. 1990a. The AIDS Litigation Project: A National Review of Court and Human Rights Commission Decisions. Part I: The Social Impact of AIDS. *JAMA* 263:1961–1970.

Gostin, L. and W. Curran. 1986. Limits of Compulsion in Controlling AIDS. *Hastings Center Report* 16:24–29.

Greenhouse, C. 1986. *Praying for Justice: Faith, Order, and Community in an American Town.* Ithaca, N.Y.: Cornell University Press.

Hawkins v. King County. 1979. 602 P.2d 361.

Hearst, N. and S. Hulley. 1988. Preventing the Heterosexual Spread of AIDS: Are We Giving Our Patients the Best Advice? *JAMA* 259:2428–2432.

Henry, K., S. Campbell, B. Jackson, H. Balfour, F. Rhame, K. Sannerud, S. Pollack, J. Sninsky, and C. Kwok. 1990. Long-Term Follow-Up of Health Care Workers with Work-Site Exposure to Human Immunodeficiency Virus. *JAMA* 263:1765.

Hilts, P. 1990. AIDS Bias Grows Faster Than Disease, Study Says. *New York Times* (June 17), p. A14.

Kathleen K. v. Robert B. 1984. 198 *California Reporter* 273.

Kegeles, S., N. Adler, and C. Irwin. 1988. Sexually Active Adolescents and Condoms: Changes Over One Year in Knowledge, Attitudes, and Use. *American Journal of Public Health* 78:460–461.

Krause, H. 1986. *Family Law.* St. Paul: West Publishing.

Lambert, B. 1990. AIDS: Keeping Track of the Infected. *New York Times* (May 13), p. 15A.

Lewis, M. 1986. Duty to Warn Versus Duty to Maintain Confidentiality: Conflicting Demands on Mental Health Professionals. *Suffolk Law Review* 20:579–615.

Luban, D. 1988. *Lawyers and Justice: An Ethical Study.* Princeton, N.J.: Princeton University Press.

Marcus, R. 1988. Surveillance of Health Care Workers Exposed to Blood from Patients Infected with the Human Immunodeficiency Virus. *New England Journal of Medicine* 319:1118–1123.

Matthews, G. and V. Neslund. 1987. The Initial Impact of AIDS on Public Health Law in the United States—1986. *JAMA* 257:344–352.

McCusker, J., A. Stoddard, K. Mayer, J. Zapka, C. Morrison, and S. Saltzman. 1988. Effects of HIV Antibody Test Knowledge on Subsequent Sexual Behaviors in a Cohort of Homosexually Active Men. *American Journal of Public Health* 78:462–467.

Mussivand v. David (544 N.E. 2d 265).

People v. Younghanz 202 *California Reporter* 907.

Potterat, J., N. Spencer, D. Woodhouse, and J. Muth. 1989. Partner Notification in the Control of Human Immunodeficiency Virus Infection. *American Journal of Public Health* 79:874–876.

Recent Reports: Unsafe Sex and Relapse. 1990. *Focus: A Guide to AIDS Research and Counselling* 5(6):4.

Regan, R. 1943. *Professional Secrecy in Light of Moral Principles*. Washington, D.C.: Augustinian Press. Cited in S. Eth. 1988. The Sexually Active, HIV Infected Patient: Confidentiality Versus the Duty to Protect. *Psychiatric Annals* 18:571–576 and 575–576.

Schoeman, F. 1980. Rights of Children, Rights of Parents, and the Moral Basis of the Family. *Ethics* 91:6–19.

Schoeman, F., ed. 1984a. *Philosophical Dimensions of Privacy*. New York: Cambridge University Press.

Schoeman, F. 1984b. Privacy and Intimate Information. In F. Schoeman, ed., *Philosophical Dimensions of Privacy*, pp. 403–418.

Schoeman, F. 1984c. Introduction. In F. Schoeman, ed., *Philosophical Dimensions of Privacy*, pp. 1–33.

Schoeman, F. 1989. Adolescent Confidentiality and Family Privacy. In G. Graham and H. LaFollette, eds., *Person to Person*, pp. 213–234. Philadelphia: Temple University Press.

Shilts, R. 1987. *And the Band Played On: Politics, People, and the AIDS Epidemic.* New York: St. Martins.

Stone, L. 1979. *The Family, Sex, and Marriage in England, 1500–1800.* New York: Harper & Row.

Tarasoff v. Regents of the University of California. 1974. 118 *California Reporter* 129.

Tarasoff v. Regents of the University of California. 1976. 17 Cal.3d 425.

United States v. Sergeant Nathaniel Johnson, Jr. 27 M.J. 798.

Wykoff, R., C. Heath, Jr., S. Hollis, S. Leonard, C. Quiller, J. Jones, M. Artzrouni, and R. Parker. 1988. Contact Tracing to Identify Human Immunodeficiency Virus Infection in a Rural Community. *JAMA* 259:3563–3566.

Zimring, F. and G. Hawkins. 1973. *Deterrence: The Legal Threat in Crime Control.* Chicago: University of Chicago Press.

11. AIDS and the Law

DONALD H. J. HERMANN

LEGISLATION AND LITIGATION addressing issues created by acquired immune deficiency syndrome (AIDS) are vast in both volume and span of subject matter. There are, however, two fundamental elements that run through the legal developments that have occurred in reaction to the spread of the human immunodeficiency virus (HIV). These are, first, the influence of and tension between various ethical considerations, including individual autonomy, personal rights, social protection, and the proper use of state power. The second has been a tension between responsible legislators and jurists, who continually insist that statutes, regulations, and judicial opinions reflect the best understanding provided by medical and scientific authorities, and those who show a willingness to practice demagoguery by placating or stimulating false and irrational fears through proposed enactments or decisions that ignore established medical evidence.

The papers in this book address a wide range of difficult ethical issues related to the AIDS crisis. Clearly, it is important to examine these issues through an ethical lens, to explore the relevance of moral or normative concepts that AIDS raises, and to evaluate the responses to AIDS from an ethical perspective. Given the nature of the issues involved here, however, one inevitably encounters complex legal questions. Although one's arguments about the ethical dimension of these issues should not necessarily be determined by legal opinions and precedent or by statutory developments, it is essential to acknowledge the legal dimensions of the ethical inquiry.

The goal of this paper is to alert readers to the broad range of legal issues explored in this book. The emphasis is on identifying areas where there have been significant legal developments that raise impor-

tant ethical questions and on highlighting those areas of legal development that have the widest significance. This paper does not pretend to
provide a comprehensive review of AIDS law. Among the sources listed
at the end of the paper are a number of legal treatises that do so.
Rather the emphasis here is on the major areas of AIDS law that have
significance to persons with HIV infection and to the general public.

I begin by considering the basic ethical and public policy issues that
arise in relation to the development of legislation or resolution of legal
disputes involving HIV. A basic complicating factor in AIDS has been
the fear and threat of discrimination against those who are HIV infected. I consider legal developments concerning AIDS- and HIV-related
discrimination. I then address a number of the more significant areas
of law that affect persons with AIDS and those that have general social
significance. Among those areas of legal development that most clearly
involve all persons with HIV infection are testing, counseling, and
informed consent; confidentiality, reporting, and warning to third parties; duty to treat and access to treatment; and insurance. Those areas
of legal development that deal with legal measures primarily aimed at
reducing the spread of HIV are the role of public coercion, the role of
civil liability, and AIDS education. I conclude with a consideration of
the special problems raised by infected health care workers, including
special duties these workers may have to their patients, the possible
obligation to inform patients of the health care worker's HIV status,
and the appropriateness of restrictions on infected health care workers'
ability to treat patients.

Individual Interests Versus Public Concerns

From the threshold issue of determination of who is HIV infected to
the question of possible restrictions imposed upon those who are infected, individual automony and civil liberties and their tension with
proposed measures to protect the public loom large.

The testing or screening of individuals for HIV infection raises the
issue of individual patient autonomy in making decisions related to
medical treatment and diagnosis. Without some clear benefit from
mandatory screening, rejection of systematic screening may not be
controversial. However, when the issue arises in relation to special
populations such as the military, prisoners, or prostitutes, the matter
becomes more complicated. For example, the mandatory screening of
armed forces personnel has been justified on the basis of the possible
need for in-the-field transfusions from one soldier to another without

the possibility of applying blood-screening tests. Another justification given is the need to reassure foreign governments that military personnel serving on bases on foreign soil pose no danger to the civilians of that country as a result of infection following sexual relations. These justifications require evaluation and exploration of less restrictive available alternatives.

The measures available to protect the public range from persuasion, using educational programs, to coercion, employing measures such as isolation or quarantine. Movement along the spectrum toward the more restrictive measures requires a constant balancing of the infringement of autonomy and civil liberties against the need for and effectiveness of the restrictive measures being considered. For instance, proposals to close bathhouses, where individuals engage in sexual activity that may transmit HIV, need to be evaluated in terms of the effectiveness of such closure in eliminating or reducing the conduct likely to transmit HIV and in terms of the chilling effect such action has on free association. Moreover, such a restrictive measure must be evaluated against such less restrictive measures as mandated safe-sex instruction in such facilities, removal of doors on private rooms to reduce the likelihood of unsafe conduct, and mandated monitoring of activity in the facility to discourage conduct likely to transmit HIV. More basic concerns are raised by proposals to quarantine HIV-infected prostitutes. These include the need to protect the freedom and civil liberties of individuals from unnecessary restrictions where such proposals focus on status rather than on behavior of individuals. There is also a need to consider fashioning alternative coercive measures, such as monitored home detention, directed at those prostitutes who continue to engage in unsafe behavior after counseling and other educational measures have been applied.

The tension between the concerns about individual autonomy and personal liberty and the protection of the public by preventing the spread of HIV and by otherwise containing AIDS is exacerbated by the threat of discrimination against those with HIV infection. Such discrimination raises fundamental concerns about individual justice and the inequitable treatment of persons that is a direct threat to individual autonomy and personal liberty.

Discrimination

Discrimination against HIV-infected individuals has been viewed as a great obstacle to adopting the most appropriate and effective legal responses to AIDS and HIV infection. The *Report of the Presidential Commission* (1988:119) concluded that "discrimination is impairing this nation's ability to limit the spread of the epidemic."

For example, the Illinois AIDS Confidentiality Act (1988) was enacted to provide confidentiality protections to persons with AIDS because of fear that they would otherwise be the subject of discrimination. At the same time, the legislature of Illinois recognized the need to have accurate information about persons with AIDS and HIV infection for public health reasons, including possible contact tracing to warn past sexual partners of persons infected with HIV. In order to assuage the fear that access to the information in such public health records might lead to discrimination by various individuals or groups, which in turn might discourage individuals from submitting to voluntary HIV-antibody testing, a distinction was drawn between records of individuals with an AIDS diagnosis and those who merely tested positive for the HIV antibody. If it is assumed that the public health purpose of contact tracing has any merit, the distinction drawn is irrational. A person with HIV antibody is just as likely to have infected former sexual contacts as a person with an AIDS diagnosis is.

Legal protection for those with AIDS or HIV infection is provided in some situations by the federal Rehabilitation Act of 1973, which provides that no otherwise qualified individual shall, solely by reason of handicap, be excluded from participation in, be denied the benefits of, or be subjected to discrimination under, any program or activity receiving federal financial assistance. As a result of a subsequent amendment made in 1974, handicap is construed very broadly to include physical and mental disabilities that substantially limit an individual's major life activities. An individual is handicapped if the person has a record of or is regarded as being, or perceived as being, disabled. The Rehabilitation Act requires that a person must be otherwise qualified; that is, the person must be capable of meeting all the performance or eligibility criteria for any position, service, or benefit at issue.

Although the United States Supreme Court has not directly ruled on whether AIDS or HIV infection is a handicap for purposes of the federal Rehabilitation Act, other federal courts have. The Supreme Court did rule in *School Board of Nassau County Florida v. Arline* (1987), a case involving a teacher infected with tuberculosis, that the protection of section 504 extends to persons with infectious diseases. The United States Court of Appeals for the Ninth Circuit in *Chalk v. United States District Court* (1988) determined that AIDS is a protected handicap under the Rehabilitation Act.

Doe v. Centinela Hospital (1988) involved the exclusion of an asymptomatic HIV-infected person from a federally funded hospital's residential drug and alcohol treatment program because of alleged fear of contagion. The hospital contended that Doe was not handicapped since he exhibited no clinical symptoms from his AIDS-related condition. In denying the hospital's motion for summary judgment, the court ruled that discrimination based solely on fear of contagion is discrimination based on handicap.

Note, however, that the federal Rehabilitation Act applies only to programs established by the federal government or programs receiving federal financial assistance.

The Americans With Disabilities Act (ADA) (1990) extends antidiscrimination protection, for persons with disabilities, to the private sector in employment, public accommodations, transportation, and public services. The Act uses the definition of a person with disability incorporated into the Rehabilitation Act of 1973. In using the section 504 definition, the ADA uses a functional definition of disability, rather than a list of every possible medical disability. Such lists have not been used in disability legislation, owing to both the difficulty of ensuring the comprehensiveness of such a list and the fact that some medical conditions may not yet be discovered or prevalent at the time legislation is passed.

The courts have consistently held that those with AIDS and those infected with HIV are covered under the section 504 definition of disability. Under these prior court interpretations it is clear that those with AIDS and those who are HIV infected will also receive protection under the ADA. However, consistent with the law that has existed under section 504, the ADA provides that any individual who poses a direct threat to the health or safety of others does not receive protection under the Act. The Act defines the term "direct threat" as "a significant risk to the health or safety of others that cannot be eliminated by reasonable accommodation."

The enactment of the Americans with Disabilities Act came only after lengthy debate in Congress over a proposal to permit food industry employers to transfer workers with HIV to other jobs. Instead the ADA was adopted with an amendment that gives the Secretary of Health and Human Services the responsibility of preparing a list of communicable diseases that are transmitted by food. This is an example of resolution of a legislative dispute between those legislators who maintain that employers, such as those in the food industry, must rely on scientific evidence for transferring workers with communicable diseases and those legislators who would instead indulge public misconceptions, fear, and prejudice.

Most states have handicap statutes that prohibit discrimination in both the private and public sectors. In more than half the states these provisions have been found to apply to persons with AIDS and HIV infection.

Concern about discrimination against persons with AIDS or HIV infection is well founded. The major areas of discrimination that have given rise to litigation include education, employment, housing, insurance, and health care. The latter two areas will be discussed in subsequent sections of this paper.

School boards have attempted to exclude HIV-infected children. Parents have, however, been successful in asserting the right of HIV-infected children to attend school. For example, in *Doe v. Dolton Elem. Sch. Dist. No. 148* (1988), parents successfully challenged a school board decision to exclude their child from education at school, relying on section 504 of the federal Rehabilitation Act of 1973.

Discrimination against persons with AIDS and HIV infection in employment has taken the forms of dismissal, demotion to positions of lower experience and skill, denial of insurance benefits, reduction in salary, and harassment. Employees of federal agencies or entities receiving federal funds have obtained protection under the federal Rehabilitation Act. Employees in the private sector have relied on state rehabilitation laws, human rights laws, and AIDS-specific antidiscrimination laws. In *Raytheon Co. v. Fair Employment and Housing Commission* (1989), the California Court of Appeals affirmed a lower court's decision that AIDS was a physical handicap under the California disability law, which provided, therefore, protection to employees from unlawful discrimination.

The West Virginia Supreme Court decision in *Benjamin v. Orkin Exterminating Company, Inc.* (1990) was the first decision by a state's highest court to find that asymptomatic HIV infection is covered as a handicap, reasoning that psychological problems faced by persons with HIV infection can themselves be considered impairments under the law.

Discrimination in housing against persons with AIDS or HIV infection has ranged from attempts at eviction, turning off utilities, refusing to make repairs, and harassment to real estate agents' directing prospective purchasers away from premises in which persons with HIV have lived. Complaints have been filed with state and local administrative bodies, as well as with courts. In *Baxter v. Belleville* (1989), the city defendant denied a special use permit to the plaintiff to open a residence for persons with HIV-related illnesses. Suit was brought alleging violation of the Fair Housing Amendments Act of 1988 and the fourteenth amendment. Following the issuance of a preliminary injunction requiring the city to grant the permit, the parties entered into a consent decree embodying the argument that HIV infection is a handicap within the meaning of the Fair Housing Amendments Act.

Testing, Counseling, and Informed Consent

Testing for HIV antibody (HIV testing) is appropriate for those who desire to know whether they are HIV infected or not. Testing is also appropriate in connection with diagnosis and treatment of a patient; this is more clearly the case since early intervention with drug therapies has proven effective.

More controversial is the use of HIV testing as a patient-screening device to alert health care personnel to the need to follow procedures to reduce the risk of infection with HIV. The Centers for Disease Control (CDC) and other public health authorities have recommended against general screening of patients for presence of HIV antibody. Instead, the CDC recommends implementation of universal precautions for infection control, which results in treating all patients as if they are HIV-antibody positive. The Occupational Safety and Health Administration (OSHA) has issued standards for enforcement of the CDC recommendations.

The use of HIV testing to screen patients for purposes of infection control is not forbidden by any state or federal statute. In most states, however, such testing for screening purposes can be implemented only with a patient's informed consent.

The use of HIV tests for surveillance and for screening without the consent, and sometimes without the knowledge, of the individual tested has occurred in a variety of social settings. Some testing has occurred in government-funded surveillance programs; for instance, there has been widespread testing of newborns in order to determine the extent of spread of HIV through the population. This testing has not given rise to litigation by parents or guardians of those tested. Some hospitals have permitted testing of pregnant women without consent and without informing test subjects of the outcome of their tests. In several instances, such testing has been halted after media exposure of the practice by particular hospitals.

The use of HIV testing to screen various populations has given rise to litigation. In *Anonymous Fireman v. City of Willoughby* (1988), screening of fire fighters was held to be unlawful because it would not reduce the already remote risk of transmission of HIV. In contrast the federal bureau of prisons and several state correctional systems are mandated to test all new inmates, all releases, and all current inmates regardless of presence of clinical indications. (See National Institute of Justice) (1988).

Prisoners have not been successful in the courts in resisting involuntary HIV testing. For example, in *Dunn v. White* (1989), a federal appeals court found that mandatory HIV testing did not violate a prisoner's first or fourth amendment rights.

Prisoners have not been successful in obtaining forced testing and segregation of other prisoners. For example, in *Glick v. Henderson* (1988), a federal appeals court found no violation of a prisoner's eighth amendment rights by a corrections department's refusal to test other prisoners for HIV antibody.

Guidelines developed by the United States Public Health Service mandate that testing for HIV antibody should be available to all who request such testing. These guidelines give priority for testing and counseling to persons who are likely to be infected. Professional ethical standards require physicians and other health care providers to provide counseling to reduce the likelihood of spread of HIV infection. A number of states, for example, Wisconsin (West 1988), require pretest and posttest counseling in relation to HIV-antibody testing.

Several states, for example, California (Cal. Health & Safety Code § 199.22), have adopted statutes or regulations requiring informed consent for HIV testing in the medical context. Informed consent and patient autonomy provide the fundamental bases for the patient-physician relationship. This right is rooted in constitutional rights to privacy and liberty and in common law rights to bodily integrity. The basic tenet of required informed consent gives competent persons control over decisions regarding their treatment, including any extraordinary diagnostic tests that may be thought to be medically indicated.

Informed consent to HIV testing means an agreement, without inducement, to undergo suggested tests for the presence of HIV antibody following receipt of a fair explanation of the test, which includes: its purpose; potential use; limitations; the meaning of test results, including the possibility of false-positive and false-negative results; the procedures to be followed, including the voluntary nature of the test; the right to withdraw consent at any time during the testing process; the right to anonymity to the extent provided by law with respect to participation in the test and disclosure of test results; and the right to confidential treatment of information identifying the subject of the test and the results of the test to the extent provided by law.

Ordinarily, routine blood testing does not require a specific consent because such tests are regarded as low-risk procedures and are included within the general consent to medical treatment. While it may be argued that HIV testing does not pose any significant risk of physical injury to the vast majority of persons, the social and personal consequences of a positive HIV test militate in favor of requiring informed consent.

The CDC has recommended that all persons be informed before being tested for the presence of HIV antibody. Some courts have held that the doctrine of informed consent does apply to taking blood for the purposes of HIV testing (*Doe v. Equifax* 1989).

The state of Illinois, which generally requires written informed consent to HIV testing, has enacted a statutory exception (Ill. Rev. Stat. ch. 111 1/2, para. 7308) permitting physicians to test a patient on the basis of a general consent to medical treatment, when in the medical judgment of the physician, HIV testing is appropriate for treatment or for diagnostic purposes. Texas goes so far as to permit nonconsensual testing if a medical procedure is to be performed on a patient that could expose health care personnel to HIV infection (Texas Civil Pac. & Rem. Code Ann. § 902(a)).

At least one court has found no need for specific consent for HIV-antibody testing where consent to blood testing is given. In *Doe v. Dyer Goods* (1989) an individual obtained a premarital blood test. Subsequently, the physician administering the test informed the individual that he had tested positive for HIV, although further testing showed the person was not HIV infected. While plaintiff did consent to have his blood withdrawn in order to have required premarital blood testing done, he did not consent to an HIV-antibody test. The court in *Doe v. Dyer Goods* first rejected plaintiff's invasion of privacy claims. The court reasoned that a defendant is subject to liability only when he has entered into a private place or invaded an individual's private seclusion. Since the plaintiff relinquished his blood sample to the physician, the court found the blood sample was not in private seclusion. Second, the court denied plaintiff's allegations of battery based upon lack of informed consent. The court noted that individuals who are mentally and physically able to discuss their medical condition and are not in an emergency must give their informed consent to a surgical operation. The court concluded plaintiff's cause of actions could not stand because a phlebotomy is not considered a surgical procedure. However, even if a phlebotomy fell into the category of surgical procedure, the court noted no proof was presented to show plaintiff was not informed of the risks of blood withdrawal. In addition, plaintiff's blood sample was found to be simply a by-product of the medical procedure to which he had consented. Finally, the court held plaintiff failed to show the performance of the HIV test violated the physician's obligation to act in the patient's best interests.

Courts have upheld federal screening programs in the Department of State (*Local 1812, Amer. Fed. of Govt Employees v. U.S. Dept. of State* (1987) and Department of Defense (*Batten v. Lehman* (1986). The justification urged at trial for these government screening programs was not to prevent HIV transmission but to ensure that personnel would not be put at risk of contracting opportunistic infection and to uphold the nation's relations abroad.

The Immigration and Naturalization Service has a program of mandatory screening for immigration into the United States and has discretion to test visitors to the country (42 C.F.R. § 34.2(b)). The World Health Organization has, however, advised against travel restrictions based on a person's serological status (WHO 1987).

Confidentiality, Reporting, and Warning Third Parties

Obligatory confidentiality is a hallmark of the health care professions. Confidentiality is paramount to appropriate and effective treatment. A patient will not speak freely about personal and intimate matters if disclosure is likely. In the AIDS context, information about an individual's HIV status and personal life-style is important, not only for personal treatment, but also for public health purposes, including epidemiological studies. Assured confidentiality is necessary to encourage voluntary participation of HIV-infected persons. The concept of confidentiality, based on the right of privacy, recognizes that the decision to share personal information rests with the patient. A concomitant duty arises on the part of the physician and of treating health care personnel to maintain the confidentiality of communications made in the course of treatment. As with most areas of law, the duty of confidentiality is not absolute, and warranted exceptions have been recognized.

The level of protection of confidentiality of HIV-related medical records varies from state to state. California is representative of those states that have provided broad protection to HIV-related records. A California statute (Cal. Health and Safety Code § 199.20) provides that no one can be compelled to identify or provide identifying characteristics of a person who has been tested for the causative agent of AIDS. The statute provides for civil and criminal liability for wrongful disclosure.

In the absence of, or in addition to, specific legislation directed at protecting the confidentiality of HIV-related medical records, protection may be provided by general statutes. These statutes (for example, Ariz. Rev. Stat. Ann. § 12-2235) provide an evidentiary privilege to be asserted for physician-patient communication on behalf of the patient in any judicial or quasi-judicial proceeding.

Where no statutory cause of action is available, an individual whose HIV-related records have been revealed to his or her detriment may have a cause of action for invasion of privacy. In addition, when a treating physician has breached confidentiality by unauthorized communication of HIV-related information, an action may lie for breach of the physician-patient confidential relationship and malpractice.

Disclosure of HIV status of infected children has raised special problems. Some states provide that school administrators are to be informed of the identity of children with AIDS or HIV infection. For example, Illinois statutes (Ill. Rev. Stat. ch. 111 1/2, para. 2211) provide that whenever a child of school age is reported to a state or local health department as having been diagnosed with AIDS or HIV infection, such department must give prompt notice of this information to the principal of the school in which the child is enrolled. Courts have generally upheld the requirements for reporting the HIV status of children enrolled in school. For example, in *Doe v. Dolton Elem. School Dist., No. 148* (1988), a federal district court upheld a school policy requiring disclosure of a child's identity to the school district, faculty, and staff.

While requiring such disclosure, the courts have, nonetheless, safeguarded the right of HIV-infected school children not to be discriminated against in their school placement. For example, in *Robertson v. Granite City Comm. Unit Sch. Dist. No. 9* (1988), a court considered the challenge to a school requirement that a child be permitted to attend school only if placed in a separate modular classroom. Instead, the court required full integration of the child into the school without any visible barrier between the child and his or her classmates. The court reasoned that to do otherwise would cause irreparable emotional and psychological harm to the child.

Although some parents have asserted a right to know whether any HIV-infected children attend the school that their own child attends, and the identity of such infected children, no court has directly considered this question and no current statute requires such disclosure.

Statutes and regulations in every state require the reporting of defined cases of AIDS to the CDC. A number of states, including Colorado (Colo. Rev. Stat. § 25-4-1402), have statutory or regulatory provisions requiring the reporting of positive HIV-antibody test results with the names of the subject. Other states, such as Illinois (Ill. Rev. Code Ann. ch. 111 1/2 § 7404), require reporting of positive HIV-antibody test results without personal identification of the test subject. The latter provisions are said to be necessary to encourage voluntary cooperation in HIV-antibody–testing programs.

Information obtained from reporting of AIDS diagnosis and HIV infection has been used as the basis for epidemiologic studies and surveillance. Some states have used this information in tracing and notifying sexual partners of infected persons to permit such partners to obtain testing and counseling.

Court decisions from various jurisdictions have announced exceptions to the physician's duty of confidentiality. Most court opinions have determined that a physician's or therapist's duty to control a dangerous patient or to reduce the risk of harm to another person outweighs the confidential nature of the physician-patient relationship. The landmark case authorizing a breach of confidentiality is the California Supreme Court decision in *Tarasoff v. Regents of the University of California* (1976), in which the court held that when a physician or therapist determines that a patient presents a serious danger of violence to another, the physician incurs an obligation to use reasonable care to protect the intended victim against such danger. According to the court, this may require the physician or therapist to warn the intended victim or others likely to apprise the victim of the danger, to notify the police, or to take whatever steps are reasonably necessary under the circumstances.

It has been argued that a physician has a duty to inform the spouse or current sexual or needle-sharing partners of an HIV-infected patient. Some states are considering legislation that would permit a physician to inform the spouse of an HIV-infected patient of the patient's condition. Litigation has been brought by an estranged wife of a patient who was not informed of her partner's seropositivity (*Doe v. Prime Health, Kansas City* 1988). It may be appropriate for a physician to inform the spouse of an HIV-infected patient about the patient's condition if the patient refuses to do so. Nevertheless, if the patient has been counseled by the physician and has satisfied the physician that he or she will inform the spouse or will not engage in behavior likely to transmit HIV to the spouse, the physician may owe no further duty to the spouse. Since HIV is not transmitted casually in the workplace or at home, there is no obligation to warn a patient's employer or family

Insurance companies have long taken the life-style of applicants into account in determining insurability and premium levels. In addition to HIV-antibody testing, some insurance companies initiated practices of life-style investigations to attempt to identify applicants who were at risk for AIDS.

In *NGRA and David Hurilbert v. Great Republic Ins.* (1988), a public interest law firm challenged the life-style-underwriting practices of an insurance company. At the time, California law banned HIV-antibody testing by insurance companies. The NGRA alleged that the insurance company had asked particular questions concerning the occupation and past health of single male applicants and had inferred sexual orientation and risk of HIV infection from the answers. The plaintiff asserted that these practices violated state civil rights laws forbidding discrimination by businesses serving the public on the basis of sex, marital status, and sexual orientation. When the trial court refused to dismiss the complaint, the company settled the case by agreeing to change its underwriting practices.

Most health insurance policies provide that an insurer will not be liable for expenses attributed to a preexisting condition, which is a medical condition in existence at the time the policy is issued. In the AIDS context, controversy has arisen whether an applicant's knowledge about his or her HIV status should be relevant for determining preexisting conditions. Advocates for persons with AIDS argue that asymptomatic HIV infection should not be considered a preexisting condition, because a preexisting condition is usually regarded as something for which treatment was being rendered prior to the application. Insurance companies assert that HIV infection is a medical condition and is therefore properly regarded as a preexisting condition. No litigation on this issue has advanced to the point of generating appellate precedent.

Some insurance companies have attempted to limit their exposure to claims by excluding AIDS-related expenses or to limit the yearly or lifetime benefits payable to a participant for such expenses. In some jurisdictions, such as New York, insurance regulations forbid companies that sell general health insurance policies from excluding coverage for particular diseases. Caps on coverage that differentiate between diseases in a disproportionate manner also violate many state regulations. Insurance companies may, however, place a ceiling over the total claims that can be asserted under a policy. In *Health Ins. Assn. of America v. Corcoran* (1988), a New York court also limited the regulatory power to require insurers to offer insurance without regard to proven actuarial factors.

members of the patient other than those with whom the patient may be engaging or likely to engage in sexual activity likely to transmit HIV.

Where a physician does decide to inform a spouse, it is likely that a court will uphold that action. A Florida Court, in *Tradup v. Mayer* (1988), upheld a physician's decision to inform a woman who was nine weeks pregnant that the father was HIV positive. The court held that the disclosure of confidential medical information was proper on the basis of emergency need.

In contrast a court in Hawaii, in *Drug Addiction Serv. v. Doe* (1st Cir. Ct. Hawaii), would not support a drug addiction clinic's decision to disclose to a client's sexual and needlesharing partner, who was also a client at the clinic, information that the client was HIV infected. The court reasoned that since all clients of the clinic were counseled not to engage in high-risk behavior and to obtain proper testing and counseling, there was no need for any clinic client to be provided information about another infected client.

Duty to Treat and Access to Treatment

Traditionally physicians have been free to accept or reject patients as they see fit, even though no other physician is available. This view was rooted in the general principle that an individual is not obligated to act affirmatively to prevent injury to another, absent special circumstances. Special circumstances have been found where there was a prior relationship between the parties, such as an ongoing physician-patient relationship, or where an individual was responsible for placing another person in a position out of which the injury to the person proximately resulted.

This common-law approach has been extended to limit the duty owed by a hospital to potential patients. Courts impose no general duty on a hospital to admit a person who presents himself or herself to a facility for treatment. The principal exception to the common-law rule is the "emergency exception," which has been codified by federal statute establishing emergency care requirements for all hospitals participating in the Medicare Program (COBRA 1985). The general emergency exception imposes liability upon hospitals for refusing to treat, on an emergency basis, seriously ill or injured patients. An emergency is generally held to be a sudden, unforeseen event calling for immediate action. Some of the opportunistic diseases associated with AIDS may produce conditions that warrant emergency care. In such a case a facility may be obligated to provide the emergency care required.

Most health care professional associations have determined that their members have an ethical duty to treat HIV-infected patients. Nevertheless, there are cases involving refusals of health care personnel to treat persons diagnosed with AIDS. For example, *Hurwitz v. Human Rights Commission* (1988) involved the refusal of a dentist to provide further treatment to a patient diagnosed with AIDS. The patient filed a complaint alleging unlawful discrimination with the New York City Commission on Human Rights. A New York court found that the dentist's office was a place of public accommodation and was prohibited from discriminating against the HIV-infected patient. The Americans With Disabilities Act (1990) provides protection to all persons from such discrimination in places of public accommodation, which include the offices of dentists and physicians.

Discriminatory activity falling short of outright refusal to treat has given rise to litigation; such discriminatory activity includes placing patients in isolation that is not medically indicated or placing food trays outside a patient's room (*Doe v. St. Francis Hosp.* 1987). Some physicians have attempted to justify their decision not to treat a patient, or to refer a patient to another provider, on the basis that they lack sufficient expertise to treat conditions associated with HIV infection. Given the availability of information on treatment alternatives for HIV patients, licensed health care practitioners should not easily evade responsibility without raising legitimate concern about their qualifications to practice. Certainly a refusal to treat or a decision to refer a patient to another provider should be viewed as medically unjustified and based on irrational fear and prejudice.

Some health care workers have refused, when directed by their employer, to provide care to an HIV-infected patient. Such a refusal may be legitimately based on the failure of a facility to observe appropriate infection control precautions. Refusals in such cases may be protected by the federal Occupational Safety and Health Act, 29 U.S.C. § 651 et seq. In the case of unionized employees, such refusal may be protected under section 7 of the National Labor Relations Act, 29 U.S.C. § 180. Where proper safety precautions are followed and where educational efforts are directed at eliminating irrational refusal to treat or care, a facility may take appropriate disciplinary action, including termination (*Steep v. Review Board of Indiana Employment Security* 1988).

HIV-infected persons have claimed a right to access to innovative pharmaceuticals approved by federal regulatory agencies, as well as a right to adequate public financing to make such access possible. Patients with AIDS have successfully sued state agencies (*Weaver v. Reagon* 1989) and hospitals (*Dallas v. Gay Alliance v. Dallas City*

Hosp. Dist. 1989) for access to azidothymidine, now called zidovutine (AZT) and aerosolized pentamidine.

A Missouri federal court in *Weaver* ordered that Medicaid coverage for AZT must be determined by the physician's assessment that the drug is medically necessary, rather than by a state-imposed diagnosis or laboratory standard. In the *Dallas* case, a Texas court prohibited a hospital from using a waiting list to control access to AZT and pentamidine, because such a process violated a state policy that provided that no person be denied treatment for fiscal reasons.

Insurance

Following licensing of the HIV-antibody test in 1985, insurance companies began requiring HIV tests for underwriting purposes for life and health insurance. The insurance companies asserted that HIV test results were relevant for actuarial determination in order to set premiums. Opponents of HIV test requirements for insurance coverage asserted these tests were wrongful and would result in inappropriate denial of medical coverage to persons with HIV infection.

Several states sought to regulate the insurance industry by limiting the use of HIV testing in making decisions about insurability. The aim of such legislation was to compel the insurance industry to bear the burden of a portion of the health costs generated by AIDS. Nevertheless, insurance industry opposition led to repeal of these laws and regulations. The California statutory ban on insurance use of HIV-antibody tests was repealed, and the determination was made by the District of Columbia, by order of Congress, and by the State Health Commissioner of Wisconsin that HIV-antibody testing is reliable enough for underwriting purposes.

In *Life Insurance Association of Massachusetts v. Commission of Insurance* (1988), the Massachusetts Supreme Judicial Court ruled that an attempt to ban HIV-antibody testing of health insurance applicants was invalid. Although the state insurance laws gave the commissioner significant discretion in regulating the operation of insurance companies, the court ruled that the statutes extended only to deceptive sales practices and to the content of policies. According to the court, the legislature did not authorize the commissioner to dictate underwriting practices.

Other legislation and regulations regarding HIV-antibody testing have been focused on such issues as maintaining confidentiality of test results, obtaining informed consent before testing, and requirement for appropriate counseling to accompany testing.

McGann v. H. & H. Music Co., et al. (1990) involved a challenge to an employer's decision to cap benefits under a self-insurance plan. The plaintiff had been covered by a group health insurance policy as part of his employee benefit plan. After the plaintiff was diagnosed with AIDS and began to claim benefits under the policy, the insurance company advised the employees to convert to a self-insured plan administered by the insurance company. The self-insured plan included a $5,000 lifetime cap on AIDS-related benefits. Plaintiff alleged the changes in policy violated the Employee Retirement Income Security Act of 1974 (ERISA), 29 U.S.C.A. § 1144(a) because the change had the purpose of depriving him of benefits he would have been entitled to under the plan as it existed before the change. The employer maintained that health benefits do not become vested under ERISA, so that a plan can be changed unilaterally by the employer. The trial court found the change in benefits did not violate ERISA even if motivated by a desire to avoid expenses associated with AIDS.

Role of Public Coercion

The majority of health care professionals and public health authorities maintain that education and counseling are the most effective means to stem transmission of HIV. Evidence suggests that educational programs are effective in changing the conduct of certain populations at high risk of HIV infection. Nonetheless, there is concern that certain individuals, knowing they are HIV infected, may disregard the risk they pose to others. Some people may deliberately engage in conduct that threatens others with HIV infection. When individuals threaten others by their behavior, the use of public coercion may be appropriate.

Three forms of legal public coercion are available: the mental health law, the public health law, and the criminal law. The mental health law requires not only a showing that an individual poses a risk of harm to others but also that the person suffers from a mental illness. In some cases HIV may trigger underlying psychosis or lead to a dementia that may qualify as a mental illness. Where such mental illness results in a person's engaging in conduct such as sexual attacks or other behavior likely to transmit HIV, involuntary mental commitment may be appropriate (*In re Commitment of B.S.* 1986).

Public health law can provide the means to isolate individuals who persist in engaging in HIV-transmitting behavior. The power to quarantine or isolate persons with communicable diseases is provided for by statutes in every state and by federal statutes. Some states have enacted statutes that specifically extend quarantine or isolation authority to persons with AIDS or HIV infection (for example, Idaho Code § § 39-601 and 39-603 (1986) and Ky. Rev. Stat., chs. 214.020 and 2124.410 (1986)). In *Jacobson v. Massachusetts* (1905), the United States Supreme Court broadly ruled that states have authority "to enact quarantine laws and health laws of every description" as a way of protecting a community against communicable disease.

HIV-infected prostitutes have been quarantined in several states. In one Florida case, a female prostitute with AIDS was confined to her home and required to wear an electronic device that would alert police if she strayed too far from the monitoring device placed in her telephone (See Institute of Medicine 1989:187–188). In another case, a male prostitute was the subject of a quarantine order that forbade him to have sexual relations without informing his partner of his condition. Violating provisions of the quarantine, which was of indefinite duration, made the prostitute subject to jail sentence and fine (See "Man Exposed to AIDS" 1987).

Quarantine of AIDS-infected prisoners has been upheld in New York. In *LaRocca v. Dalsheim* (1983), a New York Supreme Court upheld a Department of Corrections-instituted plan to segregate HIV-infected prisoners from other prisoners in order to halt the transmission of HIV. The court held that the corrections department acted reasonably in an effort to stop HIV transmission. The court found that quarantine was appropriate in the prison context but in dicta observed that medical knowledge about HIV would suggest that mass quarantine of the general public infected with HIV would not be justified.

The *Report of the Presidential Commission* (1988:78) concluded that quarantine based on HIV status alone cannot be justified: "Quarantine or isolation of HIV-infected individuals based only on status without consideration of an individual's behavior is not appropriate and should not be adopted." Instead the Commission recommended development of procedures for quarantine or isolation based on behavior.

There are a number of reasons why mass quarantine of HIV-infected persons is inappropriate. These include the medical and scientific evidence that HIV is not spread through casual contact, making segregation unnecessary and unduly restrictive; the fact that more than one million Americans are HIV infected, which makes general isolation unmanageable; the fact that infectiousness is permanent, so isolation would be limitless; and the fact that, because there is no curative treatment, there would be no way infected persons could ever regain their freedom.

Isolation or quarantine based on behavior imposes restrictions on those HIV-infected persons whose actions are likely to facilitate transmission of HIV. Several states have enacted statutes directed at recalcitrant individuals with HIV infection who persist in behaviors likely to transmit HIV (for example, Ill. Rev. Stat. ch. 111 1/2, para. 7408 (1988)).

For example, Illinois Department of Public Health Regulations (77 Ill. Admin. Reg. § 693.80(b)) provide for isolation of a "noncompliant HIV carrier" who is defined as "a person who knows or has reason to know that he or she is infected with HIV" and "is engaging in conduct or activities which place others at risk of exposure to HIV infection" as a result of specified behaviors, which include: selling or donating blood, sperm, organs, or other tissues or bodily fluids; engaging in or attempting, offering, or soliciting sexual activities likely to transmit HIV; sharing intravenous drug needles with another person; or action or statement by an individual that are clear indicators of his or her intention to place others at risk of exposure to HIV infection, such as a statement of intent to perform a specific action in order to infect another person.

These statutes generally include two important features: a showing that isolation is the least restrictive alternative or the alternative of last resort and a requirement of a court order making the findings required to authorize the respective department of public health to impose isolation.

For example, the Colorado statute (1987 Colo. Sess. Laws, chapter 208 (HB 1177)) authorizes the imposition of specified restrictive measures or orders on individuals with HIV infection only when all other efforts to protect the public health have failed. The statute further provides that orders and measures are to be applied serially, with the least intrusive measure utilized first. The burden of proof is on the state or local health department to show that specific grounds exist for the issuance of orders or measures and that the terms are not more restrictive than necessary to protect the public health.

A significant feature of the Illinois regulations governing isolation of noncompliant HIV carriers is the limiting of the order of isolation to the period for which the individual refuses to cease engaging in the behavior likely to transmit HIV. The regulations provide for obtaining a court order isolating such person in a restricted environment until such time as he or she has demonstrated a willingness and ability as shown by reported acts and statement of intention to refrain from behavior that places others at risk of exposure to HIV infection.

The *Report of the Presidential Commission* (1988) recommended that states adopt statutes that permit isolation of noncompliant HIV-infected persons. The Commission recommended, however, that the less restrictive measures available should be exhausted before more restrictive measures, such as limited isolation, are imposed. Further, the commission recommended that in exercising powers of isolation, there should be a heavy burden of proof requiring a showing that such measures are necessary and appropriate and that a factual basis exists for making the determination to isolate an individual.

The criminal law can be properly applied in certain cases of individuals deliberately engaging in behavior likely to transmit HIV. The *Report of the Presidential Commission* (1988:130) properly concluded that: "Just as other individuals in society are held responsible for their actions outside the criminal law's established parameters of acceptable behavior, HIV-infected individuals who knowingly conduct themselves in ways that pose a significant risk of transmission to others must be held accountable for their actions." Moreover, criminal prosecutions of those who deliberately act in ways likely to spread HIV will educate the public about conduct likely to spread HIV while at the same time reinforcing social norms against behavior likely to result in HIV transmission.

The range of behaviors and charges related to conduct likely to transmit HIV reveals that prosecutions have been brought for behaviors that are viewed by medical and scientific authorities as likely to facilitate transmission such as unprotected sexual intercourse, as well as behaviors that are not viewed as likely to prevent HIV transmission, such as spitting or biting.

Charges of attempted murder, attempted manslaughter, and assault are among those that most often have been brought against persons charged with conduct likely to transmit HIV. For example, in *United States v. Moore* (1987, *aff'd* 1988), a HIV-infected federal prison inmate in Minnesota was convicted of assault with a deadly and dangerous weapon for biting two prison guards upon a finding that his teeth constituted a deadly and dangerous weapon. In *Brock v. State* (1989), an appeals court reversed the conviction of an HIV-infected Alabama inmate charged with intent to commit murder for biting a corrections officer; the appeals court found that AIDS was not likely to be spread through saliva. In *State v. Sherouse* (1989), a Florida prostitute was charged with attempted manslaughter for engaging in sexual intercourse with a client after she had been informed that she had AIDS. A man in Indiana was charged with attempted murder when, with knowledge he had AIDS, he sprayed his blood on others (*State v. Haines* 1989).

Traditional criminal law offenses have not been adequate for punishing behavior of HIV-infected persons who are likely to infect others. Almost all traditional crimes involved serious problems of proving intent of the HIV-infected person to cause injury to another person or to cause that person to be infected with HIV where the charge involves a criminal attempt. There are also problems in many cases of proving that a specific act led to the infection of a victim where proof of infection is required to establish causation in order to prosecute an HIV-infected person on a homicide charge. For example, in charging a person with attempted murder for engaging in unsafe sex without informing the sexual partner, it is extremely difficult to prove the infected partner intended to transmit HIV to the other person. With murder, it is necessary to establish that the victim died as a consequence of a specific act of the defendant that transmitted HIV, which ultimately caused the victim's death.

In response to the inadequacies of the traditional criminal law in punishing and deterring conduct by HIV-infected persons that is likely to result in transmission of HIV, many state legislatures have enacted or proposed legislation making it a criminal offense for an HIV-infected person to knowingly engage in activity likely to result in the transmission of HIV. For example, the Louisiana statute (La. Rev. Stat. Ann. § 14:43.5 1990) provides that: "No person shall intentionally expose another to any acquired immune deficiency syndrome (AIDS) virus through sexual contact without the knowing and lawful consent of the victim."

The *Report of the Presidential Commission* (1988) observed that the problems in applying traditional criminal law to HIV transmission should lead to the adoption of criminal statutes specific to behavior related to transmitting HIV infection. According to the commission, an HIV-specific statute can provide clear notice of socially unacceptable standards of behavior specific to the HIV epidemic and can facilitate tailoring punishment appropriate to the specific HIV-transmitting behavior.

Role of Civil Liability

Given the pain, incapacity, and death that afflict persons with AIDS, it is not surprising that those exposed to HIV or those who have developed AIDS may sometimes feel themselves wronged and entitled to damages. The main areas of AIDS-related civil liability litigation have involved charges of medical malpractice and liability related to transmission as a result of receiving contaminated blood or blood products as a result of sexual intercourse.

The legal theories upon which liability is based are most often a breach of a statutory duty, negligence by a health care institution, or malpractice by a health care professional. The range of conduct leading to liability includes failure to obtain informed consent for HIV testing or treatment of HIV-related diseases, breach of confidentiality in the release of HIV-related medical records, and failure to enforce infection control guidelines and consequent infection of a patient or health care worker with HIV.

In the area of medical malpractice, lawsuits have been brought by patients claiming a health care provider was negligent for failing to properly diagnose and treat HIV infection (*Quintana v. United Blood Serv.* 1988). Suits have also been filed for psychological damages resulting from a negligent false diagnosis (*Bannow v. Mich. Public Health Dept.* 1989).

Health care workers have successfully brought suit where negligent disposal of contaminated material has resulted in infection with HIV. In *Prego v. City of New York* (1989), a health care worker obtained a significant recovery where she was injured as a result of a needlestick caused by negligent placement of a used syringe on a patient bed mixed in with gauze wrappings and other refuse, which it was the plantiff's job to clean up.

Transmission of AIDS through blood, including cases involving transfusions and the providing of the plasma blood product Factor-VIII to hemophiliacs, has accounted for approximately 2 to 3 percent of the reported medical cases of diagnosed AIDS.

Suits brought by persons contracting HIV infection from contaminated blood or blood products have cited several legal theories, including implied warranty, strict liability, and negligence. An action for a breach of implied warranty is based on statutes that read certain guarantees into contracts for the sale of goods. A claim based on an implied warranty for blood asserts the blood or blood product is guaranteed fit for transfusion or other patient use. An action for strict liability is based on the assertion that blood and blood products are inherently dangerous because of undetectable impurities. Underlying doctrines of strict liability and implied warranty is the theory that providers of blood and blood products are better situated to bear the loss caused by such products than the patient or recipient of such product is. To prevail in a suit for negligence, a plaintiff must show that a blood supplier failed to carry out the necessary precautions required to guarantee the purity of the blood or blood product. Suits have been brought against hospitals at which HIV-infected blood or blood products were received. In addition, suits have been brought against blood banks and manufacturers of blood products. There are, however, significant barriers to recovery in these suits. Most courts do not recognize a blood transfusion to be a sale to which warranties are attached; these court decisions are based on statutory definitions characterizing blood transfusions as services. Strict liability is also precluded by other statutes that state explicitly that the transfusion of blood will not be subject to strict liability. Similarly, some courts have found that the protection of these statutes is not limited to blood but extends to commercially manufactured blood products contaminated with HIV.

In determining the potential liability for negligence by suppliers of blood and blood products, it is necessary to distinguish between cases in which infected blood and blood products were received before the development and availability of screening tests for the HIV antibody and those cases arising after the advent of such tests.

One of the earliest cases dealing with liability for providing HIV-infected blood was *Kozup v. Georgetown University* (1988). The case involved an infant born in 1983 who contracted AIDS from a blood transfusion necessitated by its premature birth. Following the child's death, the parents sued the hospital and the blood supplier. On the theories of informed consent and battery, a federal district court in Washington, D.C., concluded that at the time of the transfusion, the risk of contracting AIDS from a blood transfusion was not known. The court indicated, however, that even if the risk had been known, the parents would not have been able to establish proximate causation since no reasonable person would have refused the transfusion.

The parents also claimed that the hospital was guilty of negligence because it had failed to offer the option of directed donation. Under directed donation, the parents would have been allowed to choose the source of the blood given to their baby. The court rejected this claim on the grounds that there was no evidence that directed donation was a local practice and no basis for a finding that it was a required standard of care. Finally, the court held that at the time of the transfusion, blood was an unavoidably unsafe product owing to the lack of a screening test for HIV.

On appeal, the district court was affirmed on all counts except the battery claim. Since the defendant hospital had failed to obtain parental consent for the transfusion, the appeals court found that a substantial question of material fact remained on the battery claim. Accordingly, it remanded the case to the trial court on that one count.

The availability of the HIV-antibody test since 1985 has permitted organizations that collect blood and plasma to screen donations for antibody to HIV in accordance with guidelines developed by the CDC. Under the guidelines, any blood or plasma that is positive on initial testing is not to be transfused or manufactured into other products capable of transmitting infectious agents. Since the proportion of false-positive results is high, the incidence of false negatives is low, and the prevalence of HIV infection in the general population is small, the antibody test is highly effective in detecting infected blood. In order to minimize the number of false-negative test results, it has been further recommended that members of groups at increased risk for AIDS refrain from donating blood and plasma.

It should be recognized that some risk still remains because blood that produces a negative reaction to the test may carry the virus. Studies have reported several cases in which the antibody has not been detected in asymptomatic individuals infected with HIV for more than six months. Since blood from such persons will not produce a positive antibody test result, physicians and providers administering blood and blood products should inform the prospective recipient of the continuing risk of infection from these products. Such informed consent may preclude liability on the part of a physician or health care provider absent a showing of negligence in the use of the screening procedure.

Because of the small but identifiable risk of HIV infection to recipients of screened blood, those providing blood should consider making available to recipients autologous and directed donations. Autologous donations involve taking blood from individuals for their future use. This procedure is highly recommended where a patient is undergoing elective surgery. Another measure that may be offered is that of directed donation by which specially identified individuals donate blood for the use of a particular patient. It is arguable that this provides no real assurance of HIV-free blood. Nevertheless, some states, such as California (Cal. Health & Safety Code § 1628), require that patients be advised of the availability of directed donations.

A number of suits have been filed relating to sexual transmission of HIV. The most widely publicized of these suits was the action brought by Marc Christian, Rock Hudson's lover (*Christian v. Sheft* 1989). The suit resulted in an award of $14.5 million for emotional distress and $7.25 million in punitive damages. The jury hearing the case found that Hudson had exhibited outrageous conduct in not disclosing his HIV infection to Christian and in his continuing to engage in unprotected sexual relations.

Recognition of tort liability for transmission of HIV and for misdiagnoses or improper treatment will provide some individuals with compensation. Moreover, such litigation may encourage others to use proper diagnostic techniques or to behave so as to limit the likelihood of transmitting HIV. Although tort damage recovery will provide some individuals, infected as a result of others' conduct, with funds to meet the medical costs and other expenses associated with their illness, a broader view suggests that the expenses associated with AIDS are best spread in the private sector by insurance and in the public sector by government funding rather than through private litigation seeking damages.

AIDS Education

While education has been a significant element of public health efforts to control infectious diseases, its role has been ancillary to biomedical intervention such as vaccination. AIDS education has, however, been a principal instrument for combating the spread of infection.

The general public needs AIDS education to develop understanding of the problems raised by AIDS and to support prevention efforts. AIDS education in schools and colleges can provide information about sexually transmitted disease and drug abuse. Uninfected persons whose behavior or circumstances put them at increased risk should be targeted for special education programs. Finally, there is a special need for outreach and education for health care personnel whose work activity puts them at risk of HIV infection.

About half of the states mandate AIDS education in public schools by statute (for example, Wash. Rev. Code §§ 402–403, 501–503 1988). The statutory mandate to provide AIDS education in the schools has taken different forms: as part of comprehensive health education (e.g., Virginia and New York); as a sexually transmitted disease (e.g., Ohio and Iowa); as part of sex education (e.g., Nevada and Kansas); as a communicable disease (e.g., North Carolina); and as special AIDS education (e.g., Oklahoma, Alabama, Maryland, and Georgia). Most states that mandate AIDS education allow parents to exempt their children from instruction.

While many public health officials and professional educators have maintained that explicit educational materials are necessary to reach much of the population at risk for HIV infection, others, including some prominent politicians, have found the explicit materials developed to be morally offensive. Consequently, legislation has been enacted that forbids the use of federal funds to provide AIDS prevention materials that "promote or encourage, directly, homosexual activities," and the educational content must not be "judged by a reasonable person to be offensive to most educated adults" (P.L. 100–607). *Gay Men's Health Crisis v. Sullivan* (1989) is a suit brought against the United States Department of Health and Human Services (HHS), claiming that the restrictions imposed by federal legislation not only inhibit the ability of organizations to produce medically accurate and effective AIDS educational programs but also infringe on the constitutional right of free expression. In a memorandum opinion and order, a U.S. District Court in New York denied a motion for summary judgment by the defendant HHS, finding the plaintiffs, the Gay Men's Health Crisis and other public organizations, and the New York State Department of Health, have standing to bring a suit alleging that regulations attached to a 1988 appropriations bill limiting the scope of AIDS education programs are discriminatory.

Challenge has also been mounted against mandatory AIDS education. Litigation has been brought by those who challenge the morality and appropriateness of state-mandated AIDS education in the schools. *Ware v. Valley St. High Sch. Dist.* (1989) involves the challenge of a religious group to New York's mandatory AIDS education program as a violation of the group's freedom of religion. The New York Court of Appeals overturned a lower court grant of summary judgment to defendants and remanded the case for trial on the claim of the plaintiffs that exposure to the state-mandated AIDS education could destroy the foundation of the religious faith of its members.

Special Problem of Infected Health Care Personnel

The duty of HIV-infected health care workers toward their patients in relation to the health care workers' own infection will vary from case to case. The CDC, for instance, views the question of whether an infected physician should perform invasive procedures to be a matter to be determined on an individual basis. The American Medical Association's position is that physicians should consult their colleagues about which activities infected physicians can pursue without creating a risk to patients.

Some have espoused the view that infected physicians have a duty, arising out of a patient's right to give informed consent to medical treatment, to inform patients of their HIV infection. However, a duty to disclose would arise only where the nature of treatment is such that it would be possible for the health care worker to transmit HIV to a patient. Such a case is presented where an infected surgeon may accidentally cut himself or herself during surgery and bleed into a patient's incision.

It has been suggested that infected health care personnel refrain from engaging in procedures that may result in transmission of HIV to a patient. The CDC recommends that such decisions be made by the health care worker in consultation with the health care worker's personal physician and the medical director and personnel health services staff of the employing hospital or institution.

Cook County Hospital, in 1987, banned a physician from performing all invasive procedures. An action was filed in *Doe v. County of Cook* by the physician alleging violation of section 504 of the federal Rehabilitation Act, 29 U.S.C. § 794. A consent decree resulted in reinstatement of the physician, who agreed to refrain from certain procedures and to adopt barrier precautions when undertaking other specified invasive procedures.

Compliance of HIV-infected health care workers with facility infectious control policies has also given rise to litigation. In *Leckelt v. Board of Commissioners of Hospital District No. 1* (1989), the court held that it would not violate section 504 of the federal Rehabilitation Act, 29 U.S.C. § 794, or state handicap discrimination law, for a hospital to discharge a health care worker for refusing to reveal his HIV-antibody status. A licensed practical nurse had obtained confidential testing after his roommate, previously a patient at the hospital, died from AIDS. The nurse refused to reveal his test result. The court held that the worker was discharged for insubordination and failure to comply with the facility's infection control program, rather than for perceived or actual impairment. The court held that a hospital was entitled to establish an infection control policy under which it could demand to know the antibody status of its personnel.

The ethical issues raised by the HIV epidemic often find expression in litigation and legislative debate. At the same time the development of AIDS law often creates serious ethical dispute. The issue of possible discrimination on the basis of HIV infection has been an undercurrent in the resolution of AIDS legal issues. The development of a body of law under federal and state handicap law and the enactment of the Americans With Disabilities Act of 1990 have involved long strides in the direction of addressing that issue. Yet, the possibility of discrimination on the basis of AIDS without effective legal redress remains a concern of those at risk for HIV infection.

Differences in perceptions about the nature of the AIDS epidemic, the possible means of infection, the appropriateness of alternative public measures that may be taken to reduce further transmission, and the relevance of ethical considerations and civil liberties concerns provide the impetus for further debate, litigation, and legislative developments.

As medical advances occur, the appropriateness of particular ethical views and legal conclusions may be challenged. For instance, earlier in the history of the AIDS epidemic, an HIV-antibody test was thought to indicate no more than exposure to the virus. Currently, a positive antibody test is thought to evidence infection. Earlier, HIV testing was thought to be relevant only for counseling about appropriate behavior. Currently, testing is viewed as necessary for early intervention with drug therapy. These medical and scientific developments directly impinge on the view of the appropriateness of counseling testing, perhaps even on the issue of screening at-risk populations in order to provide appropriate medical intervention.

There have been significant developments in the law relating to specific types of discrimination, such as in employment. There remain many areas that will require further debate and resolution. For example, the proper policy toward testing HIV-infected health care personnel and the appropriateness of restrictions on the procedures infected personnel may perform will require increased attention as reports are published of possible patient infection by exposure to infected dentists and physicians.

Other questions that are on the horizon include: the proper role of domestic partners in making decisions to withhold or terminate treatment of AIDS patients who are rendered incompetent; the appropriateness of testing of employees and limiting their work activities because of mental deficits caused by HIV infection, including dementia; the appropriateness of restrictions on insurance coverage for AIDS; and the responsibility of physicians and counselors to warn spouses and sex partners of patients who refuse to inform others of their HIV status.

Finally, one of the most important factors to be kept in mind in evaluating the appropriateness of the legal response and the adequacy of the general social response to AIDS is the shift in the demographics of AIDS. The CDC reports indicate a shift in the proportionate population of persons with AIDS from a largely white, middle-class, insured population involving gay or bisexual men and recipients of blood and blood products to a minority population with limited resources and largely uninsured. This shift may exacerbate problems of discrimination, lack of access to care, and the inadequacy of financial resources available to those persons with AIDS or HIV infection.

REFERENCES

Americans with Disabilities Act. 1990. Pub. L. No. 101–336.

Anonymous Fireman v. City of Willoughby. 1988. U.S.D.C., E.D. Ohio, *AIDS Literature Reporter* (May 27).

Bannow v. Mich. Public Health Dept. 1989. Mich. Cir. Ct., *AIDS Literature Reporter* (March 10).

Batten v. Lehman. 1986. U.S.D.C. Col. No. 85–4108 (Jan. 18).

Baxter v. Belleville. 1989. U.S.D.C., S.D. Ill., No. 89–3354 (Dec. 13).

Benjamin v. Orkin Exterminating Company, Inc. 1990. 390 S.E. 2d 814 (W. Va.).

Brock v. State. 1989. (Ala. Crim. App., LEXIS State library, Ala. file).

Chalk v. United States District Court. 1988. 840 F. 2d 701 (9th Cir.).

Christian v. Sheft. 1989. Cal. Sup. Ct. Los Angeles Cty., No. 574153, *AIDS Literature Reporter* (Feb. 4).

COBRA (Consolidated Omnibus Budget Reconciliation Act). 1985. P.L. 99–272 § 9121.

Dallas v. Gay Alliance v. Dallas City Hosp. Dist. 1989. 719 F. Supp. 1380 (N.D. Tex.).

Doe v. Centinela Hospital. 1988. 57 U.S.L.W. 2034 (C.D. Cal.).

Doe v. County of Cook. 1987. (N.D. Ill. No. 87C888).

Doe v. Dolton Elem. Sch. Dist. No. 148. 1988. 694 F. Supp. 440 (N.D. Ill.).

Doe v. Dyer Goods. 1989. 566 A.2d 889 (Pa. Super.).

Doe v. Equifax. 1989. WL57348 (E.D.Pa.).

Doe v. Prime Health, Kansas City. 1988. Dist. Ct. Johnson City, Kan. Civ. Ct. (May 17).

Doe v. St. Francis Hosp. 1987. N.Y.S. Div. of Human Rights No. 3-P-D-87-12330.

Dunn v. White. 1989. 880 F.2d 1188 (10th Cir.).

Fair Housing Amendments Act. 1988. Pub. L. No. 100-430.

Gay Men's Health Crisis v. Sullivan. 1989. WL 156303 (S.D.N.Y.).

Glick v. Henderson. 1988. 855 F.2d 536 (8th Cir.).

Health Ins. Assn. of America v. Corcoran. 1988. 140 Misc. 2d 255 (N.Y. Sup.).

Hurwitz v. Human Rights Commission. 1988. 142 Misc. 2d 214 (N.Y. Supp.).

Illinois AIDS Confidentiality Act. 1988. Ill. Rev. Stat. ch 111 1/2, para. 7301 et seq.

In re Commitment of B.S. 1986. 213 N.J. Super. 243, 517 A.2d 146.

Institute of Medicine, *Mobilizing Against AIDS,* rev. ed. Washington, D.C.: National Academy of Sciences.

Jacobson v. Massachusetts. 1905. 197 U.S. 11.

Kozup v. Georgetown University. 1988. 851 F. 2d 437 (D.C. Cir.).

LaRocca v. Dalsheim. 1983. 120 Misc. 2d 697, 467 N.Y.S. 2d 302 (N.Y. Sup. Ct.).

Leckelt v. Board of Commissioners of Hospital District No. 1. 1989. 714 F. Supp. 1377 (E.D. La.).

Life Insurance Association of Massachusetts v. Commission of Insurance. 1988. 403 Mass. 410, 530 N.E. 2d 168.

Local 1812, Amer. Fed. of Govt. Employees v. U.S. Dept. of State. 1987. 662 F. Supp. 50 (D.D.C.).

McGann v. H. & H. Music Co. et al. 1990. U.S.D.C., S.D. Tex., C.A. No. H-89-1995 (June 26).

"Man Exposed to AIDS Put Under Quarantine." 1987. *New York Times* (Feb. 13), p. B4.

National Institute of Justice. 1988. *AIDS in Correctional Facilities: Issues and Opinions,* 3d ed. Washington, D.C.: U.S. Government Printing Office.

NGRA and David Hurilbert v. Great Republic Ins. 1988. Super Ct. San. Fran. Cal., *AIDS Literature Reporter* (Oct. 18).

Prego v. City of New York. 1989. 147 A.D. 165 (N.Y. A.D. 2d Dept.).

Quintana v. United Blood Serv. 1988. Dist. Ct. Denver, Colo., *AIDS Literature Reporter* (June 10).

Raytheon Co. v. Fair Employment and Housing Commission. 1989. 212 Cal. App. 3d 1242, 261 *California Reporter* 197 (2d Dist.).

Rehabilitation Act. 1973. Section 504, 29 U.S.C. § 794. Amendment. 1974, 29 U.S.C. § 706 (7) (B)

Report of the Presidential Commission on the Human Immunodeficiency Virus Epidemic. 1988. Washington, D.C.: U.S. Government Printing Office.

Robertson v. Granite City Comm. Unit. Sch. Dist. No. 9. 1988. 684 F. Supp. 1002 (S.D. Ill.).

School Board of Nassau County Florida v. Arline. 1987. 107 S. Ct. 1123.

State v. Haines. 1989. 545 N.E. 2d 834 (Ind. Ct. App.)

State v. Sherouse. 1989. 536 So. 2d 1194 (Fla. App. Ct., 5th Dist.).

Steep v. Review Board of Indiana Employment Security Division. 1988. 521 N.E. 2d 3501 (Ind. Ct. App.).

Tarasoff v. Regents of the University of California. 1976. 17 Cal. 3d 425, 551 P. 2d 334, 131 *California Reporter* 14 *aff'g in part*, 529 P. 2d 553, 118 *California Reporter* 129.

Tradup v. Mayer. 1988. 16th Cir. Ct. Monroe Cty. Fla., *AIDS Literature Reporter* (May 13).

United States v. Moore. 1988. 669 F. Supp 289 (D. Minn.), *aff'd* 846 F.2d 1163 (8th Cir. 1988).

Ware v. Valley St. High Sch. Dist. 1989. W.L. 153177 (N.Y.).

Weaver v. Reagon. 1989. 886 F.2d 194 (8th Cir.), *affirming* 701 F. Supp. 717 (W.D. Mo. 1988).

West. 1988. Wisc. Stat. Ann. § 146.025 (2) (b).

WHO (World Health Organization). 1987. *Report of the Consultation on International Travel and HIV Infection.*

SUGGESTED READINGS

The format of this bibliography dealing with legal issues of AIDS differs from the other essays of this book in the nature of the citations and references provided. This chapter has included references to primary sources involving judicial opinions and statutory materials in the text. There are virtually no references to secondary sources or other references as provided in other chapters. In order to give readers easy access to sources that provide a nearly comprehensive description of the general area of legal development of AIDS law or to sources that provide greater analysis of particular areas of AIDS-related law, the following list of suggested readings has been developed.

Abt, C. and K. Hardy. 1990. *AIDS and the Courts.* Cambridge, Mass.: Abt Books.

Barnes, M. 1989. Toward Ghastly Death: The Censorship of AIDS Education. *Columbia Law Review* 89:698–724.

Begg, R. 1989. Legal Ethics and AIDS: An Analysis of Selected Topics. *Georgetown Journal of Legal Ethics* 3:1–56.

Bennett, W. 1988. AIDS: Education and Public Policy. *St. Louis University Public Law Review* 7:1–10.

Burris, S. 1989. Rationality Review and the Politics of Public Health. *Villanova Law Review* 34:909–932.

Clifford, K. and R. Tuculano. 1987. AIDS and Insurance: The Rationale for AIDS-related Testing. *Harvard Law Review* 100:1806–1825.

Closen, M., D. Hermann, P. Horne et al. 1989. *AIDS: Cases and Materials*. Houston: John Marshall Publishing.

Comment. 1984–85. AIDS: A New Reason to Regulate Homosexuality. *Journal of Contemporary Law* 11:315–343.

Comment. 1984–85. Current Topics in Law and Policy, Fear Itself: AIDS, Herpes, and Public Health Decisions. *Yale Law and Policy Review* 3:479–518.

Comment. 1986. AIDS: Do Children with AIDS Have a Right to Attend School? *Pepperdine Law Review* 13:1041–1061.

Comment. 1986. Quarantine: An Unreasonable Solution to the AIDS Dilemma. *University of Cincinnati Law Review* 55:217–235.

Comment 1986. Protecting the Public from AIDS: A New Challenge to Traditional Forms of Epidemic Control. *Journal of Contemporary Health Law and Policy* 2:191–214.

Comment. 1987. Enforcing the Right to a Public Education for Children Affected with AIDS. *Emory Law Journal* 36:603–648.

Comment. 1988. Prohibiting the Use of the Human Immunodeficiency Virus Antibody Test by Employers and Insurers. *Harvard Journal on Legislation* 25:275–315.

Comment. 1990. Closing the Open Door: The Legal Impact of the Human Immunodeficiency Virus Exclusion of the Legalization Program of the Immigration Reform and Control Act of 1986. *Yale Journal of International Law* 15:162–189.

Curran, W., L. Gostin, and M. Clark. 1988. *AIDS: Legal and Regulatory Policy*. Frederick, Md.: University Publishing Group.

Dalton, H., S. Burris, and Yale AIDS Law Project, eds. 1987. *AIDS and the Law*. New Haven: Yale University Press.

Dolgin, J. 1985. AIDS: Social Meanings and Legal Ramifications. *Hofstra Law Review* 14:193–209.

Dornette, W., ed. 1987. *AIDS and the Law*. New York: John Wiley.

Dunlap, M. 1989. AIDS and Discrimination in the United States: Reflections on the Nature of Prejudice in a Virus. *Villanova Law Review* 34:909–932.

Field, M. and K. Sullivan. 1987. AIDS and the Criminal Law. *Law, Medicine, and Health Care* 15:46–60.

Gostin, L. 1989. Hospitals, Health Care Professionals, and AIDS: The 'Right to Know' the Health Status of Professionals and Patients. *Maryland Law Review* 48:12–54.

Gostin, L. 1989. The Politics of AIDS: Compulsory State Powers, Public Health, and Civil Liberties. *Ohio State Law Journal* 49:1017–1058.

Gostin, L., ed. 1990. *AIDS and the Health Care System*. New Haven: Yale University Press.

Gostin, L. 1990. The AIDS Litigation Project: A National Review of Court and Human Rights Commission Decisions: Part I. *JAMA* (April 11), 263(14):1961–1974.

Gostin, L. 1990. The AIDS Litigation Project: A National Review of Court and Human Rights Commission Decisions: Part II. *JAMA* (April 18), 263(15):2086–2093.

Gostin, L. and W. Curran. 1987. Legal Control Measures for AIDS: Reporting Requirements, Surveillance, Quarantine, and Regulations of Public Meeting Places. *American Journal of Public Health* 77:214–218.

Gray, A. 1986. The Parameters of Mandatory Public Health Measures and the AIDS Epidemic. *Suffolk University Law Review* 20:505–522.

Greeley, H. 1989. AIDS and the American Health Care Financing System. *University of Pittsburgh Law Review* 51:73–166.

Hermann, D. 1986–87. AIDS: Malpractice and Transmission Liability. *University of Colorado Law Review* 58:63–107.

Hermann, D. 1987. Hospital Liability and AIDS Treatment: The Need for a National Standard of Care. *University of California at Davis Law Review* 20:441–479.

Hermann, D. 1987. Liability Related to Diagnosis and Transmission of AIDS. *Law, Medicine, and Health Care* 15:36–45.

Hermann, D. and R. Gagliano. 1989. AIDS, Therapeutic Confidentiality, and Warning Third Parties. *Maryland Law Review* 48:55–76.

Hermann, D. 1990. Criminalizing Conduct Related to HIV Transmission. *St. Louis University Public Law Review* 9:351–378.

Hermann, D. and W. Schurgin. 1990. *AIDS Legal Issues.* Deerfield, Ill.: Callaghan.

Hiam, P. 1987/88. Insurers, Consumers, and Testing: The AIDS Experience. *Law, Medicine, and Health Care* 15:212–222.

Hoffmann, J. and E. Kincaid. 1986–87. AIDS: The Challenge to Life and Health Insurers' Freedom of Contract. *Drake Law Review* 35:709–771.

Janus, E. 1988. AIDS and the Law: Setting and Evaluating Threshold Standards for Coercive Public Health Intervention. *William Mitchell Law Review* 14:503–573.

Jarvis, R., M. Closen, D. Hermann, and A. Leonard, 1990. *AIDS Law in a Nutshell.* St. Paul, Minn.: West Publishing.

Jayasuriya, D. 1988. *AIDS: Public Health and Legal Dimensions.* Boston: Martinus Nijhoff Publishers.

Joseph, P. 1988. Civil Liberties in the Crucible: An Essay on AIDS and the Future of Freedom in America. *Nova Law Review* 12:1083–1102.

Kim, R. and K. McMullin. 1988. AIDS and the Insurance Industry. *St. Louis University Public Law Review* 7:155–176.

Leonard, A. 1985. Employment Discrimination Against Persons with AIDS. *University of Dayton Law Review* 10:681–703.

Leonard, A. 1989. AIDS, Employment, and Unemployment. *Ohio State Law Journal* 49:929–964.

Lipton, K. 1986. Blood Donor Services and Liability Issues Relating to Acquired Immune Deficiency Syndrome. *Journal of Legal Medicine* 7:131–186.

Merritt, D. 1986. Communicable Diseases and Constitutional Law: Controlling AIDS. *New York University Law Review* 61:739–799.

Mohr, R. 1987. Policy, Ritual, Purity: Gays and Mandatory AIDS Testing. *Law, Medicine, and Health Care* 15:178–185.

Note. 1986. Constitutional Rights of AIDS Carriers. *Harvard Law Review* 99:1274–1292.

Note. 1986. Protecting Children with AIDS Against Arbitrary Exclusion from School. *California Law Review* 74:1373–1407.

Note. 1987. AIDS in the Classroom: Room for Reason Amidst Paranoia. *Dickinson Law Review* 91:1055–1083.

Note. 1987. Tort Liability for AIDS. *Houston Law Review* 24:957–990.

Note. 1988. Asymptomatic Infection with the AIDS Virus as a Handicap Under the Rehabilitation Act of 1973. *Columbia Law Review* 88:563–586.

Note. 1988. Discrimination in the Public Schools: Dick and Jane Have AIDS. *William and Mary Law Review* 29:881–898.

Note. 1988. Negligence as a Cause of Action for Sexual Transmission of AIDS. *University of Toledo Law Review* 19:923–945.

Note. 1988. The AIDS Pandemic: International Travel and Immigration Restrictions and the World Health Organization's Response. *Virginia Journal of International Law* 28:1043–1064.

Note. 1988. The Impact of AIDS on Immigration Law: Unresolved Issues. *Brooklyn Journal of International Law* 14:223–248.

Note. 1988. Tort Liability for the Transmission of the AIDS Virus: Damages for Fear of AIDS and Prospective AIDS. *Washington and Lee Law Review* 45:185–211.

Note. 1989. AIDS Antibody Testing and Health Insurance Underwriting: A Paradigmatic Inquiry. *Ohio State Law Journal* 49:1059–1076.

Note. 1989. Standards of Conduct, Multiple Defendants, and Full Recovery of Damages in Tort Liability for the Transmission of Human Immunodeficiency Virus. *Hofstra Law Review* 18:37–87.

Parmet, W. 1985. AIDS and Quarantine: The Revival of an Archaic Doctrine. *Hofstra Law Review* 14:53–90.

Parmet, W. 1987. AIDS and the Limits of Discrimination Law. *Law, Medicine and Health Care* 15:61–72.

Robinson, D. 1985. AIDS and the Criminal Law: Traditional Approaches and a New Statutory Proposal. *Hofstra Law Review.* 14:91–105.

Schatz, B. 1987. The AIDS Insurance Crisis: Underwriting or Overreaching. *Harvard Law Review* 100:1782–1805.

Schulman, D. 1988. AIDS Discrimination: Its Nature, Meaning, and Function. *Nova Law Review* 12:1113–1140.

Schultz, G. 1988. AIDS: Public Health and the Criminal Law. *VII St. Louis University Public Law Review* 65 7:65–113.

Sinkfield, R. and T. Houser. 1989. AIDS and the Criminal Justice System. *Journal of Legal Medicine* 10:103–125.

Sullivan, K. and M. Field. 1988. AIDS and the Coercive Power of the State. *Harvard Civil Rights–Civil Liberties Law Review* 23:139–197.

Wasson, R. 1987. AIDS Discrimination Under Federal, State, and Local Law After *Arline. Florida State University Law Review* 15:221–278.

Wood, G. 1987. The Politics of AIDS Testing. *AIDS and Public Policy Journal* (Fall-Winter), 2:35–49.

∎ Index

Access to investigational drugs: ethical issues, 6; mechanisms, 91-92

Activism: civil disobedience, 156-58, 169-83, 186n2; collaborative approach, 165-66; Community Research Inititatives (CRI) 166-67; concerns of, 158-59; die-ins or red tape, 159, 171-72; drug research successes, 181; ethics of, 12; genocide protest, 158, 174-78, 184, 186n4; legal and translegal warrants, 173-74; limitations, 182-83; militancy, 2, 6, 155-57, 181; models of protest, 162-164, 178; nonviolent disruptive tactics, 165; objectives, expectations and successes, 179-84; political and social tolerance limits, 158-59; persuasive or coercive acts, 170-72; rationale for, 160-62; resource allocation issues, 158; symbol of, 159; views of FDA process, 162, 168; *see also:* AIDS Coalition to Unleash Power (ACT UP)

Adolescents: changing sexual practices, 134; debate over explicit sex education, 148-51; educational HIV/AIDS programs, 136

AIDS Clinical Trial Group (ACTG), 90, 166-67, 186n1

AIDS Coalition to Unleash Power (ACT UP): Community Research Initiatives (CRI), 167; confrontational tactics, 160-62, 174-75; drug development and release, 90, 156, 162-66; gadfly protests, 168; National AIDS Treatment Research Agenda, 166; nonviolent disruptive action, 165; red tape demonstrations, 163, 167; symbols of, 159-60

AIDS Confidentiality Act, 280

AIDS related civil liberties: areas of litigation, 297; discrimination, 141; theories of legal liability, 297-98

American Medical Association, ethical standards, 222, 225

American Nursing Association, ethical stance on AIDS, 225

Americans with Disabilities Act (ADA 1990): AIDS/HIV infected persons, 281; antidiscrimination laws, 290

Antibody to HIV, testing for: anonymous testing, 196; asymptomatic HIV, 196; consensual, 285; critical issues, 37-40, 50-51; ethical and moral issues of, 51-55; informed consent, 195, 284-85; pretest counseling, 195; voluntary, legal issues, 280; *see also:* Screening/testing for HIV antibody

Applied ethics: AIDS crisis and, 4, 11-21; strong and weak versions, 14-16

Asymptomatic HIV: liabilities of blood donors, 300; protected handicap status, 280-82

Azidothymidine (AZT), 58, 159, 162-163, 166-167, 205, 263; Medicaid coverage, 291; placebo controlled